# Current C
# Therapy

**Series Editor**
Juan Carlos Kaski
Cardiovascular & Cell Sciences
St George's University of London
London
UK

Cardiovascular pharmacotherapy is a fast-moving and complex discipline within cardiology in general. New studies, trials and indications are appearing on a regular basis. This series created with the support of the International Society of Cardiovascular Pharmacotherapy (ISCP) is designed to establish the baseline level of knowledge that a cardiovascular professional needs to know on a day-to-day basis. The information within is designed to allow readers to learn quickly and with certainty the mode of action, the possible adverse effects, and the management of patients prescribed these drugs. The emphasis is on current practice, but with an eye to the near-future direction of treatment. This series of titles will be presented as highly practical information, written in a quick-access, no-nonsense format. The emphasis will be on a just-the-facts clinical approach, heavy on tabular material, light on dense prose. The books in the series will provide both an in-depth view of the science and pharmacology behind these drugs and a practical guide to their usage, which is quite unique. Each volume is designed to be between 120 and 250 pages containing practical illustrations and designed to improve understand and practical usage of cardiovascular drugs in specific clinical areas. The books will be priced to attract individuals and presented in a softback format. It will be expected to produce new editions quickly in response to the rapid speed of development of new CV pharmacologic agents.

More information about this series at
http://www.springer.com/series/10472

Antoni Martínez-Rubio
Juan Tamargo
Gheorghe-Andrei Dan
Editors

# Antiarrhythmic Drugs

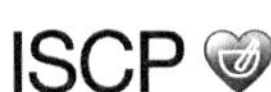


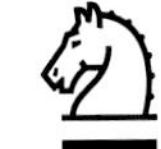

Springer

*Editors*
Antoni Martínez-Rubio
Department of Cardiology
University Hospital of Sabadell
Institut d'Investigació i
Innovació I3PT
University Autonoma of
Barcelona
Sabadell
Spain

Juan Tamargo
Department of Pharmacology
School of Medicine
Universidad Complutense
CIBERCV
Madrid
Spain

Gheorghe-Andrei Dan
"Carol Davila" University
of Medicine
Colentina University Hospital
Bucharest
Romania

Current Cardiovascular Therapy
ISBN 978-3-030-34891-5 ISBN 978-3-030-34893-9 (eBook)
https://doi.org/10.1007/978-3-030-34893-9



This Springer imprint is published by the registered company Springer Nature Switzerland AG
The registered company address is: Gewerbestrasse 11, 6330 Cham, Switzerland

# Contents

# Contributors

**Jesús Almendral** Electrophysiology Laboratory and Arrhythmia Unit, Hospital Monteprincipe, Grupo HM Hospitales, University CEU-San Pablo, Madrid, Spain

**Teresa Barrio-Lopez** Electrophysiology Laboratory and Arrhythmia Unit, Hospital Monteprincipe, Grupo HM Hospitales, University CEU-San Pablo, Madrid, Spain

**Martin Borggrefe** Department of Medicine, University Medical Center Mannheim, Mannheim, Germany

German Center for Cardiovascular Research (DZHK), Partner Site Heidelberg/Mannheim, Mannheim, Germany

**Catalin Adrian Buzea** Carol Davila University of Medicine and Pharmacy, Bucharest, Romania

Department of Cardiology, Clinical Hospital Colentina, Bucharest, Romania

**Ricardo Caballero** Department of Pharmacology, School of Medicine, Universidad Complutense, Instituto de Investigación Sanitaria Gregorio Marañón, Madrid, Spain

CIBERCV, Madrid, Spain

**Anca Rodica Dan** Department of Cardiology, Clinical Hospital Colentina, Bucharest, Romania

**Gheorghe-Andrei Dan** "Carol Davila" University of Medicine, Colentina University Hospital, Bucharest, Romania

**Eva Delpón** Department of Pharmacology, School of Medicine, Universidad Complutense, Instituto de Investigación Sanitaria Gregorio Marañón, Madrid, Spain

CIBERCV, Madrid, Spain

**Antoni Martínez-Rubio** Department of Cardiology, University Hospital of Sabadell, Institut d'Investigació i Innovació I3PT, University Autonoma of Barcelona, Sabadell, Spain

**Alina Scridon** University of Medicine, Pharmacy, Science and Technology "George Emil Palade" of Târgu Mureş, Târgu Mureş, Romania

**Mohammad-Ali Shenasa** Heart and Rhythm Medical Group, Monte Sereno, CA, USA

**Mariah Smith** Heart and Rhythm Medical Group, Monte Sereno, CA, USA

**Juan Tamargo** Department of Pharmacology, School of Medicine, Universidad Complutense, CIBERCV, Madrid, Spain

**Erol Tülümen** Department of Medicine, University Medical Center Mannheim, Mannheim, Germany

German Center for Cardiovascular Research (DZHK), Partner Site Heidelberg/Mannheim, Mannheim, Germany

# Chapter 1
# Mechanisms of Cardiac Arrhythmias

**Teresa Barrio-Lopez and Jesús Almendral**

## Electrophysiological Basis of the Arrhythmias

Cardiac myocytes are specialized cells responsible for both mechanical contraction and conduction of electrical impulses. Some myocytes demonstrate automaticity, defined by the capability of cardiac cells to undergo spontaneous diastolic depolarization and to initiate an electrical impulse in the absence of external electrical stimulation [1]. Spontaneously originated action potentials (AP) are propagated through cardiac myocytes, which are excitable, referring to their ability to respond to a stimulus with a regenerative AP [2]. Propagation of the cardiac impulse is enabled by gap junctions. Gap junctions are membrane structures composed of multiple intercellular ion channels that facilitate chemical and electrical communication between cells. Cardiac AP are

T. Barrio-Lopez · J. Almendral (✉)
Electrophysiology Laboratory and Arrhythmia Unit,
Hospital Monteprincipe, Grupo HM Hospitales,
University CEU-San Pablo, Madrid, Spain
e-mail: almendral@secardiologia.es



A. Martínez-Rubio et al. (eds.), *Antiarrhythmic Drugs*,
Current Cardiovascular Therapy,
https://doi.org/10.1007/978-3-030-34893-9_1

regionally distinct due to each myocyte type expressing different numbers and types of ion channels [3].

Usually, the sinoatrial node is the primary pacemaker of the heart, with a resting membrane potential of approximately-60 mV. $I_f$ ("funny") current plays an important role in the initiation of diastolic depolarization [4]. The aggregate activity of various currents results in a net inward flow of sodium ($Na^+$) and thus an increase in the membrane potential. When it reaches –40 mV, calcium ($Ca^{2+}$) currents (T-type $I_{Ca,T-}$ and L-type $I_{Ca,L}$) are activated, and serve as the predominant ion carriers during the AP upstroke of pacemaker cells [4] ($Ca^{2+}$-dependent). Subsequently, outward potassium ($K^+$) currents are activated and $Ca^{2+}$ currents are inactivated. The membrane potential decreases due to the outward flow of $K^+$, the major repolarizing ion of the heart. Upon reaching the resting membrane potential, the cycle is ready to repeat itself.

The resting membrane potential of muscle cells is –90 mV. Inflow of positive charge ($Ca^{2+}$ and $Na^+$) through the gap junction increases the voltage towards threshold (approximately 65 mV) [3] initiating an AP. At this point, $Na^+$ channels are triggered to open, resulting in a large but transient inward $Na^+$ current (phase 0). The $Na^+$ current is quickly inactivated, followed by a subsequent outward $K^+$ current and thereby initiating repolarization (phase 1).

The $I_{Ca,L}$ plays an important role during the AP plateau (phase 2), opposing the $K^+$ current. The $I_{Ca,L}$ is the main route for $Ca^{2+}$ influx and triggers $Ca^{2+}$ release from the sarcoplasmic reticulum, initiating contraction of the myocyte. Activation of delayed rectifier $K^+$ channels and inactivation of $Ca^{2+}$ channels leads to termination of the plateau and initiates late repolarization (phase 3). Finally, outward $K^+$ channels mediate the final repolarization (phase 4).

Following activation, the cardiac myocytes must enter a relaxation or refractory phase during which they cannot be depolarized. The refractory period is defined by the time interval following excitation during which the cell remains unexcitable. This is due to the lack of availability of depolarizing current ($Na^+$ in muscle cells). It is classified as either

TABLE 1.1 Mechanisms of cardiac arrhythmias

| **Disorders of impulse formation** | **Disorders of impulse conduction** |
|---|---|
| • Automaticity<br>– Altered normal automaticity<br>– Abnormal automaticity<br>• Triggered activity<br>– Delayed afterdepolarization (DAD)<br>– Early afterdepolarization (EAD) | • Reentry<br>– Anatomic reentry<br>– Functional reentry |

absolute or relative, depending on whether it is completely unexcitable or needs a greater stimulus than normal.

The mechanisms responsible for cardiac arrhythmias may be divided into disorders of impulse formation, disorders of impulse conduction or a combination of both (Table 1.1).

## Disorders of Impulse Formation

### *Normal Automaticity*

As previously described, some specialized heart cells (sinoatrial nodal cells, the atrioventricular (AV) node, the His-Purkinje system, some cells in both atria) [5], possess the property of automaticity. Suppression or enhancement of this activity may lead to clinical arrhythmias.

Under normal conditions, the sinoatrial nodal cells have the fastest rate of firing and the subsidiary pacemaker cells fire at slower rates. The firing rate is determined by the interaction of three factors:

- The maximum diastolic potential,
- The threshold potential at which the AP is initiated,
- The rate or slope of phase 4 depolarization.

A change in any of these may alter the rate of impulse initiation [6, 7].

Pacemaker activity is controlled by the autonomic system and can be modulated by a lot of factors, including metabolic alterations or pharmacologic substances.

Parasympathetic activity reduces the rate of the pacemaker cells by releasing acetylcholine (Ach) and hyperpolarizing the cells by increasing conductance of the $K^+$ channels. It may also decrease $I_{Ca\text{-}L}$ and If activity, which further slows the rate.

The suppressive effect of Ach is frequently used in practice for both diagnostic and therapeutic purposes. Tachycardias resulting from enhanced normal automaticity usually respond to vagal maneuvers (promoting Ach release) with a transient decrease in frequency, and a progressive return towards baseline after transiently accelerating to a faster rate upon cessation of the maneuver (this phenomenon is called "post-vagal tachycardia") [8].

Conversely, sympathetic activity increases the sinus rate. Catecholamines increase the permeability of $I_{Ca\text{-}L}$, increasing the inward $Ca^{2+}$ current. Sympathetic activity also results in enhancement of the If current [9], thereby increasing the slope of phase 4 repolarization.

Metabolic disorders as hypoxia and hypokalemia can lead to enhanced normal automatic activity as a result of $Na^+/K^+$ pump inhibition, thereby reducing the background repolarizing current and enhancing phase 4 diastolic repolarization [8].

In degenerative diseases that affect the cardiac conduction system, suppression of the sinus automaticity cells can be seen, resulting in sinus bradycardia or even sinus arrest. A subsidiary pacemaker may manifest as a result of suppression of sinus automaticity.

An essential property of normal automaticity, so characteristic that constitutes a "trademark" is the phenomenon called "overdrive suppression". Overdriving a latent pacemaker cell faster than its intrinsic rate decreases the slope of phase 4, mediated mostly by enhanced activity of the $Na^+/K^+$ exchange pump. When overdrive stimulation has ended, there is a gradual return to the intrinsic rate called the "warm-up" period. The degree of suppression and the recovery time are proportional to the rate and duration of the applied stimulation [8, 9].

This mechanism plays an important role in maintaining sinus rhythm because the sinus node continuously inhibits the activity of subsidiary pacemaker cells [6]. In patients with external pacemakers, the intrinsic rhythm may also be suppressed by this mechanism [10].

The absence of overdrive suppression may indicate that the arrhythmia mechanism is different of enhanced normal automaticity. However, the reverse is not always true because enhanced normal automatic activity may not respond to overdrive pacing or faster intrinsic rates due to entrance block [3]. Clinical examples: sinus tachycardia during exercise, fever, and thyrotoxicosis; inappropriate sinus tachycardia and AV junctional rhythms.

## *Abnomal Automaticity:* $I_{CaL}$

Atrial and ventricular myocardial cells, which in the healthy heart do not show spontaneous activity, may exhibit automaticity properties. This can happen under conditions that drive the maximum diastolic potential towards the threshold potential, which is explained by the interplay of numerous currents that together result in a net inward depolarizing current associated with a decrease in $K^+$ conductance.

The intrinsic rate of an automatic abnormal focus depends on the membrane potential; the less negative the membrane potential, the faster the automatic rate [6]. Abnormal automaticity is thought to play a role in cases of elevated extracellular $K^+$, low intracellular pH, and elevated catecholamines.

An important distinction between enhanced normal and abnormal induced automaticity is that the latter is less sensitive to overdrive suppression [11]. Under these circumstances, an ectopic automatic focus displays characteristics of other arrhythmia mechanisms [12]. Clinical examples: some atrial tachycardias, premature beats, accelerated idioventricular rhythm, some ventricular tachycardia (VT), particularly in the acute phase of myocardial infarction, associated with ischemia and reperfusion.

## *Triggered Activity*

Triggered activity (TA) is defined by impulse initiation caused by afterdepolarizations (membrane potential oscillations that occur during or immediately following a preceding AP) [13]. Afterdepolarizations occur only in the presence of a previous AP (the trigger), and when they reach the threshold potential, a new AP is generated. This may be the source of a new triggered response, leading to self-sustaining TA.

Based on their temporal relationship, two types of afterpolarizations are described: early afterdepolarizations (EADs) occur during phase 2 or 3 of the AP, and delayed afterdepolarizations (DADs) occur after completion of the repolarization phase.

### DADs

A DAD is an oscillation in membrane voltage that occurs after completion of repolarization of the AP (during phase 4). These oscillations are caused by a variety of conditions that raise the diastolic intracellular $Ca^{2+}$ concentration, which cause $Ca^{2+}$ mediated oscillations that can trigger a new AP if they reach the stimulation threshold [14].

As the cycle length decreases, the amplitude and rate of the DADs increases, and therefore DADs are expected to initiate arrhythmias when the heart rate increases (either spontaneously or during pacing). In fact, the amplitude and number of triggered responses are direct functions of both the rate and duration of overdrive pacing (easier to induce with continued stimulation). When overdrive pacing is performed during an ongoing arrhythmia, the TA can slow until it stops, or when it is not rapid enough to terminate the triggered rhythm it can cause overdrive acceleration, in contrast to the overdrive suppression seen with automatic rhythms [6].

Toxic concentration of digitalis was the first observed cause of DAD [15]. This occurs secondary to the inhibition of the Na/K pump, which promotes the release of $Ca^{2+}$ from the sarcoplasmic reticulum. Clinically, bidirectional fascicular tachycardia due to digitalis toxicity is an example of TA [16].

Catecholamines can cause DADs by causing intracellular $Ca^{2+}$ overload via an increase in $I_{Ca\text{-}L}$ and the $Na^{+}$-$Ca^{2+}$ exchange current. Ischemia-induced DADs are thought to be mediated by the accumulation of lysophosphoglycerides in the ischemic tissue [17], with subsequent elevation in $Na^{+}$ and $Ca^{2+}$. Abnormal sarcoplasmic reticulum function (e.g. mutations in ryanodine receptor) can also lead to intracellular $Ca^{2+}$ overload, facilitating clinical arrhythmias, such as catecholaminergic polymorphic VT [18] (Fig. 1.1).

An important factor for the development of DADs is the duration of the AP. Longer APs are associated with more $Ca^{2+}$ overload and facilitate DADs. Therefore, drugs that prolong AP (eg, Class IA antiarrhythmic agents) can occasionally increase DAD amplitude.

Adenosine can be used as a test for the diagnosis of DADs. Adenosine reduces the $Ca^{2+}$ inward current by inhibiting effects on adenylate cyclase and cyclic adenosine monophosphate.

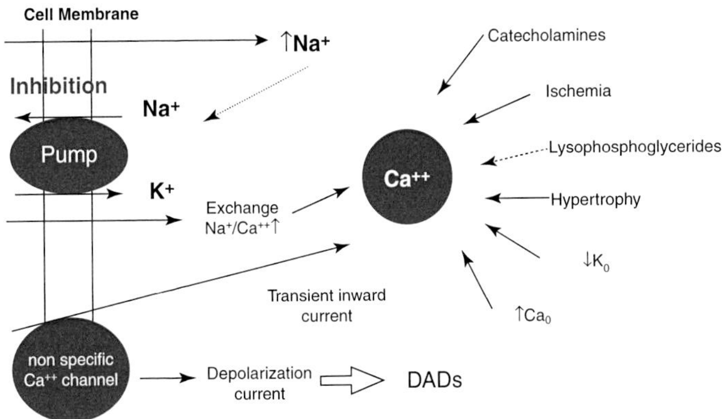


FIGURE 1.1 Mechanisms responsible for DAD (modified from Jalife et al.) [8]

Thus, it may abolish DADs induced by catecholamines, but does not alter DADs induced by $Na^+/K^+$ pump inhibition. The interruption of VT by adenosine suggests catecholamine-induced DADs as the underlying mechanism [19].

Clinical examples: some atrial tachycardias, digitalis toxicity-induced tachycardia, accelerated ventricular rhythms during ischemia, some forms of repetitive monomorphic VT, reperfusion-induced arrhythmias, ventricular outflow tract VT, exercise-induced VT (e.g. catecholaminergic polymorphic VT).

## EADs

The EADs are oscillatory potentials that occur during the AP plateau (phase 2 EADs) or during the late repolarization (phase 3 EADs). Both types may appear during similar experimental conditions, but they differ morphologically as well as in the underlying ionic mechanism. Phase 2 EADs appear to be related to $I_{Ca\text{-}L}$ current [20], while phase 3 EADs may be the result of electronic current across repolarization or the result of low $I_{K1}$ [21].

The plateau of the AP is a period of high membrane resistance [3] and little current flow. Therefore, small changes in either repolarizing or depolarizing currents can have profound effects on the AP duration and profile. A wide variety of agents and conditions can result in a decreased outward current or increased inward current and therefore establish the conditions necessary for EADs (Table 1.2.).

A fundamental condition underlying the development of EADs is AP prolongation, which manifests on the surface electrocardiogram (ECG) as QT prolongation. Some antiarrhythmic agents, principally class IA and III drugs, may become proarrhythmic because of their therapeutic effect of prolonging the AP. Many other drugs (Table 1.2.) can predispose to the formation of EADs, particularly when associated with ↓$K^+$ and/or bradycardia, additional factors that result in prolongation of the AP [8]. Several drugs have been associated with QT prolongation and *torsades de pointes* ([22],

Table 1.2 Agents and manipulations that may lead to early afterdepolarizations

| |
|---|
| – Slow rate (bradycardia, complete heart block, etc.) |
| – Mechanical stretch |
| – Hypokalemia |
| – Hypoxia |
| – Acidosis |
| – Low extracellular $K^+$ concentration |
| – Low extracellular $Ca^{2+}$ concentration |
| – Low extracellular magnesium ($Mg^{2+}$) concentration |
| – Class IA antiarrhythmic drugs (quinidine, disopyramide, procainamide) |
| – Class IC antiarrhythmic drugs (flecainide, encainide, indecainide) |
| – Class III antiarrhythmic drugs (amiodarone, sotalol, bretylium) |
| – Phenothiazines |
| – Tricyclic and tetracyclic antidepressants |
| – Erythromycin |
| – Antihistamines |
| – Cesium |
| – Amiloride |
| – Barium |

www.qtdrugs.org]. Catecholamines may enhance EADs by an increase in $Ca^{2+}$ current, however the resultant increase in heart rate along with the increase in $K^+$ current effectively reduces the APD and thus abolishes EADs [8]. Experimental studies have shown that magnesium can eliminate TA of these EAD and can provide an effective treatment of certain cases of drug induced *torsades de pointes* [23].

An EAD-mediated TA appears to be the underlying cause of arrhythmias that develop in the setting of long QT syndrome (LQTS). The true mechanism of these arrhythmias is still debated, but it is accepted that an enhanced dispersion of repolarization seen in the syndrome can create a proarrhythmic substrate [24]. There is growing interest in the effects of genetic mutations in repolarizing membrane currents in relation to the congenital LQTS associated with polymorphic ventricular tachycardia like *torsades de pointes*, and repolarization in general [22]. These tachycardias probably begin by EAD and TA, although a reentrant mechanism may also be involved in its genesis [25]. Patients with LQTS have a greater dispersion of refractoriness which could favor the presence of unidirectional block and the development of a reentrant mechanism. Several genetic mutations responsible for alterations in the flow of $K^+$ and $Na^+$ have been identified (Table 1.3) [26, 27].

EAD triggered arrhythmias are rate dependent, and in general the EAD amplitude increases at a slow rate. Therefore, this type of TA is not expected to follow premature stimulation (which is associated with an acceleration of repolarization that decreases the EAD amplitude), with the exception of a long compensatory pause following a premature stimulus, which can be even more important than bradycardia in initiating *torsades de pointes* [28]. Clinical examples: *torsades de pointes*, that is the characteristic polymorphic VT seen in patients with LQTS.

## Disorders of Impulse Conduction

### *Block*

Conduction delay and block occurs when the propagating impulse fails to conduct. Several factors determine the conduction velocity of an impulse and whether conduction is successful, such as the stimulating efficacy of the impulse and the excitability of the tissue into which the impulse is con-

TABLE 1.3 LQTS genes (modificado de Schwartz PJ et al.) [26]

| | Gene | Locus | Protein | Current (functional effect) | Frecuency (%) |
|---|---|---|---|---|---|
| LQT1 | KCQ1 | 11p.15.5 | Iks (α subunity) | ↓Iks | 40–55% |
| LQT2 | KCNH2 | 7q35-q36 | Ikr (α subunity) | ↓Ikr | 30–45% |
| LQT3 | SCN5A | 3p21-p24 | Na channel (α subunity) | ↑INa | 5–10% |
| LQT4 | ANK2 | 4q25-q27 | Arqkirin B | ↓Ncx1, Na/k, ATPasa INsP3 | <1% |
| LQT5 | KCNE1 | 21q22.1 | Iks (β subunity) | ↓Iks | <1% |
| LQT6 | KCNE2 | 21q22.1 | Ik (β subunity) | ↓Ikr | <1% |
| LQT7 | KCNE2 | 17q23 | Ik1 (α subunity) | ↓Ik1 | <1% |
| LQT8 | CACNA1C | 12p13.3 | CaV1.2 | ↓ICa | <1% |
| LQT9 | CAV3 | 3p25 | Caveolin 3 | ↓INa | <1% |
| LQT10 | SCN4B | 11q23.3 | Na (β4 subunity) | ↓INa | <1% |
| LQT11 | mAKAP | 7q21-q22 | A-kinase anchorin | ↓IKs | <1% |

(continued)

TABLE 1.3 (continued)

| | Gene | Locus | Protein | Current (functional effect) | Frecuency (%) |
|---|---|---|---|---|---|
| LQT12 | SNTA1 | 20q11.2 | Shyntophin α1 | ↓INa | <1% |
| LQT13 | KCNJ5 | 11q24 | Kir 3.4 | ↓IK | <1% |

*LQT* long-QT syndrome, *KCNQ1* potassium voltage-gated channel, *KCNH2* potassium voltage-gated channel, subfamily H, memeber 2, *SCN5A* sodium voltage-gated channel, type V, α subunity, *ANKB* ankyrin B, *KCNE1* potassium voltage-dependent channel, subfamily ISK, member 1, *KCNE2* potassium voltage-dependent channel, subfamily ISK, member 2, *KCNJ2* potassium internal rectifier channel, subfamily J, member 2, *CACNA1C* calcium voltage-dependent channel type L, 1C subunity, *CAV3* caveolin 3, *SCN4B* sodium voltage-gated channel, type IV, à subunity, *mAKAP9* A-kinase anchor protein 9, *SNTA1* syntrophina 1, *KCNJ5* potassium channel, inwardly rectifying, subfamily J, member 5.
Functional effect: (↓) loss-of-function or (↑) gain-of-function at the cellular in vitro level.

ducted [14]. Gap junction coupling plays a crucial role for the velocity and safety of impulse propagation [29].

Usually, impulses are blocked at high rates as a result of incomplete recovery from refractoriness. When an impulse arrives at tissue that is still refractory, it will not be conducted or the impulse will be conducted with aberration. This is the typical mechanism that explains several phenomena, such as block or functional bundle brunch block of a premature beat, Ashman's phenomenon during atrial fibrillation (AF), and acceleration-dependent aberration.

Bradycardia or deceleration-dependent block is suggested to be caused by a reduction in excitability at long diastolic intervals with subsequent reduction in the AP amplitude.

Many factors can alter conduction, including rate, autonomic tone, drugs (eg, calcium channel blockers, beta blockers, digitalis, adenosine/adenosine triphosphate), or degenerative processes (by altering the physiology of the tissue and the capacity to conduct impulses).

## *Reentry*

During normal electrical activity, the cardiac cycle begins in the sinoatrial node and continues to propagate until the entire heart is activated. This impulse dies out when all fibers have been depolarized and are completely refractory. However, if a group of isolated fibers is not activated during the initial wave of depolarization, they can recover excitability in time to be depolarized before the impulse dies out. They may then serve as a link to reexcite areas that were previously depolarized but have already recovered from the initial depolarization [6]. Such a process is commonly denoted as reentry, reentrant excitation, circus movement, reciprocal or echo beats, or reciprocating tachycardia (RT), referring to a repetitive propagation of the wave of activation, returning to its site of origin to reactivate that site [13].

Table 1.4 Types of reentry

| |
|---|
| – Anatomic reentry |
| – Functional reentry |
| – Leading circle |
| – Anisotropic reentry |
| – Figure of eight reentry |
| – Reflection |
| – Spiral wave (rotor) reentry |

Reentry has been divided in 2 main groups (Table 1.4.):

- Anatomical or classic reentry, where the circuit is determined by anatomical structures
- Functional reentry, which in turn includes different mechanisms. It is characterized by a lack of anatomic boundaries.

Both forms can coexist in the same setting and share biophysical mechanisms [30]. Reentry is the most common arrhythmia mechanism seen in clinical arrhythmias, both in classical or variant forms.

Prerequisites for reentry include:

- A substrate: the presence of myocardial tissue with different electrophysiological properties, conduction, and refractoriness.
- An area of block (anatomical, functional, or both): an area of inexcitable tissue around which the wavefront can circulate.
- A site with unidirectional conduction block.
- A path of slowed conduction that allows sufficient delay in the conduction of the circulating wavefront to enable the recovery of the refractory tissue proximal to the site of unidirectional block.
- A critical tissue mass to sustain the circulating reentrant wavefronts.
- An initiating trigger.

## Macroreentry/Anatomical

The classic reentry mechanism is based on an inexcitable anatomical obstacle surrounded by a circular pathway in which the wavefront can "reenter", creating fixed and stable reentrant circuits. The anatomic obstacle determines the presence of two pathways (Fig. 1.2a). When a premature impulse encounters the obstacle, it will block in one pathway (unidirectional block) and travel down the other pathway propagating until the point of block, thus initiating a reentrant circuit (Fig. 1.2b).

Initiation and maintenance of reentry will depend on the conduction velocity and refractory period of each pathway, which determines the wavelength (wavelength = conduction velocity * refractory period). For reentry to occur, the wavelength must be shorter than the length of the pathway. Conditions that decrease conduction velocity or shorten the refractory period will allow the creation of smaller circuits, facilitating the initiation and maintenance of reentry.

The excitable gap is a key concept essential to understanding the mechanism of reentry. The excitable gap refers to the excitable myocardium that exists between the head of the reentrant wavefront and the tail of the preceding wavefront (Fig. 1.3) [30]. This gap allows the reentrant wavefront to continue propagation around the circuit. The presence of an excitable gap also makes it possible for an external wavefront to enter the reentrant circuit. This can be performed using external pacing and explains the phenomena of resetting, entrainment, and termination of the tachycardia with electrical stimulation.

Clinical examples: AV reentrant tachycardia associated with a bypass tract, AV nodal reentrant tachycardia, atrial flutter (common flutter and many of the atypical flutters), bundle branch reentry VT, post-infarction VT.

## Functional Reentry

In functional reentry, the circuit is not determined by anatomic obstacles; it is defined by dynamic heterogeneities in the electrophysiologic properties of the involving tissue [2].

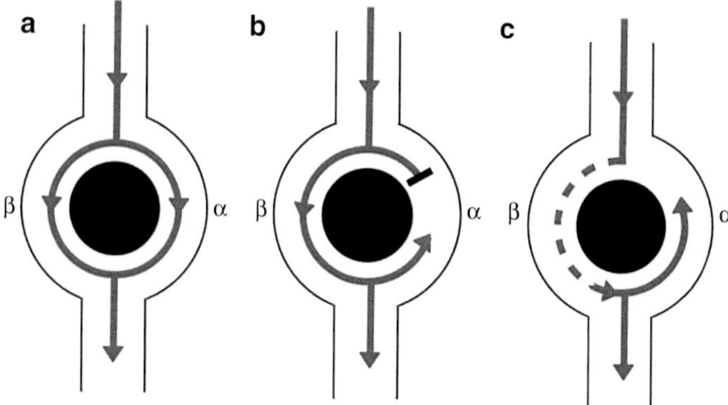


FIGURE 1.2 Schematic representation of classic reentry mechanism: (**a**) An anatomical obstacle (central cicle) causes bifurcation of wavefront (upper arrow) in two pathways (β and α). For both pathways the wavefront propagates downward if the heart rate is slow despite a zone with prolonged refractory period. (**b**) when a premature impulse reaches the structure shown in (**a**), the wavefront is blocked in the pathway with long refractory period and it progresses through the other route. The impulse accesses the blocked route in the opposite direction (retrograde), which could be blocked when accessing α occurs again. (**c**) An area of slow conduction is added to the panel (**b**) (dashed line in β pathway). Now the impulse accesses retrogradely through α pathway that is recovered from the refractory period causing impulse reentry

The size of functional reentrant circuits can vary, but they are usually small and unstable. As previously stated, functionally determined reentrant circuits can occur due to different mechanisms:

- *Leading circle reentry*
  In 1976, Allesie et al. described a reentrant mechanism in the absence of an anatomical boundary. They postulated that the impulse circulates around a central core that is maintained in a refractory state because it is constantly bombarded by impulses and travels through partially refractory tissue [31]. Leading circle was defined as “the smallest possible pathway in which the impulse can continue to circulate” [32].

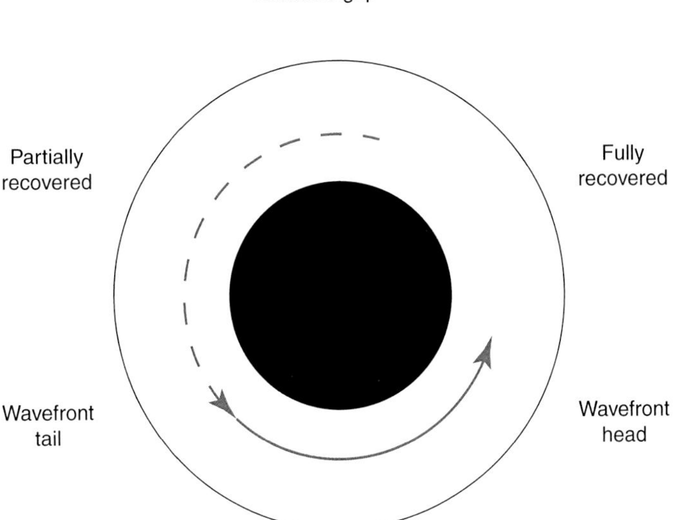


FIGURE 1.3 Schematic representation of an excitable gap

This type of reentry is less susceptible to resetting, entrainment, and termination by pacing maneuvers because there is not a fully excitable gap.

– *Anisotropic reentry*
  Anisotropic conduction relates to directionally dependent conduction velocity in cardiac muscle [33] and depends on the structure and organization of myocytes within cardiac tissue. These include the orientation of fibers and nonuniform distribution of gap junctions, with a larger number of channels poised to propagate the impulse longitudinally rather than transversely [4]. The heterogeneity in conduction velocities and repolarization properties of the anisotropic tissue can result in blocked impulses and slowed conduction that allows reentry even in small anatomical circuits [30]. Clinical examples: anisotropic reentry in atrial and ventricular muscle, which may be responsible in the setting of VT originating in surviving myocardial infarction [34].

- *Figure of eight reentry*
  This type of reentry consists of two concomitant wavefronts circulating in opposite directions (clockwise and counterclockwise) around two functional or fixed arcs of block that merge into a central common pathway. Clinical example: this type of reentry may be seen in the setting of infarction-related VT or atrial flutter in patients with prior atriotomy.
- *Reflection*
  Reflection is a unique subclass of reentry that occurs in a linear segment of tissue, where the impulse travels in both directions over the same pathway in the presence of severely impaired conduction [35].
- *Spiral wave activity (rotor)*
  Spiral waves occur in a wide variety of excitable media [36]. They represent a two-dimensional form of rotating wave propagation, which may also occur in three dimensions "scroll waves". Initially the term "rotor" described the rotating source and "spiral wave" defined the shape of the emerging wave [6]. Other terms for this phenomenon could be found in the literature, such as "vortices" or "reverberators". Spiral wave activation is organized around a core, which remains unstimulated because of the pronounced curvature of the spiral (Fig. 1.4). This curvature also limits the spiral propagation velocity, resulting in slow conduction and block [31]. In contrast to the leading circle model, there is a fully excitable gap. The tip of the wave moves along a complex trajectory and can radiate waves into the surrounding medium (known as "break-up" of a mother wave). Spirals may have completely different dynamics and can circulate with different patterns, change one to another, become stationary or continuously drift or migrate [6]. These characteristics result in both monomorphic and polymorphic patterns.
- Clinical examples: atrial and ventricular fibrillation, polymorphic VT.

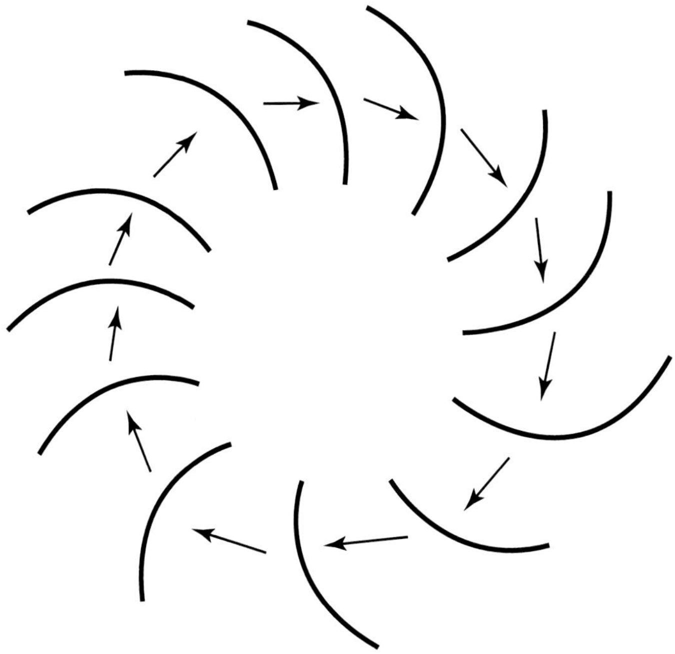

FIGURE 1.4 Schematic representation of a rotor

## Relationship to Clinical Arrhythmias

### *Bradyarrhythmias*

Bradyarrhythmias can be explained by two mechanisms:

- Failure of impulse generation. Failure of impulse generation is the failure of pacemaker cells to generate appropriate electrical impulses. In degenerative processes is frecuently seen this form of bradyarrhythmia. Although any automatic normal foci can be affected, their failure may only be seen when the superior pacemaker cell function is depressed. Thus, the failure of the sinus node will cause major or minor pauses, depending on the function of the subsidiary pacemaker cells.

- Failure of impulse propagation. The failure of impulse propagation is the failure of electrical impulses generated by pacemaker cells to conduct normally through the conduction system.

## *Tachyarrhythmias*

### Sinus Tachycardia

- Physiologic sinus tachycardia represents an enhancement of the sinus node in response to physiologic stress, and is characterized by an increased slope of phase 4 depolarization in sinus node cells.
- Inappropriate sinus tachycardia refers to a condition in which the sinus rate is increased continuously or out of proportion to the degree of physiologic stress [37] and is caused by enhanced normal automaticity.

### Focal Atrial Tachycardia

- Atrial tachycardias may be due to automaticity, TA, or reentrant mechanisms, but most of them correspond to automaticity or reentry mechanisms. They can be distinguished by their behavior in relation to various maneuvers.

### Atrial Flutter

- Atrial flutter may further be categorized into common (typical) and atypical atrial flutter.
  - Common Atrial Flutter: The wavefront in common flutter circulates in the right atrium around the tricuspid valve annulus in a counterclockwise or clockwise direction. Typical atrial flutter is the most common example of a macroreentrant circuit.
  - Atypical Atrial Flutter: In this type of flutter, the obstacle is usually related to previously performed procedures that create large anatomic barriers (atriotomy scar, suture line, or radiofrequency ablation) or facilitate

a zone of slow conduction such that reentry may occur (eg, left atrial flutter related to previous AF ablation).

### Atrial Fibrillation

- AF is the most common sustained arrhythmia. Even though its underlying mechanism is still debated, AF likely represents a complex interaction between drivers responsible for initiation and the anatomic atrial substrate required for perpetuation of the arrhythmia [38].
- The drivers are located predominantly in the pulmonary veins and can represent variable forms of focal abnormal automaticity or TA within the vein or microreentrant circuits around the vein orifices with strong autonomic potentiation [39]. Not only do they contribute to the initiation of AF, but they also participate in the maintenance of the arrhythmia [40]. Other nonpulmonary triggering foci have also been described, such as the coronary sinus, superior vena cava [41], or ligament of Marshall [42].
- Maintenance of the arrhythmia lies in a combination of electrophysiological and structural factors, which create the substrate to perpetuate AF. Different mechanisms have been postulated, including multiple wavelets of reentry or a mother rotor circuit, as well as high frequency activity in the Atria [42]. Moreover, structural and electrical remodeling of the atria over time contributes to the arrhythmogenic substrate.

### Atrioventricular Nodal Reentrant Tachycardia

- This common paroxysmal supraventricular tachycardia is caused by a classic reentrant mechanism. The presence within the AV node of two pathways with distinct electrophysiological properties makes this arrhythmia possible.
- Under normal conditions, a sinus impulse will travel through both pathways. In response to a premature stimulation, the stimulus can block in the fast pathway due to a longer refractory period and travel through the slow pathway. If conduction is slow enough, the blocked fast path-

way can have time to recover, thus setting the stage for a reentrant circuit, translating into AV nodal tachycardia when perpetuated.
- An "uncommon" form of AV nodal tachycardia can occur when activation of the circuit proceeds in the reverse direction.

Atrioventricular Junctional Tachycardia

- Atrioventricular junctional tachycardias typically occur in the setting of increased adrenergic tone or drug effect in patients with sinus node dysfunction who have undergone a previous procedure or digitalis toxicity. They can be related to enhanced normal automaticity, abnormal automaticity or TA [43].

Atrioventricular Reentrant Tachycardia Mediated by an Accessory Pathway

- The typical accessory pathway has rapid conduction and a longer refractory period in comparison to the AV node, which creates the substrate for reentry. The circuit that involves an accessory pathway is usually a large macroreentrant circuit consisting of the native conduction system, the accessory pathway, and the intervening atrial and ventricular tissue. In the orthodromic type, the most common arrhythmia related to accessory pathways, the AV node serves as the anterograde pathway and the accessory pathway as the retrograde pathway. Antidromic tachycardia occurs when activation proceeds in the reverse direction (antegrade over the accessory pathway and retrograde over the AV node), thus creating a wide QRS complex. Antidromic atrioventricular reentrant tachycardia occurs less frequently, and can be precipitated by conditions that impair antegrade conduction over the AV node with rapid conduction preserved over the AV node in a retrograde direction.
- In patients with the Wolff-Parkinson-White (WPW) syndrome and AF, rapid conduction over the accessory pathway with ventricular preexcitation may occur. Preexcitation may lead during AF to ventricular fibrillation and cardiac

arrest. The prevalence of AF in patients with WPW syndrome is unusually high in the absence of organic heart disease. While the precise mechanism remains unclear, the presence of the accessory pathway itself and retrograde activation of the atria during orthodromic supraventricular tachycardia have been postulated to play an important role in the initiation of AF [44].

Accelerated Idioventricular Rhythm

- Accelerated idioventricular rhythm is thought to be due to abnormal automaticity related to the acute phase of myocardial infarction, as well as cocaine intoxication, acute myocarditis, digoxin intoxication, and postoperative cardiac surgery [45].

Ventricular Tachycardia

- This arrhythmia has a wealth of different characteristics and behaviors. The predominant mechanisms underlying most VTs are abnormal automaticity, TA, and reentry. Reentry is the most frequent mechanism causing VT in patients with ischemic cardiomyopathy [45].

Monomorphic Ventricular Tachycardia

- In the absence of structural heart disease, most VTs are thought to correspond to TA or an automatic mechanism. However, most monomorphic VT occur in the presence of structural heart disease, with the predominant mechanism being reentry. The majority of patients within this group demonstrate VT in relation to ischemic cardiomyopathy. The postinfarction process results in a scar associated with surviving islands of cardiac myocytes. This can result in slow and discontinuous conduction and/or block in conduction through the viable tissue, likely attributable to disruption in gap junction distribution and function and poor cell-to-cell coupling [46] These changes create the ideal electrophysiologic and anatomic substrate for developing reentrant arrhythmias (slow conduction and unidirectional block).

- The second most common cause of VTs due to reentry is nonischemic cardiomyopathy. In such patients the reentrant circuit frequently involves a region of a scar near the valvular orifices or in the subepicardium. Occasionally, VTs in this setting appear to be mediated by abnormal automaticity or triggered mechanisms.
- Reentry is also the principal mechanism in VT due to arrhythmogenic right ventricular cardiomyopathy. In this condition, a reentrant circuit is formed around the characteristic fibrofatty tissue that has replaced areas of the right ventricle. A similar mechanism of VT can occur in the setting of hypertrophic cardiomyopathy (especially in the presence of an apical aneurysm), valvular heart disease, surgically repaired congenital heart diseases (large resections are needed, creating large anatomical barriers), infiltrative cardiomyopathy (eg, cardiac sarcoidosis) and neuromuscular disorders.
- Idiopathic VT. Idiopathic VT is found in structurally normal hearts and can be divided into two main groups:
  - Outflow tract tachycardia. Outflow tract tachycardias represent the most frequent idiopathic VTs. Although the pathogenesis is not fully understood, their behavior suggest that many of them are due to TA as a result of delayed afterdepolarizations.
  - Fascicular ventricular tachycardia. Fascicular VT lies in the left ventricular His-Purkinje system and although the mechanism is accepted to be a macroreentry circuit involving calcium-dependent slow response fibers of the ventricular Purkinje network [47], typically terminated by verapamil, some automatic forms of the tachycardia have also been described.

#### Polymorphic Ventricular Tachycardia and Ventricular Fibrillation

- The initiation and maintenance of these tachyarrhythmias remain unknown; however, previous work supports a similar mechanism as that suspected in AF. The initiating trigger could be mediated by TA, automaticity, or a reentrant mechanism, while maintenance may be due to different forms of functional reentries, including rotors, migrating scroll waves, or intramural or Purkinje network reentry. Elucidation of the underlying mechanism is still in its experimental phase. It is also possible that VF may be the final common endpoint of a heterogeneous group of electrical disturbances and it may not be possible to identify a single mechanism that adequately accounts for all of them [48].

– Genetically determined abnormalities predisposing to polymorphic VT:
  - LQTS: both congenital and acquired (especially via certain drugs [49]) conditions lead to a long QT interval due to lengthening of the AP plateau phase. The onset of the arrhythmia occurs due to EADs potentiated by intracellular calcium accumulation from a prolonged AP Plateau [38].
  - Brugada syndrome: genetic mutations resulting in diminished inward sodium current in the epicardium of the right ventricular outflow tract cause this syndrome. Because of the ionic alteration, the outward potassium current is unopposed at some epicardial sites, which gives rise to epicardial dispersion of repolarization that creates a vulnerable window during which a premature impulse can produce a phase 2 reentrant arrhythmia [35].
  - Short QT syndrome: genetic abnormalities that cause this syndrome lead to decreased repolarization time and decrease myocyte refractoriness, thus promoting reentrant arrhythmias [50].
  - Catecholaminergic polymorphic VT: catecholaminergic polymorphic VT is due to genetic disorders of channels and proteins (ryanodine and calsequestrin) that regulate intracellular calcium [17]. The defects cause an accumulation of intracellular calcium, which can facilitate the TA mediated by DADs. Precipitants include exercise or emotional stress as a result of increasing intracellular calcium concentration.

## References


1. Peters N, Cabo C, Wit A. Arrhythmogenic mechanisms: automaticity, triggered activity and reentry. In: Zipes DP, Jalife J, editors. Cardiac electrophysiology, from cell to bedside. 3rd ed. Philadelphia: Saunders; 2003. p. 345–55.
2. Grant A, Durrani S. Mechanisms of cardiac arrhythmias. In: Topol EJ, editor. Textbook of cardiovascular medicine. 3rd ed. Philadelphia: Lippicontt; 2007. p. 950–63.
3. Tomaselly G, Roden D. Molecular and cellular basis of cardiac electrophysiology. In: Sanjeev S, editor. Electrophysiological disorders of the heart. New York: Elsevier; 2005. p. 1–28.
4. Barbuti A, Baruscotti M, DiFrancesco D. The pacemaker current. J Cardiovasc Electrophysiol. 2007;18:342–7.
5. Matteo E, Nargeot J. Genesis and regulation of the heart automaticity. Physiol Rev. 2008;88:919–82.
6. Issa ZF, Miller JM, Zipes DP. Electrophysiological mechanisms of cardiac arrhythmias: clinical arrhythmology and electrophysiology, a companion to Brawnwald's heart disease. Philadelphia: Saunders; 2009. p. 1–26.
7. Gaztañaga L, Marchlinski FE, Betensky BP. Mecanismos de las arritmias cardiacas. Rev Esp Cardiol. 2012;65:174–85.
8. Jalife J, Delmar M, Anumonwo J, Berenfeld O, Anumonwo KJ. Basic cardiac electrophysiology for the clinician. 2nd ed. Hoboken: Wiley-Blackwell; 2009. p. 152–96.
9. DiFrancesco D. Funny channels in the control of cardiac rhythm and mode of action of selective blockers. Pharmacol Res. 2006;53:399–406.
10. Almendral J, González-Torrecilla E. Mecanismos de las arritmias cardiacas. Arritmología clínica. Madrid: Sociedad Española de Cardiología; 2007. p. 81–103.
11. Dangman KH, Hoffman BF. Studies on overdrive stimulation of canine cardiac Purkinje fibers: maximal diastolic potential as a determinant of the response. J Am Coll Cardiol. 1983;2:1183–90.
12. Rosenthal J, Ferrier G. Contribution of variable entrance and exit block in protected foci to arrhythmogenesis in isolated ventricular tissues. Circulation. 1983;67:1–8.
13. Zipes DP. Mechanisms of clinical arrhythmias. J Cardiovasc Electrophysiol. 2003;14:902–12.
14. Clusin WT. Calcium and cardiac arrhythmias: DADs, EADs, and alternans. Crit Rev Clin Lab Sci. 2003;40:227–75.

15. Rosen MR, Gelband H, Merker C, Hoffman BF. Mechanisms of digitalis toxicity. Effects of ouabain on phase four of canine Purkinje fiber transmembrane potentials. Circulation. 1973;47:681–9.
16. Wieland JM, Marchlinski FE. Electrocardiographic response of digoxin-toxic fascicular tachycardia to fab fragments: implications for tachycardia mechan- ism. Pacing Clin Electrophysiol. 1986;9:727–38.
17. Undrovinas AI FA, Makielski JC. Inward sodium current at resting potentials in single cardiac myocytes induced by the ischemic metabolite lysophosphatidylcholine. Circ Res. 1992;71:1231–41.
18. Paavola J, Vitaasalo M, Laitinen-Forsblom PJ, Pasternack M, Swan H, Tikkanen I, et al. Mutant ryanodine receptors in catecholaminergic polymorphic ventri- cular tachycardia generate delayed afterdepolarizations due to increased pro- pensity to Ca2+ waves. Eur Heart J. 2007;28:1135–42.
19. Bruce B, Lerman MD. Adenosine sensitive ventricular tachycardia: evidence suggesting cyclic AMP-mediated triggered activity. Circulation. 1986;74:270–80.
20. Yamada M, Ohta K, Niwa A, Tsujino N, Nakada T, Hirose M. Contribution of L- type Ca2+ channels to early depolarizations induced by IKr and IKs channel suppression in guinea pig ventricular myocytes. J Membr Biol. 2008;222:151–66.
21. Mitsunori M, Lin S, Xie Y, Chua SK, Joung B, Han S, et al. Genesis of phase 3 early afterdepolarizations and triggered activity in acquired long-QT syndrome. Circ Arrhythm Electrophysiol. 2011;4:103–11.
22. Drew BJ, Ackerman MJ, Funk M, Gibler WB, Kligfield P, Menon V, Philippides GJ, Roden DM, Zareba W. Prevention of torsade de pointes in hospital settings. JACC. 2010;55:934–47.
23. White CM, Xie J, Chow MS, Kluger J. Prophylactic magnesium to decrease the arrhythmogenic potential of class III antiarrhythmic agents in a Rabbit model. Pharmacotherapy. 1999;19:635–40.
24. Hiroshu M, Jiashin W. The QT syndrome: long and short. Lancet. 2008;372:750–63.
25. Cranefield PF, Aronson RS. Cardiac arrhytmias: the role of triggered activity and other mehanism. Mount Kisco. New York: Futura; 1988.
26. Schwartz PJ, Crotti L, Insolia R. Long-QT syndrome: from genetics to management. Circ Arrhythm Electrophysiol. 2012;5:868–77.

27. Kapplinger JD, Tester DJ, Salisbury BA, Carr JL, Harris-Kerr C, Pollevick GD, Wilde AA, Ackerman MJ. Spectrum and prevalence of mutations from the first 2,500 consecutive unrelated patients referred for the FAMILION long QT syndrome genetic test. Heart Rhythm. 2009;6:1297–303.
28. Kannankeril P, Roden DM, Darbar D. Drug induced long QT syndrome. Pharmacol Rev. 2010;62:760–81.
29. Rohr S. Role of gap junctions in the propagation of the cardiac action potential. Cardiovasc Res. 2004;62:309–22.
30. Kleber AG, Rudy Y. Basis mechanisms of cardiac impulse propagation and associated arrhythmias. Physiol Rev. 2004;84:431–88.
31. Cabo C, Wit A. Cellular electrophysiologic mechanisms of arrhythmias. Cardiol Clin. 1997;4:521–38.
32. Allesie MA, Bonke FJ, Schopman FJ. Circus movement in Rabbit atrial muscle as a mechanism of tachycardia. III. The "leading circle" concept. A new model of circus movement in cardiac tissue without the involvement of an anatomical obstacle. Circ Res. 1976;39:168–77.
33. Valderrábano M. Influence of anisotropic conduction properties in the propagation of the cardiac action potential. Prog Biophys Mol Biol. 2007;94:144–68.
34. Sapch MS, Josephson ME. Initiating reentry: the role of nonuniform anisotropy in small circuits. J Cardiovasc Electrophysiol. 1994;5:182–209.
35. Antzelevirch C. Basis mechanisms of reentrant arrhythmias. Curr Opin Cardiol. 2001;16:1–7.
36. Davidenko J, Kent P, Jalife J. Spiral waves in normal isolated ventricular muscle. Waves and patterns in biological systems. Physica D. 1991;49:182–97.
37. Morillo CA, Guzmán JC. Taquicardia sinusal inapropiada: actualización. Rev Esp Cardiol. 2007;60(Supl 3):10–4.
38. Marchinski F. The tachycardias. Harrison's cardiovacular medicine. New York: McGraw-Hill; 2010. p. 147–77.
39. Arora R, Verheule S, Scott L, Navarrete A, Katari V, Wilson E, et al. Arrhythmogenic substrate of the pulmonary vein assessed by high resolution optical mapping. Circulation. 2003;107:1816–21.
40. Sanders P, Nalliah CJ, Dubois R, Takahashi Y, Hocini M, Rotter M, et al. Frequency mapping of the pulmonary veins in paroxysmal versus permanent atrial fibrillation. J Cardiovasc Electrophysiol. 2006;17:965–72.

41. Tsai CF, Tai CT, Hsieh MH, Lin WS, Yu WC, Ueng KC, et al. Initiation of atrial fibrillation by ectopic beats originating from the superior vena cava. Circulation. 2000;102:67–74.
42. Okuyama Y, Miyauchi Y, Park AM, Hamabe A, Zhou S, Hayashi H, et al. High resolution mapping of the pulmonary vein and the vein of Marsharll during induce atrial fibrillation and atrial tachycardia in a canine model of pacing induced congestive heart failure. J Am Coll Cardiol. 2003;42:348–60.
43. Sanders P, Berenfeld O, Hocini M, Ja¨is P, Vaidyanathan R, Hsu LF, et al. Spectral analysis identifies sites of high frequency activity maintaining atrial fibrillation in humans. Circulation. 2005;112:789–97.
44. Centurio OA, Shimizu A, Somoto S, Konoe A. Mechanisms for the genesis of paroxysmal atrial fibrillation in the Wolff-Parkinson-White syndrome: intrinsic atrial muscle vulnerability vs. electrophysiological properties of the accessory pathway. Europace. 2008;10:294–302.
45. Rubar M, Zipes DP. Genesis of cardiac arrhythmias: electrophysiologic considerations. In: Bonow RO, Mann DL, Zipes DP, Libby P, editors. Braunwald's heart disease. A textbook of cardiovascular medicine. 9th ed. Philadelphia: Saunders Elsevier; 2011. p. 653–86.
46. Peters NS, Coromilas J, Severs NJ, Wit AL. Disturbed connexin 43 gap junction distribution correlates with the location of reentrant circuits in the epicardial border zone of healing canine infarcts that cause ventricular tachycardia. Circulation. 1997;95:988–96.
47. Ouyang F, Cappato R, Ernst S, Goya M, Volkmer M, Habe J, et al. Electroanatomical substrate of idiopathic left ventricular tachycardia: unidirectional block and macroreentry within the purkinje network. Circulation. 2002;105:462–9.
48. Issa ZF, Miller JM, Zipes DP. Other ventricular tachycardias: clinical arrhythmology and electrophysiology. A companion to Brawnwald's heart disease. Philadelphia: Saunders; 2009. p. 482.
49. Roden DM. Drug induced prolongation of the QT interval. N Engl J Med. 2004;350:1013–22.
50. Cross B, Homoud M, Link M, Foote C, Carlitski AC, Weinstock J, et al. The short QT syndrome. J Interv Card Electrophysiol. 2011;31:25–31.

# Chapter 2
# Class I Antiarrhythmic Drugs: $Na^+$ Channel Blockers

**Mohammad Shenasa, Mohammad-Ali Shenasa, and Mariah Smith**

## Abbreviations

| | |
|---|---|
| AAD | Antiarrhythmic drug |
| AF | Atrial fibrillation |
| AP | Action potential |
| APD | Action potential duration |
| ATP | Adenosine triphosphate |
| AVNRT | Atrioventricular nodal reentrant tachycardia |
| AVRT | Atrioventricular reentrant tachycardia |
| CAD | Coronary artery disease |
| CHF | Congestive heart failure |
| CPVT | Catecholaminergic polymorphic ventricular tachycardia |

M. Shenasa (✉)
Heart and Rhythm Medical Group, Monte Sereno, CA, USA

Department of Cardiovascular Services, O'Connor Hospital, San Jose, CA, USA

M.-A. Shenasa · M. Smith
Heart and Rhythm Medical Group, Monte Sereno, CA, USA



A. Martínez-Rubio et al. (eds.), *Antiarrhythmic Drugs*, Current Cardiovascular Therapy,
https://doi.org/10.1007/978-3-030-34893-9_2

| | |
|---|---|
| DAD/EAD | Delayed/early afterdepolarization |
| ECG | Electrocardiogram |
| ERP | Effective refractory period |
| ICD | Implantable cardioverter-defibrillator |
| LQT3 | Long QT 3 (syndrome) |
| LV | Left ventricular |
| LVH | Left ventricular hypertrophy |
| SCD | Sudden cardiac death |
| TdP | Torsades de Pointes |
| VF | Ventricular fibrillation |
| VT | Ventricular tachycardia |

Glossary of Abbreviations

| | |
|---|---|
| $I_{Na}$ | Sodium current |
| $I_{Na\text{-}early}$ | Early sodium current |
| $I_{Na\text{-}late}$ | Late sodium current |
| $I_{Na/K}$ | Na/K pump current |
| $I_{Na/Ca}$ | Na/Ca exchanger current |
| $I_{to1}$ | Voltage-activated $Ca^{2+}$ outward current |
| $I_{to2}$ | $Ca^{2+}$ activated transient outward current |
| $I_{Kr}$ | Rapid component of delayed rectifier potassium current |
| $I_{Kur}$ | Ultra-rapid component of delayed rectifier current |
| $I_{Ks}$ | Slow component of delayed rectifier current |
| $I_{K1}$ | Inward rectifier potassium current |

## Introduction

For several decades, sodium channel blockers, the so-called "class I antiarrhythmic drugs (AADs)", have been the frontline of antiarrhythmic therapy for the management of a variety of cardiac arrhythmias [1, 2]. Among many others, quinidine, procainamide, and lidocaine have been in use for several decades. Progress in understanding the mechanisms of arrhythmias on one hand, and understanding the mechanisms of action of AADs from the whole heart to the single ion channels on the other hand, has improved our management of arrhythmias.

In this chapter we review the old and new mechanisms of sodium channel blockers in their broad spectrum from basic to clinical, with focus on the novel indications of theses agents. We use "sodium current" and "$I_{Na}$" interchangeably.

There have been several classifications of AADs, based on their direct effect on normal and abnormal cardiac electrical systems as well as different arrhythmia mechanisms. Although each AAD has its own distinct characteristics, classifications are generally appealing for clinicians and teaching purposes.

### *Vaughan Williams*

The Vaughan Williams classification has been used widely for several decades and is based on the effect(s) of AADs or groups of agents on action potential duration (APD) and respective ionic channels [3–5].

Class I AADs constitute agents that exclusively or predominantly block the fast sodium current, although many of them may exhibit other ion channel blocking effects such as quinidine's effect on $K^+$ channels. Table 2.1 illustrates the modified Vaughan Williams classification.

### *Sicilian Gambit*

This classification is based on individual agents, which may have multiple effects.

The concept of AAD-specific arrhythmia mechanisms in relation to ion channels are well discussed in the Sicilian Gambit (Table 2.2) [6].

The electrophysiological effect of AADs may be investigated at several levels:

1. Cell membrane
2. Ion currents and ion channels
3. Gap junctions
4. Receptors
5. Pumps
6. The whole intact-heart

Table 2.1 Vaughan Williams classification of antiarrhythmic drugs [5]

| | Class I | Class II | Class III | Class IV |
|---|---|---|---|---|
| | **Drugs with direct membrane action ($Na^+$ channel blockade)** | **Sympatholytic drugs** | **Drugs that prolong repolarization** | **Calcium channel-blocking effects** |
| Ia | Moderate depressant effect on phase 0 (Suppresses excitability)<br>Slow conduction<br>Prolong repolarization<br>*Effect on phase 0 of APD*: Intermediate<br>*Effect on APD*: Marked prolongation Eg: Quinidine, procainamide, dysopyramide | Eg: metoprolol, nadolol, and several other beta-blockers | Eg: amiodarone, sotalol, dronedarone, dofetilide (Predominantly blocks $K^+$ channels but may exert weak multichannel blocking effect) | Eg: verapmil, dilitazem |

| | |
|---|---|
| Ib | Little effect on phase 0 in normal tissue<br>Depress phase 0 in abnormal fibers<br>Shorten repolarization<br>*Effect on phase 0 of APD*: Little effect<br>*Effect on APD*: Little effect or may shorten<br>Eg: Lidocaine, mexiletine, phenytoin |
| Ic | Markedly depress phase 0<br>Markedly slow conduction<br>Slight effect on repolarization<br>*Effect on phase 0 of APD*: Marked slowing<br>*Effect on APD*: Little effect<br>Eg: propafenone, flecainide |

Abbreviations: *APD* action potential duration, *Eg* example

TABLE 2.2 Sicilian Gambit chart for AADs

| Drug | Channels | | | | | | Receptors | | | | Pumps | Clinical Effects | | | ECG Effects | | |
|---|---|---|---|---|---|---|---|---|---|---|---|---|---|---|---|---|---|
| | Na Fast | Na Med | Na Slow | Ca | K | $I_f$ | α | β | $M_2$ | P | Na-K ATPase | LV funct | Sinus rate | Extra-card | PR Inter | QRS width | JT Inter |
| Lidocaine | ○ | | | | | | | | | | | → | → | ⊜ | | | ↓ |
| Mexiletine | ○ | | | | | | | | | | | → | → | ⊜ | | | ↓ |
| Tocainide | ○ | | | | | | | | | | | → | → | ● | | | ↓ |
| Moricizine | ●(I) | | | | | | | | | | | ↓ | → | ○ | | ↑ | |
| Procainamide | | ●(A) | | | ⊜ | | | | | | | ↓ | → | ● | ↑ | ↑ | ↑ |
| Disopyramide | | ●(A) | K | | ⊜ | | | | ○ | | | ↓ | → | ⊜ | ↑↓ | ↑ | ↑ |
| Quinidine | | ●(A) | | | ⊜ | | ○ | | ○ | | | → | ↑ | ⊜ | ↑↓ | ↑ | ↑ |
| Propafenone | | ●(A) | | | | | | ⊜ | | | | ↓ | ↓ | ○ | ↑ | ↑ | |
| Flecainide | | | ●(A) | | ○ | | | | | | | ↓ | → | ○ | ↑ | ↑ | |
| Encainide | | | ●(A) | | | | | | | | | ↓ | → | ○ | ↑ | ↑ | |
| Bepridil | ○ | | | ● | ⊜ | | | | | | | ? | ↓ | ○ | | | ↑ |
| Verapamil | ○ | | | ● | | | ⊜ | | | | | ↓ | ↓ | ○ | ↑ | | |
| Diltiazem | | | | ⊜ | | | | | | | | ↓ | ↓ | ○ | ↑ | | |
| Bretylium | | | | | ● | | ◩ | ◩ | | | | → | ↓ | ○ | | | ↑ |
| Sotalol | | | | | ● | | | ● | | | | ↓ | ↓ | ○ | ↑ | | ↑ |
| Amiodarone | ○ | | | ○ | ● | | ⊜ | ⊜ | | | | → | ↓ | ● | ↑ | | ↑ |
| Alinidine | | | | | ⊜ | ● | | | | | | ? | ↓ | ● | | | |
| Nadolol | | | | | | | | ● | | | | ↓ | ↓ | ○ | ↑ | | |
| Propranolol | ○ | | | | | | | ● | | | | ↓ | ↓ | ○ | ↑ | | |
| Atropine | | | | | | | | | ● | | | → | ↑ | ⊜ | ↓ | | |
| Adenosine | | | | | | | | | | □ | | ? | ↓ | ○ | ↑ | | |
| Digoxin | | | | | | | | | □ | | ● | ↑ | ↓ | ● | ↑ | | ↓ |

Relative potency of block: ○ Low ⊜ Moderate ● High
□ = Agonist ◩ = Agonist/Antagonist
A = Activated state blocker
I = Inactivated state blocker

This table is based on the mechanisms of antiarrhythmics on ion channels and arrhythmia mechanisms. Abbreviations: *card* cardiac, *funct* function, *inter* interval. With permission from Circulation 1991;84:1831–1851 [6]

## *Action Potential*

The registration of a sudden movement of sodium ions from outside the cell membrane (depolarization), into it (inward current), and followed by the slow movement of $K^+$ ions from inside the cell membrane (repolarization) to the extracellular space (outward current) [7–9]. Fig. 2.1 shows the atrial and ventricular AP with its five phases and respective ion channels.

# The Cardiac Action Potential: Role of $I_{Na}$ Current

Figure 2.1 shows the typical atrial and ventricular action potential duration (APD) as well as the respective ion currents and genes that control the ion channels. The atrial and ventricular myocardial APD as well as Purkinje cells APD are somewhat similar and distinctive from those of the sino-atrial and A-V nodal cells.

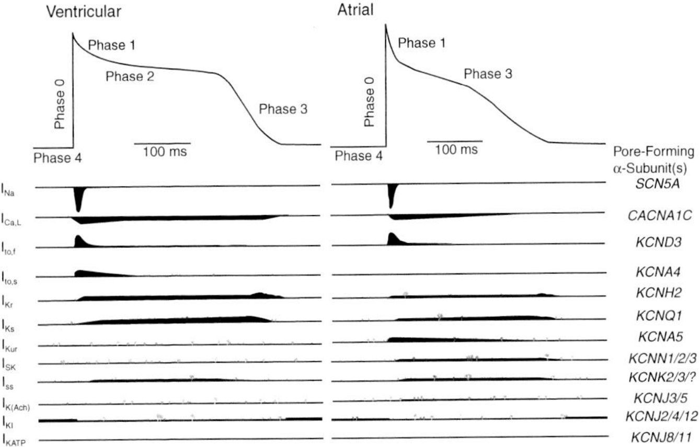


FIGURE 2.1 Illustrates atrial and ventricular AP and its respective ion channels involving different phases of APD and respective genes. With permission from Card Electrophysiol Clin 8 (2016) 257–273 [8]

The sinoatrial node has a fast phase 4 that produces spontaneous depolarization. The depolarizing current of the sinoatrial and A-V node is $Ca^{2+}$ current and L-type $Ca^{2+}$ ($I_{Ca}$) channel are discussed elsewhere in this book. Likewise, potassium ions and channels are discussed in another section.

Sodium channels are present in sinoatrial node, but for the most part, are inactivated under physiological (normal) conditions.

## Ion Channels

Channels are segments of the cell membrane that allow movement of ions across the cell membrane whether active or passive.

Ion channels are from a group of complex glycoproteins that make pores and permit the transport of cardiac ions, i.e. sodium, potassium, calcium, and chloride across the cell membrane (either inward or outward the cell). This transport takes place when the channel changes from a "closed state" to an "open state". Opening and closing ion channels are governed by voltage and voltage-operated gates, simplified as "voltage-gated" [10]. Diffusion through these protein channels is called "gating" [11]. These channels have two important features:

1. Selective permeability to certain molecules and ions such as selective $Na^+$ channel and selective $K^+$ channels.
2. Many channels can be opened (open state) or closed (closed state) under certain conditions such as chemical or electrical charges, concentrations, etc. [12]

The anatomy and function of these ion channels determine the cardiac APD [13]. The ion transport therefore depends on several factors such as the electrical and concentration gradient of a specific ion across the membrane or other triggers.

These channels further operate at different states such as active transport, inactive transport, open state, and closed state [11, 14].

## Cardiac Sodium Current ($I_{Na}$) and Channel

Voltage-gated sodium channels made of transmembrane proteins that allow the sodium ion current to travel through these channels are responsible for the rapid upstroke (phase 0) of the cardiac AP (depolarization). Sodium current is an inward current and is the major current that is present in atria, myocardial, and Purkinje cells and is responsible for depolarization, i.e. phase zero of AP (Fig. 2.1). Therefore, the sodium current is responsible for the rapid impulse conduction through atrial, His-Purkinje system, and ventricular myocardium. The sodium channel and current is controlled with multiple genes; however, the most dominant one is SCN5A. Therefore, the sodium channels are the main molecular substrate that are involved in both inherited and acquired disorders of channelopathies. The sodium current in the atria, ventricular, myocardial, and Purkinje cells are voltage dependent activated channels at −75–90 mV [14]. The main voltage-gated sodium channel that is expressed in human cardiac myocytes is $Na_v$ 1.5, which is encoded by the SCN5A gene [15–19]. Transport of $I_{Na}$ through the channels is determined by α-subunits (i.e. proteins that make the channel). The α-subunits are comprised of four serially linked homologous domains, which make the ion channels pure (Fig. 2.2) [20, 21]. These proteins are encoded and regulated by several genes, the most dominant one being SCN5A. The cardiac sodium channel gene (SCN5A) resides on the short arm of chromosome 3 (3P21) [20]. The most common subunit that controls the sodium current is α-subunit that consists of four homogenous domains as shown in Fig. 2.2 [7, 20, 22]. At the same time, there exist pathways under regulation of ion channel expression, i.e. up or down regulation of certain genes [23, 24].

Most of the sodium current transport occurs early during phase zero (phase 0) of AP ($I_{Na\text{-}early}$ or $I_{Na}$ fast). There remains a small amount of $I_{Na}$ that causes the channel to remain open during phase 2 and 3 of AP called Late $I_{Na,}$ $I_{Na\text{-}late}$ or $I_{Na}$ slow. Although $I_{Na\text{-}late}$ has little contribution under normal (healthy) conditions, it plays an important role under pathological (diseased) conditions (see section under $I_{Na\text{-}late}$ current) [25, 26].

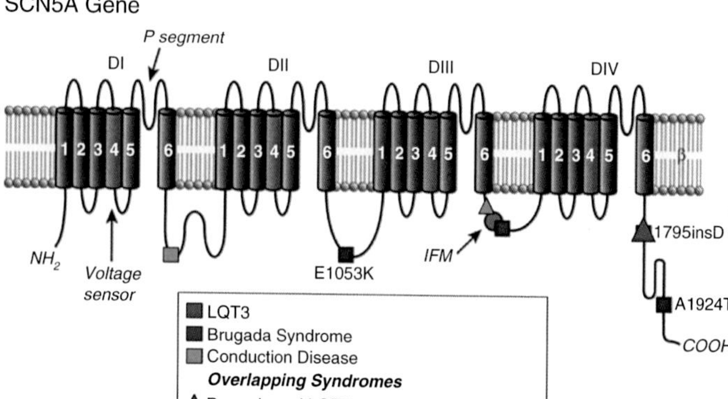


FIGURE 2.2 Illustrates the four domains of the sodium channel and SCN5A gene that are involved in various mutations and syndromes. Modified from: Hund T, Mohler PJ. Biophysics of Normal and Abnormal Cardiac Sodium Channel Function. In: Cardiac Electrophysiology: From Cell to Bedside (2014) Elsevier, Philadelphia, USA. With permission [20]

Sodium channels open fast in response to the onset of depolarization phase 0. When the voltage reaches −70 to −60 mV (the threshold of activation), the sodium ions move very rapidly into the cells. At the same time, depolarization triggers fast inactivation and sodium channels close.

## The Biology of Cardiac Sodium Channels

1. Biophysical properties of the voltage-gated sodium currents [27].
2. *Biochemical (proteins that make the channel)*: The effects of different classes of AADs have been investigated using the patch clamp (single channel) technique over the past two decades or more on the $Na^+$ channels and its modulators [28]. Channel proteins and their genetic structures have diverse properties that are divided into two main subunits.

(a) *Alpha (α) subunits*: The α-subunit is a dominant one and determines the formation of ion pores and is sufficient to produce a normally functional sodium channel.

So far, nine sodium channel protein structures that make the α-subunits have been identified; Na $V_1$.1 to Na $V_1$.9 [29–31]. Relevant to cardiac sodium channels are $Na_v$ 1.5 and its gene SCN5A that is involved in some of the cardiac channelopathies and related syndromes such as Brugada syndrome, Long QT 3 (LQT3) syndrome, idiopathic VF, and J-wave syndrome that are discussed later in this chapter (Fig. 2.3).

## Voltage-Gated Sodium Channels

- *Use-dependence Effect of Sodium Blocking Agents*: Most sodium channel blocking agents affect membrane excitability and conduction velocity in a use-dependent fashion.

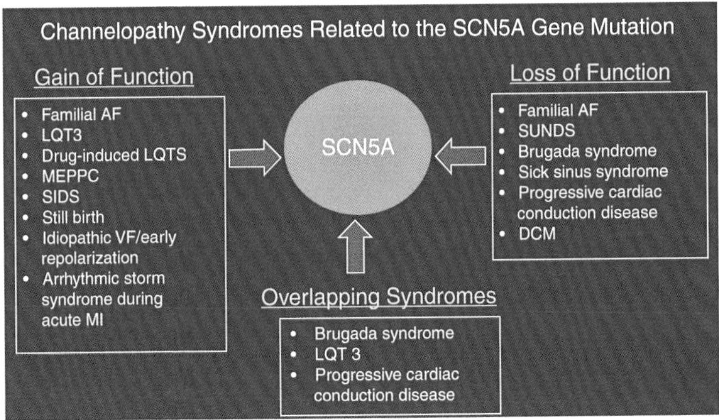


FIGURE 2.3 Shows the SCN5A mutations related to different channelopathy syndromes. Abbreviations: *AF* atrial fibrillation, *DCM* dilated cardiomyopathy, *LQTS* long QT syndrome, *MEPPC* multifocal ectopic Purkinje-related premature contractions, *MI* myocardial infarction, *SIDS* sudden infant death syndrome, *SUNDS* sudden unexplained nocturnal death syndrome

- *Frequency Dependence*: Most class I AADs demonstrate frequency-dependence, i.e. the effect is more pronounced at higher rates. However, there exists some differences between the three classes of sodium channel blockers in their frequency-response effect [32].
- *Effect of Sodium Blocking Agents*: Characterized by increase in refractoriness of the cardiac tissue at fast rates for sodium channel blockers (class I), whereas slower heart rates (lower frequency rates) are mostly observed in class III agents such as Sotalol [33].

## Late $Na^+$ Current

The sodium current is composed of two components:

1. Peak or early sodium current ($I_{Na\text{-}early}$) occurs during the phase zero of AP and is a rapid inward current that takes approximately 1–2 msec.
2. The late sodium current ($I_{Na\text{-}late}$) takes place in phase 2 and early phase 3 of AP and lasts approximately 100–300 msec. An increase in the $I_{Na\text{-}late}$ prolongs APD, and blockade of the $I_{Na\text{-}late}$ shortens APD. Most $I_{Na}$ blockers exhibit both early and late $I_{Na}$ blocking effects, however, at different magnitudes. Ranolazine, a late sodium channel blocker, exhibits 5–9 times higher late than early $Na^+$ blocking effects. $I_{Na\text{-}late}$ channel blockers dissociate from the channel faster than $I_{Na\text{-}early}$, and is probably why they exhibit less proarrhythmic effect compared to $I_{Na\text{-}early}$ blockers [25, 34, 35].

## General Electrophysiological and Electropharmacological Effects of $Na^+$ Channel Blockers

1. All class I agents have direct membrane effects and exhibit local anesthetic effects.
2. Slowing of rapid phase zero APD results in decrease in excitability.

3. Prolongation of conduction velocity (slowing conduction time).
4. Sodium channel blockers suppress both voltage-dependent and time-dependent recovery of excitability. Effects of these agents on voltage-dependent properties (kinetics) are more pronounced in ischemic tissue than normal tissue.
5. Suppression of time-dependent property by Na-channel blockers prolongs tissue refractorincss, and if such effect sustains longer than the repolarization phase it will cause post-repolarization refractoriness.
6. In cardiac fibers that demonstrate spontaneous automaticity, the sodium channel blockers exhibit increased slowing of the spontaneous diastolic depolarization [36, 37].
7. Sodium channel blockers can suppress excitability and prolong conduction and refractoriness. Therefore, may be effective on a variety of arrhythmias with diverse mechanisms and substrates.
8. Sodium ion channel blockers also eliminate the triggers, such as PAC and PVCs. It is also important to realize, as it was shown in the CAST trial, that elimination of triggers such as PVCs do not always translate to elimination of mechanisms of arrhythmias nor substrate modifications; risk predictors are not always the same as efficacy predictors. Thus, CAST showed failure of PVC elimination to improve outcome.

*Effect of Na+ channel blockers on electrocardiographic and intracardiac intervals* (Table 2.3).

## Class Ia AAD: Quinidine, Procainamide, Disopyramide, and Ajmaline

As discussed earlier, according to the Vaughan Williams classification, Class I AADs are subdivided into three classes: Ia, Ib and Ic based on their effect on APD (Table 2.1). Class Ia agents mainly affect the phase 0 of APD and thus prolong

TABLE 2.3 The effect of sodium channel blocking agents on electrocardiogram and intracardiac intervals

| Agent | Sinus rate | PR interval | QRS duration | QT interval | AH interval | HV interval |
|---|---|---|---|---|---|---|
| *Class Ia* | | | | | | |
| Quinidine | ↑ or — | ↓ or variable | ↑ | ↑ | ↓ | ↑ |
| Procainamide | — | Variable | ↑ | ↑ | ↑ or — | ↑ |
| Disopyramide | ↑ or — | Variable | ↑ | ↑ | Variable | ↑ |
| Ajmaline | — | — | ↑ | ↑ | Variable | ↑ |
| *Class Ib* | | | | | | |
| Lidocaine | — | — | No change | ↓ | ↓ or variable | Prolongs |
| Mexiletine | — | — | No change | ↓ | Variable | ↑ or variable |
| *Class Ic* | | | | | | |
| Propafenone | ↓ or variable | ↑ | ↑ | ↑ | ↑ | ↑ |
| Flecainide | ↓ or variable | ↑ | ↑ | ↑ | ↑ | ↑ |

Variable: May prolong or shorten, ↑ Prolongs, ↓ Shortens, "—" No change conduction time, and also prolong repolarization to some degree. The prototypes of this class are quinidine, procainamide, and disopyramide.

## *Quinidine*

- *Effects of quinidine on the ECG* (Table 2.3).
- *Electrophysiologic and antiarrhythmic properties of quinidine (*Table 2.4*). Pharmacokinetic properties of quinidine (*Table 2.5*)* [38].
- *Drug interactions* (Table 2.6).
- *Novel indications of sodium channel blockers of quinidine*: Recent reports suggest that low dose quinidine (<600 mg/day) was effective in preventing ventricular arrhythmia recurrences and storm in patients with Brugada syndrome [39–43]. Mizusawa, et al. reported on the effects of low-dose quinidine in VT in patient with Brugada syndrome [44]. High dose quinidine ($\geq$ 1 g/day; needed to block the transient rapid outward potassium current ($I_{to}$)) was also found to be effective in ventricular tachyarrhythmias and VT storm in patients with Brugada syndrome [39, 45–47]. This effect is only tested in a limited number of patients with Brugada syndrome who have implantable cardioverter-defibrillators (ICDs) [39, 45, 48–50].

  Belhassen, et al. reported that quinidine was effective in preventing induction of VF in 22/25 (88%) patients with Brugada syndrome [48].

  The mechanisms of quinidine's efficacy in patients with Brugada syndrome and ventricular tachyarrhythmias are believed (in part) to be due to blockade of rapid inward $I_{Na}$. Quinidine, besides its direct effect on $I_{Na}$ channel blocker, also exhibits $I_{to}$ inhibition [44].

  Interestingly, quinidine selectively blocks $I_{to}$ current more in the epicardial than endocardial region of the right ventricle. This may explain, in part, its efficacy against ventricular arrhythmias in Brugada syndrome [40, 51, 52].

Table 2.4 Effects of sodium channel blockers on electrophysiological variables

| Agent | APD | Vmax | CT | Rate dependence | | Atrial ERP | Ant ERP-AVN | Ant ERP-HPS | ERP-VM | Ret ERP-AVN | Ret ERP-HPS | Ant ERP-AP | Ret ERP-AP |
|---|---|---|---|---|---|---|---|---|---|---|---|---|---|
| | | | | All rates | Fast rates | | | | | | | | |
| *Class Ia* | | | | | | | | | | | | | |
| Quinidine | ↑ | ↓ | ↓ | ++ | | ↑ | Variable | ↑ | ↑ | ↑ | ↑ | ↑ | ↑ |
| Procainamide | ↑ | ↓ | ↓ | ++ | | ↑ | Variable | ↑ | ↑ | ↑ | ↑ | ↑ | ↑ |
| Disopyramide | ↑ | ↓ | ↓ | ++ | | ↑ | Variable | ↑ | ↑ | ↑ | ↑ | ↑ | ↑ |
| Ajmaline | ↑ | ↓ | ↑ | — | — | ↑ | Variable | ↑ | ↑ | ↑ | ↑ | ↑ | ↑ |
| *Class Ib* | | | | | | | | | | | | | |
| Lidocaine | ↓ | ↓ | ↓ | | ++ | — | Varible | ↑ | Variable | — | — | — | — |
| Mexiletine | ↓ | ↓ | ↓ | | ++ | — | Variable | Variable | — | — | — | — | — |
| *Class Ic* | | | | | | | | | | | | | |
| Propafenone | ↑ | ↓ | ↑ | ++ | | ↑ | ↑ | ↑ | ↑ | ↑ | ↑ | ↑ | ↑ |
| Flecainide | ↑ | ↓ | ↑ | ++ | | ↑ | ↑ | ↑ | ↑ | ↑ | ↑ | ↑ | ↑ |

Abbreviations: *APD* action potential duration, *CT* conduction time, *ERP* early refractory period

TABLE 2.5 Dosage and pharmacokinetic properties of sodium channel blockers

| | Class Ia | | | Class Ib | | Class Ic | |
|---|---|---|---|---|---|---|---|
| | **Quinidine** | **Procainamide** | **Disopyramide** | **Lidocaine** | **Mexiletine** | **Propafenone** | **Flecainide** |
| Daily dose | 600–1600 mg | Oral: 1000–4000 mg IV: 0.5–1 mg/kg/min | 250–750 mg | IV: 3–5 mg/kg (25–50 mg/min) | 450–900 mg | 450–900 mg | 200–400 mg |
| Absorption | >90% | >90% | 80–90% | — | >90% | 80–90% | 90% |
| Bioavailability | 70–80% | 75–90% | 70–90% | — | >80% | 13–55% | 90–95% |
| Peak blood level (hours) | 1–3 h | 1–2 h | 0.5–2 h | — | 2–4 h | 2–5 h | 3–4 h |
| Protein binding | 85–95% | 15% | 20–60% | 70% | 60–70% | 90–95% | 40–60% |
| Mean half-life | 7–18 h | 3–5 h | 7–9 h | 1–2 h[a] | 10 h[b] | 10–32 h | 20 h |
| Metabloism and elimination | Hepatic: 50–90% renal: 10–30% | Hepatic: 40–70% renal: 30–60% | Hepatic: 11–37% renal: 36–77% | Hepatic: 90% | Hepatic: 80–90% renal: <20% | Hepatic: 99% | Renal: 85% |
| Volume of distribution (L/kg) | 2–3 | 1.5–2.5 | 0.5–1.5 | 1 | 6–9 | 3 | 10 |

(continued)

Table 2.5 (continued)

| | Class Ia | | | Class Ib | | Class Ic | |
|---|---|---|---|---|---|---|---|
| | **Quinidine** | **Procainamide** | **Disopyramide** | **Lidocaine** | **Mexiletine** | **Propafenone** | **Flecainide** |
| Plasma concentration (μg/mL) | 2–6 | 4–10 | 2–5 | 1.5–5 | 1–2 | <1 | 0.2–1 |
| Active metabolites | 4-OH-Quinidine | NAPA | Mono-N-dealkyl disopyramide | MEGX, GX[b] | – | 5-OH-propafenone | Meta-O-Dealkylated flecainide |
| Safety in pregnancy (class) | C | C | C | B | C | C | C |

Abbreviations: *h* hours, *NAPA* N-Acetyl procainamide, *MEGX* monoethylglycylxylidide

[a]In patients with HF, half-life may increase to 10–12

[b]15–17 h in patients with acute myocardial infarction

Table 2.6 Sodium channel blocker drug interactions

| | Cardiac drugs | | | | | Non-cardiac drugs | |
|---|---|---|---|---|---|---|---|
| | Digoxin | β blockers | $Ca^{2+}$ blockers | Warfarin | Amiodarone | Cimetidine | Phenytoin |
| *Class Ia* | | | | | | | |
| Quinidine | ↑ | ↑[b] | ↑[b] | ↑[a] | ↑ | ↑ | ↓ |
| Procainamide | — | ↑[b] | ↑[b] | — | ↑ | ↑ | — |
| Disopyramide | — | ↑[b] | ↑[b] | ↓ | — | — | ↓ |
| *Class Ib* | | | | | | | |
| Lidocaine | — | ↑ | — | — | — | ↑ | — |
| Mexiletine | — | — | — | — | — | ↓ | ↑ |
| *Class Ic* | | | | | | | |
| Propafenone | ↑ | ↑ | ↓ | ↑ | — | ↑ | — |
| Flecainide | ↑ | ↓ | ↓ | — | ↑ | ↑ | — |

↑ increase, ↓ Decrease, "—" no change
[a]By decreasing clotting factors
[b]Cardiodepressent effect

Quinidine is also effective in patients with short QT (SQT) syndrome by prolonging the QT interval and preventing ventricular arrhythmias [53–55]. The SQT interval is due to the gain of function in $I_{Kr}$ and is related to the mutation in the HERG gene. The SQT syndrome is often seen in combination with familial AF; therefore, quinidine is effective for both conditions. In these cases, quinidine normalizes the QT interval and renders VF as non-inducible [54]. Similarly, quinidine has been shown to be effective in patients with J-wave/early repolarization syndrome [56–59]. Procainamide, propafenone, flecainide, and disopyramide may induce or unmask ST segment elevation in patients with concealed J-wave syndrome [60–62].

- *Adverse effects of quinidine*:
  - *Cardiac*: Quinidine has long been known to prolong QT interval and thus induces TdP known as quinidine syncope (1–3%). The mechanism of quinidine-induced TdP is assumed to be due to EAD [63, 64]. The QT prolongation effect of quinidine is more effective at slower heart rates (bradycardia-dependent).

## *Procainamide*

- *Effects of procainamide on the ECG* (Table 2.3).
- *Electrophysiogical properties of procainamide* (Table 2.4).
- *Phamacokinetic properties of procainamide* (Table 2.5).
- *Oral dosing* (Table 2.5): Due to the short half-life of procainamide, multiple dosages per 24 h are required. Thus, a total dose of 1000–4000 mg per day may be administered. Long acting (slow release of procainamide) is also available and may be administered at twice a day intervals.
- *Novel indications of procainamide to unmask "concealed" Brugada ECG patterns in patients suspected of Brugada Syndrome*: In Europe, IV ajmaline is used to unmasked concealed or suspected Brugada syndrome (1 mg/kg) [65], whereas in the United States, IV procainamide is used for this purpose [61, 66–68].

## *Disopyramide*

- *Effects of disopyramide on the ECG* (Table 2.3).
- *Electrophysiogical properties of disopyramide* (Table 2.4).
- *Phamacokinetic properties and dosage of Disopyramide* (Table 2.5).
- *Drug interactions* (Table 2.6).
- *Indication*: Disopyramide is effective against atrial and ventricular arrhythmias as well as effective in patients with paroxysmal and persistent AF. It is also effective against sinus node reentry tachycardia, atrial flutter, atrial tachycardia, AVNRT, and AVRT. Intravenous disopyramide is effective in controlling AF in patients with Wolff-Parkinson-White Syndrome [69]. Disopyramide has been used in the past to control a variety of ventricular arrhythmias such as PVCs, couplets, non-sustained and sustained VT; however, it has been less frequently used in recent years. Effects of disopyramide in post-infarction phase have been investigated and showed that although disopyramide reduced ventricular extrasystoles, it did not show a significant decrease in VT and VF or a reduction in cardiac mortality [70]
- *Use of disopyramide in patients with HCM and AF*: Disopyramide, due to its negative inotropic effect as well as ventricular relaxation property, is effective in reducing the LV outflow tract gradually. As AF is the most common arrhythmia in patients with HCM, disopyramide is also effective in controlling AF in these patients (300–600 mg daily; others have used 250–750 mg daily [71]) [72]. However, due to its significant cardiac and non-cardiac side effects, long-term use is limited. Sherrid et al., reported on a multicenter study of efficacy and safety of disopyramide in obstructive HCM and reported in this large cohort (118 patients) that disopyramide appeared effective in reducing the symptoms in 78 (66%) of the patients. In the remaining 40 (34%) patients, disopyramide did not adequately reduce their symptoms [73]. Several reports suggest the use of disopyramide for controlling AF in patients with HCM. However, due to its vagolytic effect, disopyramide

may increase the ventricular rate in these patients. Therefore, it should be used concomitantly with A-V nodal slowing agents such as beta-blockers or calcium antagonists. Interestingly, disopyramide did not increase the risk of proarrhythmia in these patients [73]. Needless to say, the QT/QTc interval should be monitored during disopyramide therapy in these patients [74]. In summary, disopyramide is effective in selected patients with HCM; however, due to its potential proarrhythmic and torsadogenic effect, careful monitoring is recommended and should generally be used after a beta-blocker trial before considering surgical or alcohol septal ablation [73, 75].

According to the most recently published guidelines, due to disopyramides vagolytic property, should be used in combination with an A-V nodal blocking agent to avoid rapid ventricular response [74].

## *Ajmaline*

Ajmaline is a derivative of the Rauwolfia plant and is not approved in the United States

- *Electrophysiogical properties of ajmaline* (Table 2.4).
- *Phamacokinetic properties and dosage of ajmaline* (Table 2.5).
- *Novel Indications of Ajmaline*: Aside from its usual indication for acute termination of supraventricular or ventricular arrhythmias, ajmaline is used for diagnostic purposes of:

  1. Blocking the accessory pathway in patients with Wolff-Parkinson-White syndrome [76–78]
  2. Unmasking the Brugada ECG signs in individuals suspected of this syndrome [79].
  3. Unmasking the latent His-Purkinje system disease.

- Life-threatening ventricular arrhythmias have been reported during ajmaline tests in patients with Brugada syndrome. The incidence is about 1.8% of patients in a large cohort [80, 81]

## Class Ib AAD: Lidocaine, Mexiletine

### *Lidocaine*

- *Effects of lidocaine on the ECG* (Table 2.3).
- *Electrophysiologic and antiarrhythmic properties of lidocaine* (Table 2.4).
- *Pharmacokinetic properties of lidocaine* (Table 2.5).
- *Drug interactions* (Table 2.6).

### *Mexiletine*

- *Effects of mexiletine on the ECG* (Table 2.3).
- *Electrophysiologic and antiarrhythmic properties of mexiletine (*Table 2.4*). Pharmacokinetic properties of mexiletine* (Table 2.5).
- *Drug interactions* (Table 2.6).
- *Novel indication of mexiletine*: Since mexiletine does not prolong repolarization, it has been used safely in patients with LQT syndrome; specifically LQT3 in which the SCN5A gene involved that controls the $I_{Na+}$ current [82–84]. Indeed, mexiletine shortens the QT and QTc interval and therefore reduces indices of malignant arrhythmic events in patients with LQT syndrome. Torsadogenic effects of mexiletine are rare. Another interesting finding is the blockade of mexiletine of the $I_{Na\text{-}late}$ and its potential use in patients with Timothy syndrome [85].

## Class Ic AAD: Propafenone and Flecainide

### *Propafenone (Table 2.1)*

- *Effects of propafenone on the ECG* (Table 2.3).
- *Electrophysiologic and antiarrhythmic properties of propafenone* (Table 2.4) [43].

- *Pharmacokinetic properties of propafenone* (Table 2.5).
- *Drug interactions* (Table 2.6).
- *Efficacy of propafenone in patients with AF*: Propafenone's use-dependent property makes it effective against AF and atrial flutter [86, 87]. The recommended dose of propafenone for AF is 150–300 mg three times daily. The average efficacy at 1 year is 40–75% [88]. Propafenone is currently approved for use in patients with paroxysmal and persistent AF [63].

  Propafenone prolongs anterograde and retrograde A-V nodal conduction. Thus, this makes it effective in the prevention and termination of arrhythmias that are A-V node-dependent, i.e. AVNRT and AVRT. Propafenone also reduces excitability, spontaneous automaticity, and triggered activity. It also has mild $I_{Kr}$ blocking effect as well as a weak beta-blocker effect; however, it is higher than flecainide. Propafenone also prolongs and blocks both anterograde and retrograde conduction of the accessory pathways; thus it is effective against patients with recurrent AVRT [89, 90].
- *Efficacy of propafenone in patients with ventricular arrhythmias*: Propafenone prolongs ventricular conduction time at a greater degree than refractoriness. This imbalance may be the mechanism of propafenones proarrhythmia that facilitates (promotes) ventricular tachyarrhythmias [89, 90]. Propafenone is effective in reducing PVCs, couplets, and non-sustained VT. Efficacy for sustained VT in chronic phase of MI is based on electrophysiological testing and is moderate, i.e. 40%.
- *Proarrhythmic effects of propafenone*: Like flecainide and other class Ic agents, propafenone poses significant ventricular proarrhythmias, especially in patients with CAD, ischemia, presence of myocardial scar, reduced LV systolic function, as well as LVH. Propafenone may increase ventricular response in patients with atrial flutter. This effect is due to propafenone slowing atrial flutter rate and thus allowing more flutter wave conduction to the ventricle [91, 92].

## *Flecainide*

- Effects of flecainide on the ECG (Table 2.3).
- *Electrophysiologic and antiarrhythmic properties of flecainide* (Table 2.4) [43].
- *Pharmacokinetic properties of flecainide* (Table 2.5).
- *Drug interactions* (Table 2.6) [93, 94].
- *Dosage* (Table 2.7).
- *Indication*: Flecainide is effective in reducing PVCs, ventricular couples, and non-sustained VT. Initial experience found flecainide effective against sustained monomorphic VT based on Holter and electrophysiological testing; however, due to its proarrhythmic effect, it is less used (see guidelines) [95]. No data supports the reduction of sudden cardiac death (SCD) with flecainide or propafenone. Flecainide for sustained monomorphic VT in patients with CAD based on electrophysiological studies and program stimulation is not very effective: the VT often remains inducible (Fig. 2.4).
- *Ventricular arrhythmias*: Flecainide is effective in reducing PVCs, non-sustained, and sustained VT; however, it carries the risk of proarrhythmias. Conceptually, any agent that prolongs conduction time changes the balance between conduction time and refractoriness and hence may cause increased likelihood of facilitating reentry. This was well documented in the case of propafenone, and is similar to flecainide [89, 90]. Fig. 2.4 shows exercise induced VT in a patient with CAD (see Fig. 2.4 legend for explanation). Indication for the use of flecainide in patients with VT is summarized in Table 2.7 from the 2015 ESC Guidelines.

  Almost all class I AADs effects are reversible with isoproterenol [96].
- *Novel indication of flecainide*: Interesting data is emerging on the use and effectiveness of flecainide in patients with catecholaminergic polymorphic ventricular tachycardia (CPVT) [97–104]. Although the treatment of choice for patients with CPVT is beta-blockers and ICDs, only one study has reported flecainide-inhibited ryanodine receptor-mediated calcium release in two

Table 2.7 Available AADs for the treatment of ventricular arrhythmias [95]

| AADs (Vaughan Williams class) | Dose (mg/day) | Common or important adverse effects | Indication | Cardiac contra-indications and warnings |
|---|---|---|---|---|
| Quinidine | 600–1600 | Nausea, diarrhea, auditory and visual disturbance, confusion, hypotension, thrombocytopenia, hemolytic anemia, anaphylaxis, QRS and QT prolongation, TdP | VT, VF, SQTS, Brugada syndrome | Severe sinus node disease (unless a pacemaker is present); severe AV conduction disturbances (unless a pacemaker is present); severe intraventricular conduction disturbances; previous myocardial infarction; CAD; HF; reduced LVEF; hypotension; inherited Long QT Syndrome; concomitant treatments associated with QT interval prolongation |
| Procainamide | 1000–4000 | Rash, myalgia, vasculitis, hypotension, lupus, agranulocytosis, bradycardia, QT prolongation, TdP | VT | Severe sinus node disease (unless a pacemaker is present); severe AV conduction disturbances (unless a pacemaker is present); severe intraventricular conduction disturbances: previous myocardial infarction; CAD; HF; reduced LVEF; hypotension; reduced LVEF, Brugada syndrome |

| | | | | |
|---|---|---|---|---|
| Disopyramide | 250–750 | Negative inotrope, QRS prolongation, AV block, pro-arrhythmia (atrial monomorphic VT, occasional TdP), anticholinergic effects | VT, PVC | Severe sinus node disease (unless a pacemaker is present); severe AV conduction disturbances (unless a pacemaker is present); severe intraventricular conduction disturbances; previous myocardial infarction; CAD; HF; reduced LVEF; hypotension |
| Mexiletine | 450–900 | Tremor, dysarthria, dizziness, gastrointestinal disturbance, hypotension, sinus bradycardia | VT, LQT3 | Sinus node dysfunction (unless a pacemaker is present); severe AV conduction disturbances (unless a pacemaker is present); severe HF; reduced LVEF; inherited LQTS (other than LQTS3); concomitant treatments associated with QT-interval prolongation |

(continued)

Table 2.7 (continued)

| AADs (Vaughan Williams class) | Dose (mg/day) | Common or important adverse effects | Indication | Cardiac contra-indications and warnings |
|---|---|---|---|---|
| Propafenone | 450–900 | Negative inotrope, gastrointestinal disturbance, QRS prolongation, AV block, sinus bradycardia, pro-arrhythmia (atrial monomorphic VT, occasional TdP) | VT, PVC | Severe sinus bradycardia and sinus node dysfunction (unless a pacemaker is present); (without the concomitant use of AV-blocking agents); severe AV-conduction disturbances (unless a pacemaker is present); severe intraventricular conduction disturbances; previous myocardial infarction; CAD; HF; reduced LVEF; haemodynamically valvular heart disease; Brugada syndrome; inherited LQTS (other than LQTS3); concomitant treatments associated with QT interval prolongation |

| | | | | |
|---|---|---|---|---|
| Flecainide | 200–400 | Negative inotrope, QRS widening, AV block, sinus bradycardia, pro-arrhythmia (atrial flutter, monomorphic VT, occasional TdP), increased incidence of death after myocardial infarction | VT, PVC | Sinus node dysfunction (unless a pacemaker is present); AF/flutter (without the concomitant use of AV-blocking agents); severe AV conduction disturbances (unless a pacemaker is present); severe intraventricular conduction disturbances; previous myocardial infarction; CAD; HF; reduced LVEF; haemodynamically valvular heart disease; Brugada syndrome; inherited LQTS (other than LQTS3); concomitant treatments associated with QT-interval prolongation |

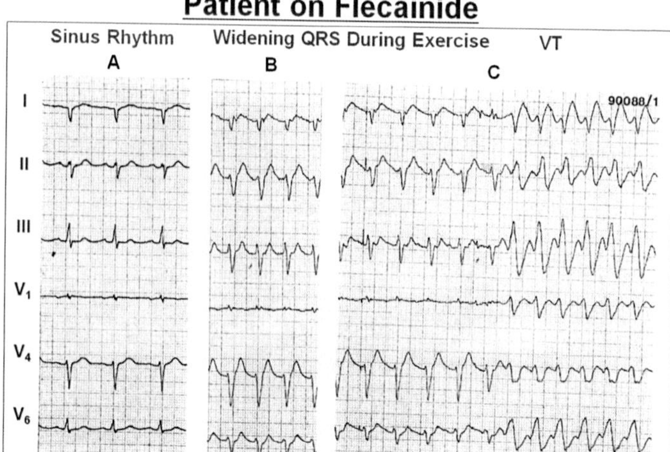


FIGURE 2.4 Exercise-induced VT in a patient with CAD on 300 mg of flecainide. (**a**) Baseline sinus rhythm with a narrow QRS morphology. (**b**) Sinus rhythm with a wider QRS duration under flecainide. (**c**) Progressive prolongation of the QRS duration and initiation of sustained monomorphic VT during exercise testing

patients with CPVT [105]. Van der Werf, et al. reported that flecainide, with a median dose of 150 mg daily, prevented exercise-induced ventricular arrhythmias in 2/3 (76%) of the patients with CPVT [100].

Flecainide may be used to unmask SCN5A related Brugada syndrome [106]. In a cohort of 22 patients, Wolpert, et al. reported on the intravenous use of flecainide and ajmaline on unmasking Brugada syndrome [107]. Flecainide unmasked 15 of the 22 patients and ajmaline unmasked 100%. Some reports suggest that flecainide may be useful in LQT-related SCN5A mutations. Interestingly, it was found that flecainide normalized the ventricular repolarization [108]. Recent reports suggested that flecainide alone or in combination with digoxin, was highly effective in converting fetal SVT to sinus rhythm [109–113]. The dosage administered was 100 mg 4 times daily for the first 2–3 days and then changed to 300 mg/d. The median time to conversion was 3 days (1–7 days).

- *Proarrhythmic effect of flecainide*:

  As flecainide exhibits negligible effect on anterograde A-V nodal conduction, when used in patients with atrial flutter, the drugs prolong atrial flutter cycle length [114] and allow a faster conduction via A-V node with 1:1 and 2:1 A-V conduction causing rapid ventricular response; therefore, flecainide should be used concomitantly with slow A-V nodal conduction agents like calcium antagonists or beta blockers [115]. Ventricular proarrhythmic effects of flecainide include sustained monomorphic VT, TdP, and incessant VT. Also, flecainide induces QRS prolongation during exercise and exercise-induced VT as shown in Fig. 2.4. An increase in the QRS duration by 15–20% is a recognized pharmacologic effect of flecainide; however, several cases have reported that as the QRS duration gets longer during exercise, sustained VT emerges, i.e. exercise-induced VT during flecainide therapy [116]. There is an exception that flecainide is effective in patients with CPVT and exercise-induced arrhythmias. Overall, the use of flecainide worldwide is still low. The Euro-Heart survey on AF shows that 17% and 13% of patients with paroxysmal and persistent AF respectively have been treated with class Ic AAD (flecainide and propafenone) [117].

  Contraindications of both propafenone and flecainide include CAD with and without myocardial ischemia, LV systolic dysfunction, and significant evidence of A-V conduction system disease.

## Other Drug and Substance Interactions

Grapefruit interacts with many cardiovascular and AADs namely quinidine, disopyramide, and propafenone. Since grapefruit decreases the activity of CYP3A4, any pharmacological agent that metabolizes through this enzyme may cause the blood levels of the drug to rise, resulting in the risk of adverse events [118–121]. For further detail of other substances, see Table 2.6 [122].

## Selective Sodium Channel Blockers

The concept of ion-channel selective agents has emerged as an interesting and appealing notion in avoiding global cardiac effect, potential arrhythmogenesis, and proarrhythmic effects [123, 124]. There exists evidence that atrial channel selectivity is expressed in the atria [125]. Among the selective $I_{Na}$ channel blockers are vernakalant and ranolazine. Both have significant atrial-selective blocking properties, which are effective against atrial arrhythmias, specifically AF and atrial flutter. Both agents also demonstrate sodium channel blocking effects in experimental models of pulmonary veins [126, 127].

Sodium channels are highly selective for sodium ions to travel across the cell membrane in a voltage-dependent manner [128]. The sodium channel selectivity is significantly higher than the potassium channel selectivity [129]. There are several factors that influence their selectivity such as voltage, pH, and other modulators and modifiers.

In general, sodium channel blockers have high binding affinity to the early ($I_{Na\text{-}early}$) phase than late ($I_{Na\text{-}late}$) phase. Ranolazine predominantly blocks the $I_{Na\text{-}late}$ phase and thus has less proarrhythmic effect. Also, late sodium currents exhibit a rapid unbinding to the sodium channel as compared to early sodium current [130]. Interestingly, recent data demonstrates that permanent AF increases the number of late $Na^+$ currents in the atria; thus, it is conceivable that ranolazine, a late sodium current blocker, is effective in patients with AF [125, 131–134].

Sodium channel blocking agents have a direct frequency-dependent effect; therefore, their efficacy will be increased during high-rate arrhythmias such as AF. Furthermore, sodium channels demonstrate higher affinity to AADs in their activated/inactivated states compared to their closed state. Late sodium channel blockers ($I_{Na\text{-}late}$) dissociate faster from ion channels than early sodium channel blockers ($I_{Na\text{-}early}$). This may, in part, explain lower proarrhythmic effect of these agents [128].

The limitations of selective ion-channel blockers are as follows:

1. At higher concentrations, they lose selectivity properties. This selectivity may work in normal tissue; however, remodeled tissue may be different.
2. Some agents like ranolazine exhibit differential effect on the $I_{Na}$ channels of the atria as compared to the ventricle.
3. They still carry the risk of proarrhythmias
4. Studies on selective ion-channel blockers are done on healthy tissue preparations in the absence of autonomic, hemodynamic, and structural changes.

Interestingly, both amiodarone and ranolazine are multi-channel blockers; however, they exert an atrial selective sodium channel blocking effect [125, 135–137].

## Genetics of Sodium Channel Dysfunction and Blockers

### *Molecular Genetics of Arrhythmias and Channelopathies Related to Sodium Channel Blockers and their Mutations*

It is quite important to briefly discuss this topic, as more evidence is emerging on the relation of sodium channels and channelopathies to many genetic syndromes related to sodium channels. These concepts are well discussed in the following references [92, 138–143].

As discussed earlier, it is now well established that ion channels operate under genetic control and that certain genes encode proteins for healthy sodium channel function. The site of each gene on chromosomes is called the *locus*, and when genetic information on the DNA sequence is translated to the respective protein(s) via a transcript code with mRNA, it is then passed through the next generation (from the parent). Many of these genes are gender specific and may be dominant or recessive (Mendelian pattern). Several factors affect and determine these mutations including environmental (i.e. radiation, drugs, and chemicals) or other unknown factors. Any errors or modification in their process may cause abnormal mutations, which may lead to the development of specific diseases. Some mutations in the sodium channels are related to Brugada Syndrome, LQT3 Syndrome, dilated cardiomyopathy, AF, and sick sinus syndrome [21, 91, 144].

## Sodium Channel Mutations and Related Channelopathies

The term channelopathies refers to a group of genetic abnormalities and mutations of ion channels that produce cardiac arrhythmias [145–147]. The most common is the SCN5A mutation related to sodium channels that produce the arrhythmia syndromes listed below and are listed in Table 2.8 and Fig. 2.3 [149, 153].

These genetic mutations may cause either loss [154] or gain of function or both [17] (Fig. 2.3).

Loss of Function

1. Brugada syndrome [154–156]
2. Sudden unexplained nocturnal death syndrome [157]
3. Familial AF.
4. Atrial standstill.
5. Sick sinus syndrome [158]
6. Cardiac conduction disease.
7. Progressive cardiac conduction disease [154, 159–162]
8. Congenital A-V block.
9. Dilated cardiomyopathy [163–166]: 16 mutations have been reported.

Gain of Function

1. LQT3 syndrome.
2. Drug-induced LQTs.
3. Familial AF.

Table 2.8 Genetic-related sodium channel arrhythmias [140, 148, 149]

| Arrhythmia syndrome | Affected ion channel | Protein | Gene | Chromosomal locus | Gain/ loss of function | Gender dominance | Inheritance |
|---|---|---|---|---|---|---|---|
| Brugada syndrome | Sodium $Na_V$ 1.5 | B1–3: α-subunit B4–B7: β-subunit | SCN5A | 3p21–p24 | Loss | Male | Autosomal dominant |
| LQT3 syndrome | Sodium $Na_V$ 1.5 | α-subunit | SCN5A | 3p21–p24 | Gain | Female | Autosomal dominant or recessive (rarely), sporadic, acquired |
| Idiopathic VF [150] | Sodium $Na_V$ 1.5 | α-subunit | SCN5A | 3p21–p24 | Gain | Male | Autosomal dominant |
| Familial AF | Sodium $Na_V$ 1.5 | α-subunit | SCN5A | 10q22–24 4q25 Others [151] | Gain and loss | Male | Autosomal dominant |
| Sick sinus syndrome | Sodium $Na_V$ 1.5 | α-subunit | SCN5A | 3p21–p24 | Loss | — | Autosomal dominant or recessive |

(continued)

Table 2.8 (continued)

| Arrhythmia syndrome | Affected ion channel | Protein | Gene | Chromosomal locus | Gain/ loss of function | Gender dominance | Inheritance |
|---|---|---|---|---|---|---|---|
| PCCD syndrome | Sodium $Na_V$ 1.5 | α-subunit | SCN5A | 3p21–p24 | Loss | – | Autosomal dominant |
| Dilated Cardiomyopathy [152] | Sodium $Na_V$ 1.5 | α-subunit | SCN5A | 3p22–p25 | Loss | Male | Autosomal dominant (adult) Autosomal recessive (pediatric) |
| Sudden infant death syndrome | Sodium $Na_V$ 1.5 | α-subunit | SCN5A | – | Gain | Male | Autosomal recessive, sporadic |

Early repolarization syndrome, several genes may be operational

Since J-wave and early repolarization is a syndrome, there will be overlap of J-wave syndrome with other channelopathies; thus, more than one ion channel may be involved. In some of the mutations in early repolarization syndrome (type 6), SCN5A is involved

Abbreviations: *AF* atrial fibrillation, *LQT3* long QT 3 syndrome, *PCCD* progressive cardiac conduction defect, *VF* ventricular fibrillation

4. Multifocal ectopic Purkinje-related premature contractions [167]
5. Sudden infant death syndrome [24]
6. Stillbirth.
7. Idiopathic VF/early repolarization [150, 168]
8. Arrhythmic storm syndrome during acute myocardial infarction [169]

## Sodium Ion Channelopathies and Related Syndromes (Table 2.8 and Fig. 2.3)

Most of these syndromes are related to the SCN5A gene mutation. These are divided into two categories, loss of function, and gain of function [170]. Furthermore, there are a few syndromes that have common genetic mutations such as LQT3 syndrome, Brugada syndrome, and progressive cardiac conduction defect [141, 160, 171–174]. Laurent G, et al. recently reported a new SCN5A-related cardiac channelopathy that presents as multifocal ectopic Purkinje-related premature contractions [167].

*Progressive Cardiac Conduction Disease Syndrome*: This syndrome is due to the mutation of SCN5A gene of the $Na_V$ 1.5 channel. It is an inherited arrhythmia disorder and is due to loss of function [175]. Recent studies suggest that autoimmune response may express the sodium channel $Na_v$ 1.5 and produce AV block [176, 177]. So far, 11 forms of mutations have been described. This syndrome overlaps with other sodium channelopathies such as Brugada syndrome, LQT3, and DCM (Fig. 2.3) [160, 178, 179].

*Genetic Forms of AF*: There is now compelling evidence that a genetic form of AF exists, [180] either as a standalone or part of a broader spectrum of other genetic arrhythmia syndromes such as Brugada syndrome, LQT syndrome, and SQT syndrome [181–185]. Several genes and their mutations are associated with genetic forms of AF such as mutations in sodium channels related to SCN5A, SCN1B-2B and many others [149, 186–188].

Aside from ventricular tachyarrhythmias and SCD, AF is the most common arrhythmia associated with Brugada syndrome [189]. The incidence varies from 20–50% according to different geographical regions [190]. Besides Brugada syndromes, AF may also exist in other cardiac channelopathies such as LQT, SQT and CPVT [191].

*LQT3 syndrome*: LQT3 syndrome is due to an increased function in the late sodium current that prolongs APD [192]. The gene responsible in LQT3 syndrome is related to SCN5A mutation and is either autosomal dominant or a recessive inheritance pattern [179, 193]. Therefore, LQT3-related arrhythmia blockade of the late sodium current by ranolazine is effective against arrhythmias related to LQT3 [194]. Ranolazine, by decreasing $I_{Na\text{-}late}$, shortens APD and abolishes arrhythmias related to LQT3 [194].

Other genetic-related sodium channel arrhythmias are summarized in Table 2.8.

Management of cardiac sodium channelopathies includes [195]:

1. Risk stratification of patients and their relatives. This depends on the severity of the symptoms, phenotypes (ECG findings), and genotypes, i.e. identifying genetic profile and mutations.
2. Pharmacological therapy such as beta-blockers, quinidine, ranolazine, and flecainide (see section on novel indication of class I agents).
3. ICDs in high-risk patients.
4. Surgical left cardiac sympathetic denervation [196, 197].

## AAD Drug-Induced Arrhythmias: Proarrhythmia, Arrhythmogenesis, or Arrhythmia Aggravation

Proarrhythmia (Latin) or arrhythmogenesis (Greek) is defined as aggravation of an existing arrhythmia or development of new arrhythmias that were not present before therapy due to a pharmacological agent (cardiac or non-cardiac) or a non-pharmacological intervention [198]. Proarrhythmia has been far recognized [199]; however, this effect has become more obvious since the CAST and other respective trials [200]. In general, cardiac tissue is anisotropic (non-uniform), particularly in myocardial disease, ischemia, and infarction, which increases anisotropic conduction. The most common form and serious proarrhythmia is TdP due to QT prolongation [201]. In general, TdP is usually initiated with a long-short RR interval sequence [202]. AADs exacerbate the occurrence of serious VT in this setting [203]. An important complication of pharmacological agents, whether cardiac or non-cardiac, is their torsadogenic effect. The mechanisms of drug-induced TdP remain controversial. Most studies suggest that ventricular arrhythmias due to TdP are related to EAD-triggered activity, and it may change to reentrant mechanisms. Multiple factors play a role including genetics, gender, and other mechanisms. Focal or reentry mechanisms are contemplated. It is most likely that both are operational [204, 205].

Virtually all class I agents have the risk of proarrhythmia and TdP. The incidence varies significantly depending on the method that is used for evaluation of proarrhythmia, i.e. invasive vs non-invasive methods and interplay of AADs with arrhythmia substrate (Figs. 2.5 and 2.6).

Class Ia and Ic AADs are among the pharmacological agents that have a high risk of drug-induced TdP (disopyramide, procainamide, quinidine, propafenone, flecainide). Drug-induced LQT Syndrome is also considered an acquired form of LQT Syndrome [206]. Genetic predisposition is an important factor that promotes drug-induced QT prolongation [207, 208]. A comprehensive review of this subject is published by Camm, et al. [209]

Ventricular proarrhythmic effect of class I agents includes increasing the ventricular response in patients with AF and flutter as well as sustained monomorphic VT, incessant VT, polymorphic VT, VF, TdP, and others.

A recent report has been published by Riad et al. on drug-induced QT prolongation. Patients were divided into four risk profiles: no risk, conditional risk, possible risk and known risk [210].

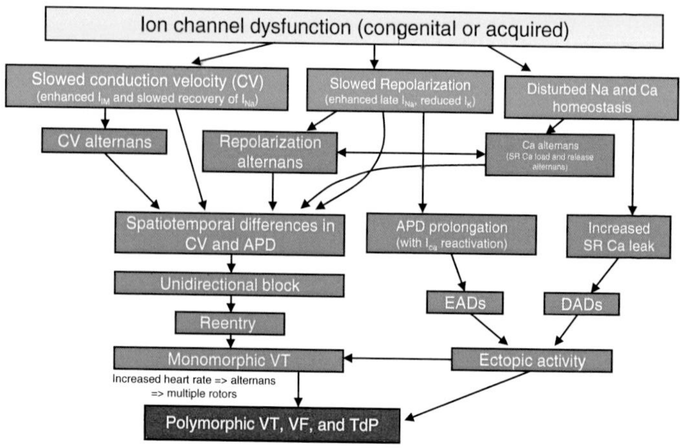


FIGURE 2.5 Interplay of different ion channel dysfunctions related to channelopathies, ventricular arrhythmias and SCD. With permission from Wagner S, et al. Circ Res 2015;116:1956–1970 [15]. Abbreviations: *APD* action potential duration, *Ca alternans* Calcium alternans, *DADs* delayed afterdepolaizations, *EADs* early afterdepolarizations, *SR* sinus rhythm, *TdP* torsades de pointes, *VF* ventricular fibrillation, *VT* ventricular tachycradia

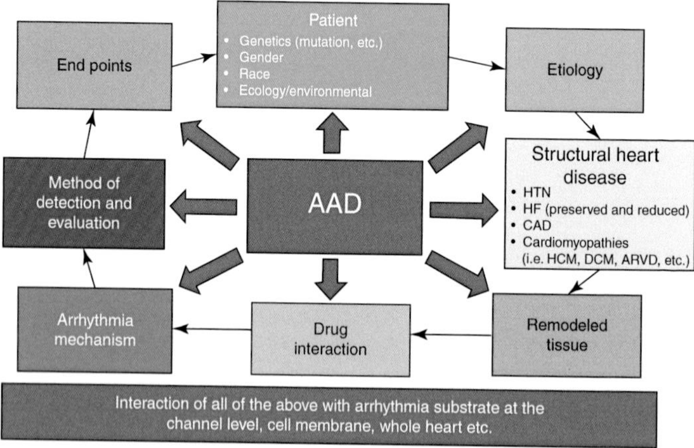


FIGURE 2.6 Relationship of AADs to Clinical Pathophysiology. Abbreviations: *AAD* antiarrhythmic drug, *ARVD* arrhythmogenic right ventricular dysplasia, *CAD* coronary artery disease, *DCM* dilated cardiomyopathy, *etc.* etcetera, *HCM* hypertrophic cardiomyopathy, *HF* heart failure, *HTN* hypertension

There are several risk factors for drug-induced proarrhythmias that are determined elsewhere [201, 208, 211–219].

Prevention of Sodium Channel Blocker Proarrhythmia [220]:

1. Elimination of the predisposing factors such as bradycardia, electrolyte imbalance, cardiac, and non-cardiac agents that promote TdP.
2. Modification of underlying heart disease such as HF, impaired renal function, hepatic disease, etc.
3. Appropriate monitoring in patients at risk of proarrhythmia and TdP such as ECG monitoring for QT prolongation, etc. [221, 222]
4. Appropriate patient teaching and use of digital devices to obtain urgent rhythms.

## Sodium Ion Channel Remodeling

There is some evidence, although controversial, about sodium channel remodeling. This mostly occurs in patients with HF, ischemia and infarction, and AF. However, in the remodeled tissue, more than one ion channel is often involved, particularly in patients with persistent and permanent AF [223]. Sodium channel remodeling creates abnormalities that favor occurrence of reentry and EADs. Reverse remodeling hopefully will correct arrhythmias related to sodium channel remodeling [224]. Amiodarone, a multichannel blocker which also blocks the sodium current, has been reported to be effective against AF-induced remodeling [225]. Sodium channels are reduced in remodeled atria during atrial tachycardia in experimental models and in patients with long-standing AF. Under these conditions the sodium channels are down-regulated [226–229].

## The Ideal Antiarrhythmic Agent

A "wish list" of an ideal AAD includes:

1. Being effective in prevention of arrhythmias.
2. Induce reverse-remodeling.

3. Prevent and reverse inflammation and fibrosis.
4. Exhibit both ion-channel as well as systemic effect (system pharmacology).
5. Minimal to no adverse effect including cardiac and systemic, i.e. no proarrhythmic consequences.
6. No drug interaction
7. Affordable

At present, such expectations are far from reality.

## Nontraditional Sodium Channel Blockers

1. Vanoxerine is an oral multichannel blocker that also affects the sodium current and has been reported in a randomized trial that it is effective in converting patients with recent onset of AF and atrial flutter to sinus rhythm. Piccini, et al. reported on using a single oral dose of Vanoxerine (400 mg). In 18 out of 26 patients (69%) who received Vanoxerine for atrial arrhythmias converted to sinus rhythm; however, the trial was prematurely terminated due to increased risk of TdP [230]
2. Another agent is Relaxin, which has been tested as an anti-fibrosis agent and was found to improve the sodium current in a rat model of AF [231]
3. WenXin KeLi is a traditional Chinese medicine which has significant multichannel blocking effects, including late and early sodium current [232]
4. There is evidence that suggest that fish oil and n-3 PUFA blocks the sodium channels [233, 234]. Furthermore, limited evidence suggests that fatal arrhythmias may be prevented in high-risk subjects by fish oil n-3 fatty acid intake [235, 236]
5. Conflicting results exist on the efficacy of angiotensin converting enzyme (ACE) inhibitors and angiotensin receptor blockers (ARBs) in patients with AF. This is in part due to the complexity on the mechanisms of AF as well as the relation to structural heart disease. For example, it may be effective in patients with hypertension-related AF due to HF and probably not to other etiologies.

Previous trials have failed to show significant improvement on the efficacy of these agents in patients with AF. The hypothesis is that these agents may have an antifibrotic effect [237, 238]. Two large trials did not show any beneficial effects on reducing AF by valsartan and Irbesartan [239, 240]. Similarly, ACEs and ARBs did not prevent recurrence of AF after catheter ablation [241]. In summary, there is conflicting data regarding the use of ACEs and ARBs. They only work to prevent angiotensin-mediated fibrotic remodeling. Treatment, which has to be given before remodeling, is so advanced that nothing can be done. At the same time, patients have to be at high enough risk for fibrosis that an effect is detectable over the time frame of observation.

## Guidelines on the Use of Sodium Channel Blockers (EHRA/ESC; AHA/ACC/HRS; CCS)

Guidelines for the use of sodium channel blockers by EHRA/ESC are summarized in Table 2.7 [242–244]. Fig. 2.7 shows the algorithms for using AADs in patients with AF.

## Summary

1. The cardiac sodium channels are voltage-dependent channels that consist of four homologous domains, which are regulated mostly by SCN5A genes.
2. AADs that block or modulate the sodium current have a diverse effect on atrial, ventricular, and specialized conduction system. They also exhibit different effects, normal (healthy) and abnormal (pathological substrate) hearts.
3. Abnormalities in cardiac sodium channels, respective genes, and their mutations are responsible for a variety of "channelopathies" and related syndromes such as Brugada Syndrome, LQT3, progressive cardiac conduction defect, and many others.

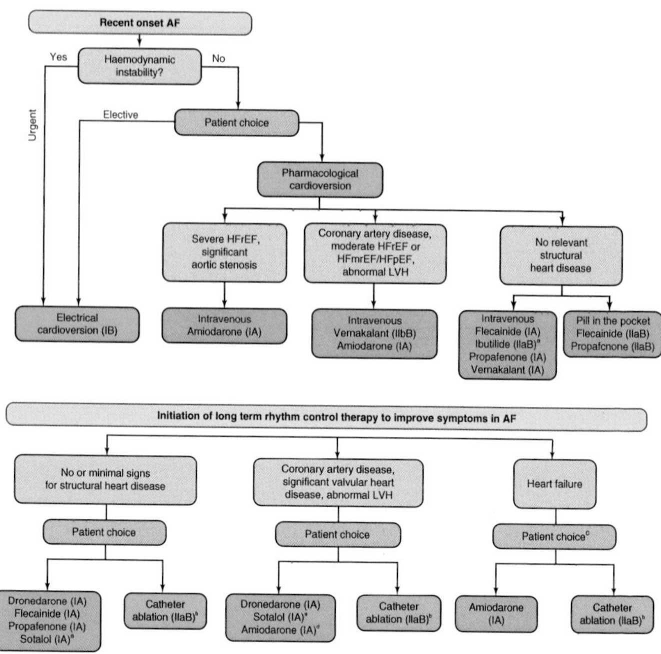


FIGURE 2.7 Algorithm for using AADs in patients with AF. (**a**) Recent onset AF, (**b**) Initiation

4. Precaution should be exercised in patients with systemic disease such as HF, renal, and hepatic failure.
5. The concept of AF is constantly evolving; therefore, response to chronic therapy may change over time [245].
6. Sodium channel blockers or class I AADs, especially class Ic agents, remain the most common AAD used for the control of a variety of arrhythmias; however, caution must be used to exercise the potential proarrhythmic events, i.e. TdP.
7. Recent observations suggest that there are novel indications for several class I agents including quinidine for Brugada syndrome and mexiletine for LQT3 and the like.
8. Class I AADs are among the first class of drugs that came into clinical practice and remain among the major indications for cardiac arrhythmias per the current guidelines,

and more novel indications related to the sodium current and channels will emerge.

## Future Directions

1. Development of novel channel selective agents (sodium channel specific targets) [246]. Due to negative impact of large randomized trials on AADs on VAs and sudden death, the pharmaceutical companies were not interested to invest in developing new AADs; however, with the new frontiers in drugs, devices, and pharmacogenetics, new agents may be developed and expedited by the FDA [247, 248]
2. Development of screening methods to identify responders, non-responders, and proarrhythmic effects with respect to the channels, substrates, and pharmacological agents [249]
3. Gene therapy for channelopathy-related arrhythmias [250]
4. Identification of genetic modifiers.
5. Correlation with genotype-phenotype and detection of high-risk carriers.
6. More detailed insight into the gender/racial, geographic, socioeconomic, circadian variations, and response to medications should be implemented in drug therapy guidelines [251]
7. Identification of the level of penetrance of all related genes and mutations and the role of genetics [252]
8. Identification of factors that precipitate upregulation or down-regulation of genetic function [24]
9. Genomic medicine, pharmacogenomics, and proteomics [253–255]
10. Role of Receptors.
11. Role of MicroRNA [256, 257]
12. Development of substrate-based pharmacological agents such as anti-fibrosis and anti-inflammation.
13. Pharmacological agents that modulate the gap junction (normalize gap junction conduction) [258].

14. Identification of genetic factors related to the risk of drug-induced arrhythmias (the most common one is TdP) [259–261].
15. Stem cell therapy and regenerative medicine relative to arrhythmias and antiarrhythmics.
16. Spinal cord stimulation in the management of drug refractory arrhythmias and storms [262]
17. Personalized and precision medicine [263]
18. Most importantly, considering the effect of AADs on patients, specifically system biology and pharmacology.
19. A gene-specific approach should be implemented more for both risk stratification and selection of AADs [144]

For further information the readers are referred to the following references [176, 264–266]

**Acknowledgements** We wish to thank Sarah Janell Honoré for her superb assistance in the preparation of this manuscript.

Disclosures

The authors do not report any disclosures.

Conflict of Interest

None.

## References

1. Roden DM. Anti-arrhythmic drugs. In: Brunton L, Chabner B, Knollman B, editors. Goodman & Gilman's: the pharmacological basis of therapeutics. New York: McGraw Hill; 2011.
2. Fuster V, Harrington RA, Narula J, Eapen ZJ. Hurst's the heart. 13th ed. New York: McGraw Hill; 2011.
3. Williams EMV. A classification of antiarrhythmic actions reassessed after a decade of new drugs. J Clin Pharmacol. 1984;24(4):129–47. https://doi.org/10.1002/j.1552-4604.1984.tb01822.x.

4. Williams V. Significance of classifying antiarrhythmic action since the cardiac arrhythmia suppression trial. J Clin Pharmacol. 1991;31:123–35.
5. Williams V. Subgroups of class 1 antiarrhythmic drugs. Eur Heart J. 1984;5(2):96–8.
6. The Sicilian Gambit. A new approach to the classification of antiarrhythmic drugs based on their actions on arrhythmogenic mechanisms. Circ. 1991;84:1831–51.
7. Grant AO. Cardiac ion channels. Circ Arrhythm Electrophysiol. 2009;2(2):185–94. https://doi.org/10.1161/CIRCEP.108.789081.
8. Nerbonne JM. Molecular basis of functional myocardial potassium channel diversity. Card Electrophysiol Clin. 2016;8(2):257–73. https://doi.org/10.1016/j.ccep.2016.01.001.
9. Marban E. Cardiac channelopathies. Nature. 2002;415(6868):213–8.
10. Lehmann-Horn F, Jurkat-Rott K. Voltage-gated ion channels and hereditary disease. Physiol Rev. 1999;79:1317–72.
11. Hall J. Transport of substances through cell membranes. In: Hall J, editor. Guyton and Hall textbook of medical physiology. 13th ed. Amsterdam: Elsevier; 2015.
12. Sheets M, Hanck D. Voltage-dependent open-state inactivation of cardiac sodium channels: gating current studies with anthopleurin-A toxin. J Gen Physiol. 1995;106:617–40.
13. Shih H. Anatomy of the action potential in the heart. Tex Heart Inst J. 1994;21:30–41.
14. Jalife J, Delmar M, Anumonwo J, Berenfeld O, Kalifa J. Basic cardiac electrophysiology for the clinician. Hoboken: Wiley-Blackwell; 2009.
15. Wagner S, Maier LS, Bers DM. Role of sodium and calcium dysregulation in tachyarrhythmias in sudden cardiac death. Circ Res. 2015;116(12):1956–70. https://doi.org/10.1161/CIRCRESAHA.116.304678.
16. Abriel H, Rougier JS, Jalife J. Ion channel macromolecular complexes in cardiomyocytes: roles in sudden cardiac death. Circ Res. 2015;116(12):1971–88. https://doi.org/10.1161/CIRCRESAHA.116.305017.
17. Abriel H. Cardiac sodium channel Na(v)1.5 and interacting proteins: physiology and pathophysiology. J Mol Cell Cardiol. 2010;48(1):2–11. https://doi.org/10.1016/j.yjmcc.2009.08.025.
18. Rook MB, Evers MM, Vos MA, Bierhuizen MF. Biology of cardiac sodium channel Nav1.5 expression. Cardiovasc Res. 2012;93(1):12–23. https://doi.org/10.1093/cvr/cvr252.

19. Perez-Riera AR, Daminello Raimundo R, Akira Watanabe R, Luiz de Figueiredo J, Carlos de Abreu L. Cardiac sodium channel, its mutations and their spectrum of arrhythmia phenotypes. J Hum Growth Dev. 2016;26(3):281–96. https://doi.org/10.7322/jhgd.119236.
20. Hund T, Mohler PJ. Biophysics of normal and abnormal cardiac sodium channel function. In: Cardiac electrophysiology: from cell to bedside. Philadelphia: Elsevier; 2014.
21. Wilde AA, Brugada R. Phenotypical manifestations of mutations in the genes encoding subunits of the cardiac sodium channel. Circ Res. 2011;108(7):884–97. https://doi.org/10.1161/CIRCRESAHA.110.238469.
22. Amin AS, Tan HL, Wilde AA. Cardiac ion channels in health and disease. Heart Rhythm. 2010;7(1):117–26. https://doi.org/10.1016/j.hrthm.2009.08.005.
23. Rosati B, McKinnon D. Regulation of ion channel expression. Circ Res. 2004;94(7):874–83. https://doi.org/10.1161/01.RES.0000124921.81025.1F.
24. Van Norstrand DW, Tester DJ, Ackerman MJ. Overrepresentation of the proarrhythmic, sudden death predisposing sodium channel polymorphism S1103Y in a population-based cohort of African-American sudden infant death syndrome. Heart Rhythm. 2008;5(5):712–5. https://doi.org/10.1016/j.hrthm.2008.02.012.
25. Noble D, Noble PJ. Late sodium current in the pathophysiology of cardiovascular disease: consequences of sodium-calcium overload. Heart. 2006;92(Suppl 4):iv1–5. https://doi.org/10.1136/hrt.2005.078782.
26. Antzelevitch C, Nesterenko V, Shryock JC, Rajamani S, Song Y, Belardinelli L. The role of late $I_{Na}$ in development of cardiac arrhythmias. Handb Exp Pharmacol. 2014;221:137–68. https://doi.org/10.1007/978-3-642-41588-3_7.
27. Fozzard H, Hanck D. Structure and function of voltage dependent sodium channels: comparison of brain II and cardiac isoforms. Physiol Rev. 1996;76:887–926.
28. Balser JR. Structure and function of the cardiac sodium channels. Cardiovasc Res. 1999;42:327–38.
29. Catterall WA. Voltage-gated sodium channels and electrical excitability of the heart. In: Cardiac electrophysiology: from cell to bedside. Amsterdam: Elsevier; 2014.

30. Catterall WA. From ionic currents to molecular review mechanisms- the structure and function of voltage-gated sodium channels. Neuron. 2000;26:13–25.
31. Goldin A, Barchi R, Caldwell J, Hofmann F, Howe J, Hunter J, Kallen R, Mandel G, Meisler M, Netter Y, Noda M, Tamkun M, Waxman S, Wood J, Catterall WA. Nomenclature of voltage-gated sodium channels. Neuron. 2000;28:365–8.
32. Weirich J, Antoni H. Differential analysis of the frequency dependent effects of class I-J Cardiovasc Pharma-1990-Weirich & Antoni. J Cardiovasc Pharmacol. 1990;15:998–1009.
33. Hondeghem L, Snyders D. Class III antiarrhythmic agents have a lot of potential but a long way to go: reduced effectiveness and dangers of reverse use dependence. Circ. 1990;81(2):686–90.
34. Shryock JC, Song Y, Rajamani S, Antzelevitch C, Belardinelli L. The arrhythmogenic consequences of increasing late INa in the cardiomyocyte. Cardiovasc Res. 2013;99(4):600–11. https://doi.org/10.1093/cvr/cvt145.
35. Belardinelli L, Giles WR, Rajamani S, Karagueuzian HS, Shryock JC. Cardiac late Na(+) current: proarrhythmic effects, roles in long QT syndromes, and pathological relationship to CaMKII and oxidative stress. Heart Rhythm. 2015;12(2):440–8. https://doi.org/10.1016/j.hrthm.2014.11.009.
36. Campbell T. Differing electrophysiological effects of class IA, IB and IC antiarrhythmic drugs on guinea-pig sinoatrial node. Br J Pharmacol. 1987;91:395–401.
37. Williams V. Disopyramide. Ann N Y Acad Sci. 1984;432:189–200.
38. Podrid PJ, Kowey P. Specific Antiarrhythmic Drugs. In: Cardiac arrhythmia: mechanisms, diagnosis, and management. Philadelphia: Williams & Wilkins; 1995. p. 369.
39. Marquez MF, Bonny A, Hernandez-Castillo E, De Sisti A, Gomez-Flores J, Nava S, Hidden-Lucet F, Iturralde P, Cardenas M, Tonet J. Long-term efficacy of low doses of quinidine on malignant arrhythmias in Brugada syndrome with an implantable cardioverter-defibrillator: a case series and literature review. Heart Rhythm. 2012;9(12):1995–2000. https://doi.org/10.1016/j.hrthm.2012.08.027.
40. Antzelevitch C, Fish JM. Therapy for the Brugada syndrome. Handb Exp Pharmacol. 2006;171:305–30.

41. Belhassen B. Is quinidine the ideal drug for Brugada syndrome? Heart Rhythm. 2012;9(12):2001–2. https://doi.org/10.1016/j.hrthm.2012.08.037.
42. Marquez MF, Salica G, Hermosillo AG, Pastelin G, Gomez-Flores J, Nava S, Cardenas M. Ionic basis of pharmacological therapy in Brugada syndrome. J Cardiovasc Electrophysiol. 2007;18(2):234–40. https://doi.org/10.1111/j.1540-8167.2006.00681.x.
43. Hermida JS, Denjoy I, Clerc J, Extramiana F, Jarry G, Milliez P, Guicheney P, Di Fusco S, Rey JL, Cauchemez B, Leenhardt A. Hydroquinidine therapy in Brugada syndrome. J Am Coll Cardiol. 2004;43(10):1853–60. https://doi.org/10.1016/j.jacc.2003.12.046.
44. Mizusawa Y, Sakurada H, Nishizaki M, Hiraoka M. Effects of low-dose quinidine on ventricular tachyarrhythmias in patients with Brugada syndrome low-dose quinidine therapy as an adjunctive treatment. J Cardiovasc Pharmacol. 2006;47:359–64.
45. Adler A, Viskin S. Clinical features of genetic cardiac diseases related to potassium channelopathies. Card Electrophysiol Clin. 2016;8(2):361–72. https://doi.org/10.1016/j.ccep.2016.02.001.
46. Al-Ahmad A, Shenasa M, Shenasa H, Soleimanieh M. Incessant ventricular tachycardia and fibrillation. Card Electrophysiol Clin. 2014;6(3):613–21. https://doi.org/10.1016/j.ccep.2014.05.010.
47. Belhassen B, Glick A, Viskin S. Excellent long-term reproducibility of the electrophysiologic efficacy of quinidine in patients with idiopathic ventricular fibrillation and Brugada syndrome. Pacing Clin Electrophysiol. 2009;32(3):294–301.
48. Belhassen B, Glick A, Viskin S. Efficacy of quinidine in high-risk patients with Brugada syndrome. Circ. 2004;110(13):1731–7. https://doi.org/10.1161/01.CIR.0000143159.30585.90.
49. Viskin S, Wilde AA, Guevara-Valdivia ME, Daoulah A, Krahn AD, Zipes DP, Halkin A, Shivkumar K, Boyle NG, Adler A, Belhassen B, Schapachnik E, Asrar F, Rosso R, Fadreguilan EC, Veltman C, Veerakul G, Marquez M, Juneja R, Daoulah AN, Caorsi WR, Cuesta A, Jensen HK, Hamad AK, Spears D, Lozano IF, Urda VC, Peinado R, Panduranga P, Emkanjoo Z, Bergfeldt L, Janousek J. Quinidine, a life-saving medication for Brugada syndrome, is inaccessible in many countries. J Am Coll Cardiol. 2013;61(23):2383–7. https://doi.org/10.1016/j.jacc.2013.02.077.

50. Shen T, Yuan B, Geng J, Chen C, Zhou X, Shan Q. Low-dose quinidine effectively reduced shocks in Brugada syndrome patients with an implantable cardioverter defibrillator: a Chinese case series report. Ann Noninvasive Electrocardiol. 2017;22(1):e12375. https://doi.org/10.1111/anec.12375.
51. Marquez M, Salica G, Hermosillo AG, Pastelin G, Cardenas M. Drug therapy in Brugada syndrome. Curr Drug Targets Cardiovasc Haematol Disord. 2005;5(5):409–17.
52. Wilde AA, Postema PG, Di Diego JM, Viskin S, Morita H, Fish JM, Antzelevitch C. The pathophysiological mechanism underlying Brugada syndrome: depolarization versus repolarization. J Mol Cell Cardiol. 2010;49(4):543–53. https://doi.org/10.1016/j.yjmcc.2010.07.012.
53. Giustetto C, Schimpf R, Mazzanti A, Scrocco C, Maury P, Anttonen O, Probst V, Blanc JJ, Sbragia P, Dalmasso P, Borggrefe M, Gaita F. Long-term follow-up of patients with short QT syndrome. J Am Coll Cardiol. 2011;58(6):587–95. https://doi.org/10.1016/j.jacc.2011.03.038.
54. Wolpert C, Schimpf R, Giustetto C, Antzelevitch C, Cordeiro J, Dumaine R, Brugada R, Hong K, Bauersfeld U, Gaita F, Borggrefe M. Further insights into the effect of quinidine in short QT syndrome caused by a mutation in HERG. J Cardiovasc Electrophysiol. 2005;16(1):54–8. https://doi.org/10.1046/j.1540-8167.2005.04470.x.
55. Gaita F, Giustetto C, Bianchi F, Schimpf R, Haissaguerre M, Calo L, Brugada R, Antzelevitch C, Borggrefe M, Wolpert C. Short QT syndrome: pharmacological treatment. J Am Coll Cardiol. 2004;43(8):1494–9. https://doi.org/10.1016/j.jacc.2004.02.034.
56. Haissaguerre M, Derval N, Sacher F, Jesel L, Deisenhofer I, de Roy L, Pasquie JL. Sudden cardiac arrest associated with early repolarization. N Engl J Med. 2008;358:2016–23.
57. Antzelevitch C, Yan GX. J wave syndromes. Heart Rhythm. 2010;7(4):549–58. https://doi.org/10.1016/j.hrthm.2009.12.006.
58. Yan G, Antzelevitch C. Cellular basis for the Brugada syndrome and other mechanisms of arrhythmogenesis associated with ST-segment elevation. Circ. 1999;100:1660–6.
59. Gussak I, Antzelevitch C, Bjerregaard P, Towbin J, Chaitman B. The Brugada syndrome: clinical, electrophysiologic and genetic aspects. J Am Coll Cardiol. 1999;33(1):5–15. https://doi.org/10.1016/s0735-1097(98)00528-2.

60. Shimizu W, Antzelevitch C, Suyama K, Kurita T, Taguchi A, Aihara N. Effect of sodium channel blockers on ST segment, QRS duration, and corrected QT interval in patients with Brugada syndrome. J Cardiovasc Electrophysiol. 2000;11:1320–9.
61. Brugada R, Brugada J, Antzelevitch C, Kirsch GE, Potenza D, Towbin JA, Brugada P. Sodium channel blockers identify risk for sudden death in patients with ST-segment elevation and right bundle branch block but structurally normal hearts. Circ. 2000;101:510–5.
62. Morita H, Morita T, Nagase S, Banba K, Nishi N, Tani Y, Watanabe A. Ventricular arrhythmia induced by sodium channel blocker in patients with Brugada syndrome. J Am Coll Cardiol. 2003;42:1624–31. https://doi.org/10.1016/S0735-1097(03)01124-0.
63. Kirchhof P, Benussi S, Kotecha D, Ahlsson A, Atar D, Casadei B, Castella M, Diener HC, Heidbuchel H, Hendriks J, Hindricks G, Manolis AS, Oldgren J, Popescu BA, Schotten U, Van Putte B, Vardas P, ESC Scientific Document Group. 2016 ESC Guidelines for the management of atrial fibrillation developed in collaboration with EACTS: The Task Force for the management of atrial fibrillation of the European Society of Cardiology (ESC) Developed with the special contribution of the European Heart Rhythm Association (EHRA) of the ESCEndorsed by the European Stroke Organisation (ESO). Eur Heart J. 2016;37(38):2893–962. https://doi.org/10.1093/eurheartj/ehw210.
64. Roden DM. Cellular basis of drug-induced torsades de pointes. Br J Pharmacol. 2008;154(7):1502–7. https://doi.org/10.1038/bjp.2008.238.
65. Roten L, Derval N, Sacher F, Pascale P, Wilton SB, Scherr D, Shah A, Pedersen ME, Jadidi AS, Miyazaki S, Knecht S, Hocini M, Jais P, Haissaguerre M. Ajmaline attenuates electrocardiogram characteristics of inferolateral early repolarization. Heart Rhythm. 2012;9(2):232–9. https://doi.org/10.1016/j.hrthm.2011.09.013.
66. Postema PG, Wolpert C, Amin AS, Probst V, Borggrefe M, Roden DM, Priori SG, Tan HL, Hiraoka M, Brugada J, Wilde AA. Drugs and Brugada syndrome patients: review of the literature, recommendations, and an up-to-date website (http://www.brugadadrugs.org). Heart Rhythm. 2009;6(9):1335–41. https://doi.org/10.1016/j.hrthm.2009.07.002.

67. Somani R, Krahn AD, Healey JS, Chauhan VS, Birnie DH, Champagne J, Sanatani S, Angaran P, Gow RM, Chakrabarti S, Gerull B, Yee R, Skanes AC, Gula LJ, Leong-Sit P, Klein GJ, Gollob MH, Talajic M, Gardner M, Simpson CS. Procainamide infusion in the evaluation of unexplained cardiac arrest: from the cardiac arrest survivors with preserved ejection fraction registry (CASPER). Heart Rhythm. 2014;11(6):1047–54. https://doi.org/10.1016/j.hrthm.2014.03.022.
68. Fish JM, Antzelevitch C. Role of sodium and calcium channel block in unmasking the Brugada syndrome. Heart Rhythm. 2004;1(2):210–7. https://doi.org/10.1016/j.hrthm.2004.03.061.
69. Fujimura O, Klein GJ, Sharma AD, Yee R, Szabo T. Acute effect of disopyramide on atrial fibrillation in the Wolff-Parkinson-white syndrome. J Am Coll Cardiol. 1989;13(5):1133–7. https://doi.org/10.1016/0735-1097(89)90275-1.
70. Zainal N, Griffiths JW, Carmichael DJS, Besterman EMM, Kidner PH, Gillham AD, Summers GD. Oral disopyramide for the prevention of arrhythmias in patients with acute myocardial infarction admitted to open wards. Lancet. 1977;310(8044):887–9. https://doi.org/10.1016/S0140-6736(77)90829-7.
71. Psotka MA, Lee BK. Atrial fibrillation: antiarrhythmic therapy. Curr Probl Cardiol. 2014;39(10):351–91. https://doi.org/10.1016/j.cpcardiol.2014.07.004.
72. Ito M, Onodera S, Hashimoto J, Noshiro H, Shinoda S, Nagashima M, Suzuki H. Effect of disopyramide on initiation of atrial fibrillation and relation to effective refractory period. Am J Cardiol. 1989;63:561–6.
73. Sherrid MV, Barac I, McKenna WJ, Elliott PM, Dickie S, Chojnowska L, Casey S, Maron BJ. Multicenter study of the efficacy and safety of disopyramide in obstructive hypertrophic cardiomyopathy. J Am Coll Cardiol. 2005;45(8):1251–8. https://doi.org/10.1016/j.jacc.2005.01.012.
74. Reiffel J, Estes M, Waldo A, Prystowsky E, DiBianco R. A consensus report on antiarrhythmic drug use. Clin Cardiol. 1994;17:103–16.
75. Sherrid MV, Arabadjian M. A primer of disopyramide treatment of obstructive hypertrophic cardiomyopathy. Prog Cardiovasc Dis. 2012;54(6):483–92. https://doi.org/10.1016/j.pcad.2012.04.003.
76. Wellens HJJ, Bär FW, Gorgels AP, Vanagt EJ. Use of ajmaline in patients with the Wolff-Parkinson-White syndrome to disclose short refractory period of the accessory pathway. In: Smeets

JLRM, Doevendans PA, Josephson ME, Kirchhof C, Vos MA, editors. Professor Hein J.J. Wellens: 33 years of cardiology and arrhythmology. Dordrecht: Springer; 2000. p. 215–9. https://doi.org/10.1007/978-94-011-4110-9_20.

77. Khalilullah M, Sathyamurthy I, Singhal NK. Ajmaline in WPW syndrome: an electrophysiologic study. Am Heart J. 1980;99(6):766–71. https://doi.org/10.1016/0002-8703(80)90627-4.
78. Wellens HJJ, Bär FW, Dassen WRM, Brugada P, Vanagt EJ, Farré J. Effect of drugs in the wolff-parkinson-white syndrome. Am J Cardiol. 1980;46(4):665–9. https://doi.org/10.1016/0002-9149(80)90518-4.
79. Rolf S. The ajmaline challenge in Brugada syndrome: diagnostic impact, safety, and recommended protocol. Eur Heart J. 2003;24(12):1104–12. https://doi.org/10.1016/s0195-668x(03)00195-7.
80. Conte G, Sieira J, Sarkozy A, de Asmundis C, Di Giovanni G, Chierchia GB, Ciconte G, Levinstein M, Casado-Arroyo R, Baltogiannis G, Saenen J, Saitoh Y, Pappaert G, Brugada P. Life-threatening ventricular arrhythmias during ajmaline challenge in patients with Brugada syndrome: incidence, clinical features, and prognosis. Heart Rhythm. 2013;10(12):1869–74. https://doi.org/10.1016/j.hrthm.2013.09.060.
81. Nault I, Champagne J. How safe is ajmaline challenge in patients with suspected Brugada syndrome? Heart Rhythm. 2013;10(12):1875–6. https://doi.org/10.1016/j.hrthm.2013.10.047.
82. Mazzanti A, Maragna R, Faragli A, Monteforte N, Bloise R, Memmi M, Novelli V, Baiardi P, Bagnardi V, Etheridge SP, Napolitano C, Priori SG. Gene-specific therapy with mexiletine reduces arrhythmic events in patients with long QT syndrome type 3. J Am Coll Cardiol. 2016;67(9):1053–8. https://doi.org/10.1016/j.jacc.2015.12.033.
83. Badri M, Patel A, Patel C, Liu G, Goldstein M, Robinson VM, Xue X, Yang L, Kowey PR, Yan G-X. Mexiletine prevents recurrent torsades de pointes in acquired long QT syndrome refractory to conventional measures. JACC Clin Electrophysiol. 2015;1(4):315–22. https://doi.org/10.1016/j.jacep.2015.05.008.
84. Shimizu W, Antzelevitch C. Sodium channel block with mexiletine is effective in reducing dispersion of repolarization and preventing torsade de pointes in LQT2 and LQT3 models of the long-QT syndrome. Circ. 1997;96:2038–47.

85. Gao Y, Xue X, Hu D, Liu W, Yuan Y, Sun H, Li L, Timothy KW, Zhang L, Li C, Yan GX. Inhibition of late sodium current by mexiletine: a novel pharmotherapeutical approach in timothy syndrome. Circ Arrhythm Electrophysiol. 2013;6(3):614–22. https://doi.org/10.1161/CIRCEP.113.000092.
86. Chimienti M, Cullen M, Casadei G. Safety of long-term flecainide and propafenone in the management of patients with symptomatic paroxysmal atrial fibrillation: report from the Flecainide and Propafenone Italian Study Investigators. Am J Cardiol. 1996;77:60A–75A.
87. Antman EM, Beamer AD, Cantillon C, McGowan N, Goldman L, Friedman P. Long-term oral propafenone therapy for suppression of refractory atrial fibrillation and atrial flutter. J Am Coll Cardiol. 1988;12:1005–11.
88. Shenasa M, Shenasa H, Rouhani S. Atrial fibrillation in different clinical subsets. In: Shenasa M, Camm J, editors. Management of atrial fibrillation. Oxford: Oxford University Press; 2015. p. 25–73.
89. Kus T, Dubuc M, Lambert C, Shenasa M. Efficacy of propafenone in preventing ventricular tachycardia: inverse correlation with rate-related prolongation of conduction time. J Am Coll Cardiol. 1990;16(5):1229–37.
90. Marchlinski F. Sorting out the mechanisms of antiarrhythmic drug action. J Am Coll Cardiol. 1990;16(5):1238–9.
91. Napolitano C, Bloise R, Monteforte N, Priori SG. Sudden cardiac death and genetic ion channelopathies: long QT, Brugada, short QT, catecholaminergic polymorphic ventricular tachycardia, and idiopathic ventricular fibrillation. Circ. 2012;125(16):2027–34. https://doi.org/10.1161/CIRCULATIONAHA.111.055947.
92. Schwartz PJ, Ackerman MJ, George AL Jr, Wilde AA. Impact of genetics on the clinical management of channelopathies. J Am Coll Cardiol. 2013;62(3):169–80. https://doi.org/10.1016/j.jacc.2013.04.044.
93. Shea P, Lal R, Kim S, Schechtman K, Ruffy R. Flecainide and amiodarone interaction. J Am Coll Cardiol. 1986;7:1127–30.
94. Roden D, Woosley RL. Drug therapy: flecainide. N Engl J Med. 1986;315(1):36–41.
95. Priori SG, Blomstrom-Lundqvist C, Mazzanti A, Blom N, Borggrefe M, Camm J, Elliott PM, Fitzsimons D, Hatala R, Hindricks G, Kirchhof P, Kjeldsen K, Kuck KH, Hernandez-Madrid A, Nikolaou N, Norekval TM, Spaulding C, Van Veldhuisen DJ. 2015 ESC guidelines for the management of patients with ventricular arrhythmias and the prevention of

sudden cardiac death: the task Force for the management of patients with ventricular arrhythmias and the prevention of sudden cardiac death of the European Society of Cardiology (ESC) endorsed by: Association for European Paediatric and Congenital Cardiology (AEPC). Eur Heart J. 2015;36(41):2793–867. https://doi.org/10.1093/eurheartj/ehv316.

96. Jazayeri MR, Vanwyhe G, Avitall B, McKinnie J, Tchou P, Akhtar M. Isoproterenol reversal of antiarrhythmic effects in patients with inducible sustained ventricular tachyarrhythmias. J Am Coll Cardiol. 1989;14(3):705–11. https://doi.org/10.1016/0735-1097(89)90114-9.
97. Bannister ML, Thomas NL, Sikkel MB, Mukherjee S, Maxwell C, MacLeod KT, George CH, Williams AJ. The mechanism of flecainide action in CPVT does not involve a direct effect on RyR2. Circ Res. 2015;116(8):1324–35. https://doi.org/10.1161/CIRCRESAHA.116.305347.
98. Smith GL, MacQuaide N. The direct actions of flecainide on the human cardiac ryanodine receptor: keeping open the debate on the mechanism of action of local anesthetics in CPVT. Circ Res. 2015;116(8):1284–6. https://doi.org/10.1161/CIRCRESAHA.115.306298.
99. van der Werf C, Zwinderman AH, Wilde AA. Therapeutic approach for patients with catecholaminergic polymorphic ventricular tachycardia: state of the art and future developments. Europace. 2012;14(2):175–83. https://doi.org/10.1093/europace/eur277.
100. van der Werf C, Kannankeril PJ, Sacher F, Krahn AD, Viskin S, Leenhardt A, Shimizu W, Sumitomo N, Fish FA, Bhuiyan ZA, Willems AR, van der Veen MJ, Watanabe H, Laborderie J, Haissaguerre M, Knollmann BC, Wilde AA. Flecainide therapy reduces exercise-induced ventricular arrhythmias in patients with catecholaminergic polymorphic ventricular tachycardia. J Am Coll Cardiol. 2011;57(22):2244–54. https://doi.org/10.1016/j.jacc.2011.01.026.
101. Jacquemart C, Ould Abderrahmane F, Massin MM. Effects of flecainide therapy on inappropriate shocks and arrythmias in catecholaminergic polymorphic ventricular tachycardia. J Electrocardiol. 2012;45(6):736–8. https://doi.org/10.1016/j.jelectrocard.2012.05.002.

102. Watanabe H, van der Werf C, Roses-Noguer F, Adler A, Sumitomo N, Veltmann C, Rosso R, Bhuiyan ZA, Bikker H, Kannankeril PJ, Horie M, Minamino T, Viskin S, Knollmann BC, Till J, Wilde AA. Effects of flecainide on exercise-induced ventricular arrhythmias and recurrences in genotype-negative patients with catecholaminergic polymorphic ventricular tachycardia. Heart Rhythm. 2013;10(4):542–7. https://doi.org/10.1016/j.hrthm.2012.12.035.
103. Pellizzon OA, Kalaizich L, Ptacek LJ, Tristani-Firouzi M, Gonzalez MD. Flecainide suppresses bidirectional ventricular tachycardia and reverses tachycardia-induced cardiomyopathy in Andersen-Tawil syndrome. J Cardiovasc Electrophysiol. 2008;19(1):95–7. https://doi.org/10.1111/j.1540-8167.2007.00910.x.
104. Padfield GJ, AlAhmari L, Lieve KV, AlAhmari T, Roston TM, Wilde AA, Krahn AD, Sanatani S. Flecainide monotherapy is an option for selected patients with catecholaminergic polymorphic ventricular tachycardia intolerant of beta-blockade. Heart Rhythm. 2016;13(2):609–13. https://doi.org/10.1016/j.hrthm.2015.09.027.
105. Watanabe H, Chopra N, Laver D, Hwang HS, Davies SS, Roach DE, Duff HJ, Roden DM, Wilde AA, Knollmann BC. Flecainide prevents catecholaminergic polymorphic ventricular tachycardia in mice and humans. Nat Med. 2009;15(4):380–3. https://doi.org/10.1038/nm.1942.
106. Meregalli PG, Ruijter JM, Hofman N, Bezzina CR, Wilde AA, Tan HL. Diagnostic value of flecainide testing in unmasking SCN5A-related Brugada syndrome. J Cardiovasc Electrophysiol. 2006;17(8):857–64. https://doi.org/10.1111/j.1540-8167.2006.00531.x.
107. Wolpert C, Echternach C, Veltmann C, Antzelevitch C, Thomas GP, Spehl S, Streitner F, Kuschyk J, Schimpf R, Haase KK, Borggrefe M. Intravenous drug challenge using flecainide and ajmaline in patients with Brugada syndrome. Heart Rhythm. 2005;2(3):254–60. https://doi.org/10.1016/j.hrthm.2004.11.025.
108. Windle J, Geletka R, Moss A, Zareba W, Atkins D. Normalization of ventricular repolarization with flecainide in long QT syndrome patients with SCN5A-DeltaKPQ mutation. Ann Noninvasive Electrocardiol. 2001;6(2):153–8.

109. Strizek B, Berg C, Gottschalk I, Herberg U, Geipel A, Gembruch U. High-dose flecainide is the most effective treatment of fetal supraventricular tachycardia. Heart Rhythm. 2016;13(6):1283–8. https://doi.org/10.1016/j.hrthm.2016.01.029.
110. Sridharan S, Sullivan I, Tomek V, Wolfenden J, Skovranek J, Yates R, Janousek J, Dominguez TE, Marek J. Flecainide versus digoxin for fetal supraventricular tachycardia: comparison of two drug treatment protocols. Heart Rhythm. 2016;13(9):1913–9. https://doi.org/10.1016/j.hrthm.2016.03.023.
111. Van Hare GF. Flecainide vs digoxin for fetal supraventricular tachycardia: comparison of 2 drug protocols. Heart Rhythm. 2016;13(9):1920–1. https://doi.org/10.1016/j.hrthm.2016.03.045.
112. Vigneswaran TV, Callaghan N, Andrews RE, Miller O, Rosenthal E, Sharland GK, Simpson JM. Correlation of maternal flecainide concentrations and therapeutic effect in fetal supraventricular tachycardia. Heart Rhythm. 2014;11(11):2047–53. https://doi.org/10.1016/j.hrthm.2014.07.031.
113. Cuneo BF, Benson DW. Use of maternal flecainide concentration in management of fetal supraventricular tachycardia: a step in the right direction. Heart Rhythm. 2014;11(11):2054–5. https://doi.org/10.1016/j.hrthm.2014.08.017.
114. Crijns HJ, van Gelder IC, Lie KI. Supraventricular tachycardia mimicking ventricular tachycardia during flecainide treatment. Am J Cardiol. 1988;62(17):1303–6. https://doi.org/10.1016/0002-9149(88)90282-2.
115. Camm J. Antiarrhythmic drugs for the maintenance of sinus rhythm: risks and benefits. Int J Cardiol. 2012;155(3):362–71. https://doi.org/10.1016/j.ijcard.2011.06.012.
116. Ranger S, Talajic M, Lemery R, Roy D, Nattel S. Amplification of flecainide-induced ventricular conduction slowing by exercise. Circ. 1989;79:1000–6.
117. Nieuwlaat R, Capucci A, Camm AJ, Olsson SB, Andresen D, Davies DW, Cobbe S, Breithardt G, Le Heuzey JY, Prins MH, Levy S, Crijns HJ, European Heart Survey Investigators. Atrial fibrillation management: a prospective survey in ESC member countries: the euro heart survey on atrial fibrillation. Eur Heart J. 2005;26(22):2422–34. https://doi.org/10.1093/eurheartj/ehi505.
118. Bailey DDG, Dresser GK. Interactions between grapefruit juice and cardiovascular drugs. Am J Cardiovasc Drugs. 2004;4(5):281–97. https://doi.org/10.2165/00129784-200404050-00002.

119. Fuhr U. Drug interactions with grapefruit juice. Drug safety. 1998;18(4):251–72.
120. Roden D. Antiarrhythmic drugs: from mechanisms to clinical practice. Heart. 2000;84:339–46.
121. Zitron E, Scholz E, Owen RW, Luck S, Kiesecker C, Thomas D, Kathofer S, Niroomand F, Kiehn J, Kreye VA, Katus HA, Schoels W, Karle CA. QTc prolongation by grapefruit juice and its potential pharmacological basis: HERG channel blockade by flavonoids. Circ. 2005;111(7):835–8. https://doi.org/10.1161/01.CIR.0000155617.54749.09.
122. Jaillon P. Antiarrhythmic drug interactions: are they important? Eur Heart J. 1987;8(Suppl A):127–32.
123. Colatsky T, Follmer C, Starmer CF. Channel specificity in antiarrhythmic drug action mechanism of potassium channel block and its role in suppressing and aggravating cardiac arrhythmias. Circ. 1990;82:2235–42.
124. Ravens U. Potassium channels in atrial fibrillation: targets for atrial and pathology-specific therapy? Heart Rhythm. 2008;5(5):758–9. https://doi.org/10.1016/j.hrthm.2007.11.008.
125. Burashnikov A, Antzelevitch C. Atrial-selective sodium channel blockers: do they exist? J Cardiovasc Pharmacol. 2008;52(2):121–8. https://doi.org/10.1097/FJC.0b013e31817618eb.
126. Sicouri S, Glass A, Belardinelli L, Antzelevitch C. Antiarrhythmic effects of ranolazine in canine pulmonary vein sleeve preparations. Heart Rhythm. 2008;5(7):1019–26. https://doi.org/10.1016/j.hrthm.2008.03.018.
127. Sicouri S, Belardinelli L, Carlsson L, Antzelevitch C. Potent antiarrhythmic effects of chronic amiodarone in canine pulmonary vein sleeve preparations. J Cardiovasc Electrophysiol. 2009;20(7):803–10. https://doi.org/10.1111/j.1540-8167.2009.01449.x.
128. Ravens U, Poulet C, Wettwer E, Knaut M. Atrial selectivity of antiarrhythmic drugs. J Physiol. 2013;591(Pt 17):4087–97. https://doi.org/10.1113/jphysiol.2013.256115.
129. Cahalan M, Begenisich T. Sodium channel selectivity: dependence on internal permeant ion concentration. J Gen Physiol. 1976;68:111–25.
130. Comtois P, Sakabe M, Vigmond EJ, Munoz M, Texier A, Shiroshita-Takeshita A, Nattel S. Mechanisms of atrial fibrillation termination by rapidly unbinding Na+ channel blockers: insights from mathematical models and experimental corre-

lates. Am J Physiol Heart Circ Physiol. 2008;295(4):H1489–504. https://doi.org/10.1152/ajpheart.01054.2007.

131. Shenasa M. Ranolazine: electrophysiologic effect efficacy, and safety in patients with cardiac arrhythmias. Card Electrophysiol Clin. 2016;8:467–79.
132. Burashnikov A, Petroski A, Hu D, Barajas-Martinez H, Antzelevitch C. Atrial-selective inhibition of sodium-channel current by Wenxin Keli is effective in suppressing atrial fibrillation. Heart Rhythm. 2012;9(1):125–31. https://doi.org/10.1016/j.hrthm.2011.08.027.
133. Antzelevitch C, Burashnikov A. Atrial-selective sodium channel block as a novel strategy for the management of atrial fibrillation. J Electrocardiol. 2009;42(6):543–8. https://doi.org/10.1016/j.jelectrocard.2009.07.007.
134. Ehrlich JR, Biliczki P, Hohnloser SH, Nattel S. Atrial-selective approaches for the treatment of atrial fibrillation. J Am Coll Cardiol. 2008;51(8):787–92. https://doi.org/10.1016/j.jacc.2007.08.067.
135. Burashnikov A, Di Diego JM, Zygmunt AC, Belardinelli L, Antzelevitch C. Atrium-selective sodium channel block as a strategy for suppression of atrial fibrillation: differences in sodium channel inactivation between atria and ventricles and the role of ranolazine. Circ. 2007;116(13):1449–57. https://doi.org/10.1161/CIRCULATIONAHA.107.704890.
136. Burashnikov A, Di Diego JM, Sicouri S, Ferreiro M, Carlsson L, Antzelevitch C. Atrial-selective effects of chronic amiodarone in the management of atrial fibrillation. Heart Rhythm. 2008;5(12):1735–42. https://doi.org/10.1016/j.hrthm.2008.09.015.
137. Burashnikov A, Di Diego JM, Zygmunt AC, Belardinelli L, Antzelevitch C. Atrial-selective sodium channel block as a strategy for suppression of atrial fibrillation. Ann N Y Acad Sci. 2008;1123:105–12.
138. Dubyak GR. Ion homeostasis, channels, and transporters: an update on cellular mechanisms. Adv Physiol Educ. 2004;28(1–4):143–54. https://doi.org/10.1152/advan.00046.2004.
139. Glaaser IW, Kass RS, Clancy CE. Mechanisms of genetic arrhythmias: from DNA to ECG. Prog Cardiovasc Dis. 2003;46(3):259–70. https://doi.org/10.1016/s0033-0620(03)00073-2.

140. Schulze-Bahr E. Arrhythmia predisposition. J Am Coll Cardiol. 2006;48(9):A67–78. https://doi.org/10.1016/j.jacc.2006.07.006.
141. Webster G, Berul CI. An update on channelopathies: from mechanisms to management. Circ. 2013;127(1):126–40. https://doi.org/10.1161/CIRCULATIONAHA.111.060343.
142. Wilde AA, Bezzina CR. Genetics of cardiac arrhythmias. Heart. 2005;91(10):1352–8. https://doi.org/10.1136/hrt.2004.046334.
143. Antzelevitch C. Molecular genetics of arrhythmias and cardiovascular conditions associated with arrhythmias. J Cardiovasc Electrophysiol. 2003;14(11):1259–72. https://doi.org/10.1046/j.1540-8167.2003.03316.x.
144. Ruan Y, Liu N, Priori SG. Sodium channel mutations and arrhythmias. Nat Rev Cardiol. 2009;6(5):337–48. https://doi.org/10.1038/nrcardio.2009.44.
145. Cerrone M, Cummings S, Alansari T, Priori SG. A clinical approach to inherited arrhythmias. Circ Cardiovasc Genet. 2012;5(5):581–90. https://doi.org/10.1161/CIRCGENETICS.110.959429.
146. Kass RS. The channelopathies: novel insights into molecular and genetic mechanisms of human disease. J Clin Invest. 2005;115(8):1986–9. https://doi.org/10.1172/JCI26011.
147. Abriel H, Zaklyazminskaya EV. A modern approach to classify missense mutations in cardiac channelopathy genes. Circ Cardiovasc Genet. 2012;5(5):487–9. https://doi.org/10.1161/CIRCGENETICS.112.964809.
148. Tsai CT, Lai LP, Hwang JJ, Lin JL, Chiang FT. Molecular genetics of atrial fibrillation. J Am Coll Cardiol. 2008;52(4):241–50. https://doi.org/10.1016/j.jacc.2008.02.072.
149. Tfelt-Hansen J, Winkel BG, Grunnet M, Jespersen T. Inherited cardiac diseases caused by mutations in the Nav1.5 sodium channel. J Cardiovasc Electrophysiol. 2010;21(1):107–15. https://doi.org/10.1111/j.1540-8167.2009.01633.x.
150. Watanabe H, Nogami A, Ohkubo K, Kawata H, Hayashi Y, Ishikawa T, Makiyama T, Nagao S, Yagihara N, Takehara N, Kawamura Y, Sato A, Okamura K, Hosaka Y, Sato M, Fukae S, Chinushi M, Oda H, Okabe M, Kimura A, Maemura K, Watanabe I, Kamakura S, Horie M, Aizawa Y, Shimizu W, Makita N. Electrocardiographic characteristics

and SCN5A mutations in idiopathic ventricular fibrillation associated with early repolarization. Circ Arrhythm Electrophysiol. 2011;4(6):874–81. https://doi.org/10.1161/CIRCEP.111.963983.

151. Roberts JD, Gollob MH. A contemporary review on the genetic basis of atrial fibrillation. Methodist Debakey Cardiovasc J. 2014;10(1):18–24.
152. Mestroni L, Brun F, Spezzacatene A, Sinagra G, Taylor MR. Genetic causes of dilated cardiomyopathy. Prog Pediatr Cardiol. 2014;37(1–2):13–8. https://doi.org/10.1016/j.ppedcard.2014.10.003.
153. Remme CA. Cardiac sodium channelopathy associated with SCN5A mutations: electrophysiological, molecular and genetic aspects. J Physiol. 2013;591(17):4099–116. https://doi.org/10.1113/jphysiol.2013.256461.
154. Chockalingam P, Clur SA, Breur JM, Kriebel T, Paul T, Rammeloo LA, Wilde AA, Blom NA. The diagnostic and therapeutic aspects of loss-of-function cardiac sodium channelopathies in children. Heart Rhythm. 2012;9(12):1986–92. https://doi.org/10.1016/j.hrthm.2012.08.011.
155. Schulze-Bahr E, Eckardt L, Breithardt G, Seidl K, Wichter T, Wolpert C, Borggrefe M, Haverkamp W. Sodium channel gene (SCN5A) mutations in 44 index patients with Brugada syndrome: different incidences in familial and sporadic disease. Hum Mutat. 2003;21(6):651–2. https://doi.org/10.1002/humu.9144.
156. Kapplinger JD, Tester DJ, Alders M, Benito B, Berthet M, Brugada J, Brugada P, Fressart V, Guerchicoff A, Harris-Kerr C, Kamakura S, Kyndt F, Koopmann TT, Miyamoto Y, Pfeiffer R, Pollevick GD, Probst V, Zumhagen S, Vatta M, Towbin JA, Shimizu W, Schulze-Bahr E, Antzelevitch C, Salisbury BA, Guicheney P, Wilde AA, Brugada R, Schott JJ, Ackerman MJ. An international compendium of mutations in the SCN5A-encoded cardiac sodium channel in patients referred for brugada syndrome genetic testing. Heart Rhythm. 2010;7(1):33–46. https://doi.org/10.1016/j.hrthm.2009.09.069.
157. Vatta M, Dumaine R, Varghese G, Richard T, Shimizu W, Aihara N, Nademanee K, Brugada R, Brugada J, Veerakul G, Li H, Bowles NE, Brugada P, Antzelevitch C, Towbin JA. Genetic and biophysical basis of sudden unexplained nocturnal death syndrome (SUNDS), a disease allelic to Brugada syndrome. Hum Mol Genet. 2002;11(3):337–46.

158. Fenske S, Krause SC, Hassan SI, Becirovic E, Auer F, Bernard R, Kupatt C, Lange P, Ziegler T, Wotjak CT, Zhang H, Hammelmann V, Paparizos C, Biel M, Wahl-Schott CA. Sick sinus syndrome in HCN1-deficient mice. Circ. 2013;128(24):2585–94. https://doi.org/10.1161/CIRCULATIONAHA.113.003712.
159. Zhang ZS, Tranquillo J, Neplioueva V, Bursac N, Grant AO. Sodium channel kinetic changes that produce brugada syndrome or progressive cardiac conduction system disease. Am J Physiol Heart Circ Physiol. 2007;292(1):H399–407. https://doi.org/10.1152/ajpheart.01025.2005.
160. Probst V, Allouis M, Sacher F, Pattier S, Babuty D, Mabo P, Mansourati J, Victor J, Nguyen JM, Schott JJ, Boisseau P, Escande D, Le Marec H. Progressive cardiac conduction defect is the prevailing phenotype in carriers of a brugada syndrome SCN5A mutation. J Cardiovasc Electrophysiol. 2006;17(3):270–5. https://doi.org/10.1111/j.1540-8167.2006.00349.x.
161. Schott J-J, Alshinawi C, Kyndt F, Probst V, Hoorntje TM, Hulsbeek M, Wilde AAM, Escande D, Mannens MMAM, Le Marec H. Cardiac conduction defects associate with mutations in SCN5A. Nat Genet. 1999;23(1):20–1.
162. Royer A, van Veen TA, Le Bouter S, Marionneau C, Griol-Charhbili V, Leoni AL, Steenman M, van Rijen HV, Demolombe S, Goddard CA, Richer C, Escoubet B, Jarry-Guichard T, Colledge WH, Gros D, de Bakker JM, Grace AA, Escande D, Charpentier F. Mouse model of SCN5A-linked hereditary Lenegre's disease: age-related conduction slowing and myocardial fibrosis. Circ. 2005;111(14):1738–46. https://doi.org/10.1161/01.CIR.0000160853.19867.61.
163. WP MN, Ku L, Taylor MR, Fain PR, Dao D, Wolfel E, Mestroni L, Familial Cardiomyopathy Registry Research Group. SCN5A mutation associated with dilated cardiomyopathy, conduction disorder, and arrhythmia. Circ. 2004;110(15):2163–7. https://doi.org/10.1161/01.CIR.0000144458.58660.BB.
164. Burkett EL, Hershberger RE. Clinical and genetic issues in familial dilated cardiomyopathy. J Am Coll Cardiol. 2005;45(7):969–81. https://doi.org/10.1016/j.jacc.2004.11.066.
165. Hershberger RE, Siegfried JD. Update 2011: clinical and genetic issues in familial dilated cardiomyopathy. J Am Coll Cardiol. 2011;57(16):1641–9. https://doi.org/10.1016/j.jacc.2011.01.015.
166. Fatkin D. Guidelines for the diagnosis and management of familial dilated cardiomyopathy. Heart Lung Circ. 2011;20(11):691–3. https://doi.org/10.1016/j.hlc.2011.07.008.

167. Laurent G, Saal S, Amarouch MY, Beziau DM, Marsman RF, Faivre L, Barc J, Dina C, Bertaux G, Barthez O, Thauvin-Robinet C, Charron P, Fressart V, Maltret A, Villain E, Baron E, Merot J, Turpault R, Coudiere Y, Charpentier F, Schott JJ, Loussouarn G, Wilde AA, Wolf JE, Baro I, Kyndt F, Probst V. Multifocal ectopic Purkinje-related premature contractions: a new SCN5A-related cardiac channelopathy. J Am Coll Cardiol. 2012;60(2):144–56. https://doi.org/10.1016/j.jacc.2012.02.052.
168. Wan X, Chen S, Sadeghpour A, Wang Q, Kirsch GE. Accelerated inactivation in a mutant Na1 channel associated with idiopathic ventricular fibrillation. Am J Physiol Heart Circ Physiol. 2001;280:H354–60.
169. Hu D, Viskin S, Oliva A, Carrier T, Cordeiro JM, Barajas-Martinez H, Wu Y, Burashnikov E, Sicouri S, Brugada R, Rosso R, Guerchicoff A, Pollevick GD, Antzelevitch C. Novel mutation in the SCN5A gene associated with arrhythmic storm development during acute myocardial infarction. Heart Rhythm. 2007;4(8):1072–80. https://doi.org/10.1016/j.hrthm.2007.03.040.
170. Delisle BP, Anson BD, Rajamani S, January CT. Biology of cardiac arrhythmias: ion channel protein trafficking. Circ Res. 2004;94(11):1418–28. https://doi.org/10.1161/01.RES.0000128561.28701.ea.
171. Sarkozy A, Brugada P. Sudden cardiac death and inherited arrhythmia syndromes. J Cardiovasc Electrophysiol. 2005;16(Suppl 1):S8–20. https://doi.org/10.1111/j.1540-8167.2005.50110.x.
172. Remme CA, Verkerk AO, Nuyens D, van Ginneken AC, van Brunschot S, Belterman CN, Wilders R, van Roon MA, Tan HL, Wilde AA, Carmeliet P, de Bakker JM, Veldkamp MW, Bezzina CR. Overlap syndrome of cardiac sodium channel disease in mice carrying the equivalent mutation of human SCN5A-1795insD. Circ. 2006;114(24):2584–94. https://doi.org/10.1161/CIRCULATIONAHA.106.653949.
173. Grant AO, Carboni MP, Neplioueva V, Starmer CF, Memmi M, Napolitano C, Priori S. A spontaneous mutation identifies a residue critical for closed-state inactivation of cardiac sodium channels. Circ. 2001;104(suppl II):II–310.
174. Havakuk O, Viskin S. A tale of 2 diseases: the history of long-QT syndrome and brugada syndrome. J Am Coll Cardiol. 2016;67(1):100–8. https://doi.org/10.1016/j.jacc.2015.10.020.

175. Gourraud JB, Kyndt F, Fouchard S, Rendu E, Jaafar P, Gully C, Gacem K, Dupuis JM, Longueville A, Baron E, Karakachoff M, Cebron JP, Chatel S, Schott JJ, Le Marec H, Probst V. Identification of a strong genetic background for progressive cardiac conduction defect by epidemiological approach. Heart. 2012;98(17):1305–10. https://doi.org/10.1136/heartjnl-2012-301872.
176. Korkmaz S, Zitron E, Bangert A, Seyler C, Li S, Hegedus P, Scherer D, Li J, Fink T, Schweizer PA, Giannitsis E, Karck M, Szabo G, Katus HA, Kaya Z. Provocation of an autoimmune response to cardiac voltage-gated sodium channel NaV1.5 induces cardiac conduction defects in rats. J Am Coll Cardiol. 2013;62(4):340–9. https://doi.org/10.1016/j.jacc.2013.04.041.
177. Lee HC, Huang KT, Wang XL, Shen WK. Autoantibodies and cardiac arrhythmias. Heart Rhythm. 2011;8(11):1788–95. https://doi.org/10.1016/j.hrthm.2011.06.032.
178. Kovach JR, Benson DW. Conduction disorders and Nav1.5. Card Electrophysiol Clin. 2014;6(4):723–31. https://doi.org/10.1016/j.ccep.2014.07.008.
179. Tester DJ, Valdivia C, Harris-Kerr C, Alders M, Salisbury BA, Wilde AA, Makielski JC, Ackerman MJ. Epidemiologic, molecular, and functional evidence suggest A572D-SCN5A should not be considered an independent LQT3-susceptibility mutation. Heart Rhythm. 2010;7(7):912–9. https://doi.org/10.1016/j.hrthm.2010.04.014.
180. Lin H, Dolmatova EV, Morley MP, Lunetta KL, McManus DD, Magnani JW, Margulies KB, Hakonarson H, del Monte F, Benjamin EJ, Cappola TP, Ellinor PT. Gene expression and genetic variation in human atria. Heart Rhythm. 2014;11(2):266–71. https://doi.org/10.1016/j.hrthm.2013.10.051.
181. Amin AS, Boink GJ, Atrafi F, Spanjaart AM, Asghari-Roodsari A, Molenaar RJ, Ruijter JM, Wilde AA, Tan HL. Facilitatory and inhibitory effects of SCN5A mutations on atrial fibrillation in brugada syndrome. Europace. 2011;13(7):968–75. https://doi.org/10.1093/europace/eur011.
182. Muggenthaler M, Behr ER. Brugada syndrome and atrial fibrillation: pathophysiology and genetics. Europace. 2011;13(7):913–5. https://doi.org/10.1093/europace/eur094.
183. Giustetto C, Cerrato N, Gribaudo E, Scrocco C, Castagno D, Richiardi E, Giachino D, Bianchi F, Barbonaglia L, Ferraro

A. Atrial fibrillation in a large population with brugada electrocardiographic pattern: prevalence, management, and correlation with prognosis. Heart Rhythm. 2014;11(2):259–65. https://doi.org/10.1016/j.hrthm.2013.10.043.

184. Smith JG, Melander O, Sjogren M, Hedblad B, Engstrom G, Newton-Cheh C, Platonov PG. Genetic polymorphisms confer risk of atrial fibrillation in patients with heart failure: a population-based study. Eur J Heart Fail. 2013;15(3):250–7. https://doi.org/10.1093/eurjhf/hfs176.
185. Lubitz SA, Rienstra M. Genetic susceptibility to atrial fibrillation: does heart failure change our perspective? Eur J Heart Fail. 2013;15(3):244–6. https://doi.org/10.1093/eurjhf/hft005.
186. Gollob M, Jones D, Krahn A, Danis L, Gong X, Shao Q, Liu X, Veinot J, Tang A, Stewart A, Tesson F. Somatic mutations in the connexin 40 gene (GJA5) in atrial fibrillation. N Engl J Med. 2006;354:2677–88.
187. Darbar D, Kannankeril PJ, Donahue BS, Kucera G, Stubblefield T, Haines JL, George AL Jr, Roden DM. Cardiac sodium channel (SCN5A) variants associated with atrial fibrillation. Circ. 2008;117(15):1927–35. https://doi.org/10.1161/CIRCULATIONAHA.107.757955.
188. Ellinor PT, Nam EG, Shea MA, Milan DJ, Ruskin JN, MacRae CA. Cardiac sodium channel mutation in atrial fibrillation. Heart Rhythm. 2008;5(1):99–105. https://doi.org/10.1016/j.hrthm.2007.09.015.
189. Francis J, Antzelevitch C. Atrial fibrillation and Brugada syndrome. J Am Coll Cardiol. 2008;51(12):1149–53. https://doi.org/10.1016/j.jacc.2007.10.062.
190. Rodriguez-Manero M, Namdar M, Sarkozy A, Casado-Arroyo R, Ricciardi D, de Asmundis C, Chierchia GB, Wauters K, Rao JY, Bayrak F, Van Malderen S, Brugada P. Prevalence, clinical characteristics and management of atrial fibrillation in patients with Brugada syndrome. Am J Cardiol. 2013;111(3):362–7. https://doi.org/10.1016/j.amjcard.2012.10.012.
191. Enriquez A, Antzelevitch C, Bismah V, Baranchuk A. Atrial fibrillation in inherited cardiac channelopathies: from mechanisms to management. Heart Rhythm. 2016;13(9):1878–84. https://doi.org/10.1016/j.hrthm.2016.06.008.
192. Horne AJ, Eldstrom J, Sanatani S, Fedida D. A novel mechanism for LQT3 with 2:1 block: a pore-lining mutation in Nav1.5 significantly affects voltage-dependence of activa-

tion. Heart Rhythm. 2011;8(5):770–7. https://doi.org/10.1016/j.hrthm.2010.12.041.
193. Moss AJ, Kass RS. Long QT syndrome: from channels to cardiac arrhythmias. J Clin Invest. 2005;115(8):2018–24. https://doi.org/10.1172/JCI25537.
194. Moss AJ, Zareba W, Schwarz KQ, Rosero S, McNitt S, Robinson JL. Ranolazine shortens repolarization in patients with sustained inward sodium current due to type-3 long-QT syndrome. J Cardiovasc Electrophysiol. 2008;19(12):1289–93. https://doi.org/10.1111/j.1540-8167.2008.01246.x.
195. Chockalingam P, Wilde A. The multifaceted cardiac sodium channel and its clinical implications. Heart. 2012;98(17):1318–24. https://doi.org/10.1136/heartjnl-2012-301784.
196. Schwartz PJ, Priori SG, Cerrone M, Spazzolini C, Odero A, Napolitano C, Bloise R, De Ferrari GM, Klersy C, Moss AJ, Zareba W, Robinson JL, Hall WJ, Brink PA, Toivonen L, Epstein AE, Li C, Hu D. Left cardiac sympathetic denervation in the management of high-risk patients affected by the long-QT syndrome. Circ. 2004;109(15):1826–33. https://doi.org/10.1161/01.CIR.0000125523.14403.1E.
197. Silver ES, Liberman L, Chung WK, Spotnitz HM, Chen JM, Ackerman MJ, Moir C, Hordof AJ, Pass RH. Long QT syndrome due to a novel mutation in SCN5A: treatment with ICD placement at 1 month and left cardiac sympathetic denervation at 3 months of age. J Interv Card Electrophysiol. 2009;26(1):41–5. https://doi.org/10.1007/s10840-009-9428-1.
198. Horowitz L, Zipes D, Bigger JT, Campbell R, Morganroth J, Podrid PJ, Rosen MR, Woosley RL. Proarrhythmia, arrhythmogenesis or aggravation of arrhythmia-a status report, 1987. Am J Cardiol. 1987;59(11):54E–6E.
199. Josephson ME. Antiarrhythmic agents and the danger of proarrhythmic events. Ann Intern Med. 1989;111(2):101–3. https://doi.org/10.7326/0003-4819-111-2-101.
200. Echt D, Liebson PR, Mitchell B, Peters R, Obias-Manno D, Barker A, Arensberg D, Baker A, Friedman L, Greene L, Huther M, Richardson D. Mortality and morbidity in patients receiving encainide, flecainide, or placebo: the cardiac arrhythmia suppression trial. N Engl J Med. 1991;324(12):781–8.
201. Fenichel R, Malik M. Drug-induced torsades de pointes and implications for drug development. J Cardiovasc Electrophysiol. 2004;15(4):475–95.

202. Liu J, Laurita KR. The mechanism of pause-induced torsades de pointes in long QT syndrome. J Cardiovasc Electrophysiol. 2005;16(9):981–7. https://doi.org/10.1111/j.1540-8167.2005.40677.x.
203. Kay GN, Plumb VJ, Arciniegas JG, Henthorn R, Waldo A. Torsades de pointes: the long-short initiating sequence and other clinical features: observations in 32 patients. J Am Coll Cardiol. 1983;2(5):806–17.
204. Vandersickel N, de Boer TP, Vos MA, Panfilov AV. Perpetuation of torsades de pointes in heterogeneous hearts: competing foci or re-entry? J Physiol. 2016;594(23):6865–78. https://doi.org/10.1113/JP271728.
205. El-Sherif N, Chinushi M, Caref EB, Restivo M. Electrophysiological mechanism of the characteristic electrocardiographic morphology of torsades de pointes tachyarrhythmias in the long-QT syndrome. Detailed analysis of ventricular tridimensional activation patterns. Circ. 1997;96(12):4392–9. https://doi.org/10.1161/01.cir.96.12.4392.
206. Viskin S, Justo D, Halkin A, Zeltser D. Long QT syndrome caused by noncardiac drugs. Prog Cardiovasc Dis. 2003;45(5):415–27. https://doi.org/10.1053/pcad.2003.00101.
207. Yap YG, Camm AJ. Drug induced QT prolongation and torsades de pointes. Heart. 2003;89:1363–72.
208. Roden DM, Viswanathan PC. Genetics of acquired long QT syndrome. J Clin Invest. 2005;115(8):2025–32. https://doi.org/10.1172/JCI25539.
209. Camm AJ, Malik M, Yap YG. Acquired long QT syndrome. Hoboken: Wiley-Blackwell; 2004.
210. Riad FS, Davis AM, Moranville MP, Beshai JF. Drug-induced QTc prolongation. Am J Cardiol. 2017;119(2):280–3. https://doi.org/10.1016/j.amjcard.2016.09.041.
211. Locati EH, Zareba W, Moss A, Schwartz PJ, Vincent M, Lehmann MH, Towbin JA, Priori SG, Napolitano C, Robinson JL, Andrews M, Timothy K, Hall W. Age- and sex-related differences in clinical manifestations in patients with congenital long-QT syndrome. Circ. 1998;97:2237–44.
212. Roden DM, Johnson JA, Kimmel SE, Krauss RM, Medina MW, Shuldiner A, Wilke RA. Cardiovascular pharmacogenomics. Circ Res. 2011;109(7):807–20. https://doi.org/10.1161/CIRCRESAHA.110.230995.

213. Lin CY, Lin YJ, Lo LW, Chen YY, Chong E, Chang SL, Chung FP, Chao TF, Hu YF, Tuan TC, Liao JN, Chang Y, Chien KL, Chiou CW, Chen SA. Factors predisposing to ventricular proarrhythmia during antiarrhythmic drug therapy for atrial fibrillation in patients with structurally normal heart. Heart Rhythm. 2015;12:1490–500. https://doi.org/10.1016/j.hrthm.2015.04.018.
214. Behr ER, Roden D. Drug-induced arrhythmia: pharmacogenomic prescribing? Eur Heart J. 2013;34(2):89–95. https://doi.org/10.1093/eurheartj/ehs351.
215. Roden DM. Drug-induced prolongation of the QT interval. N Engl J Med. 2004;350(10):1013–22. https://doi.org/10.1056/NEJMra032426.
216. Padfield GJ, Escudero CA, De Souza AM, Steinberg C, Gibbs KA, Puyat JH, Lam PY, Sanatani S, Sherwin E, Potts JE, Sandor G, Krahn AD. Characterization of myocardial repolarization reserve in adolescent females with anorexia nervosa. Circ. 2016;133:557–65. https://doi.org/10.1161/CIRCULATIONAHA.115.016697.
217. Frommeyer G, Eckardt L. Drug-induced proarrhythmia: risk factors and electrophysiological mechanisms. Nat Rev Cardiol. 2016;13(1):36–47. https://doi.org/10.1038/nrcardio.2015.110.
218. Schimpf R, Veltmann C, Papavassiliu T, Rudic B, Goksu T, Kuschyk J, Wolpert C, Antzelevitch C, Ebner A, Borggrefe M, Brandt C. Drug-induced QT-interval shortening following antiepileptic treatment with oral rufinamide. Heart Rhythm. 2012;9(5):776–81. https://doi.org/10.1016/j.hrthm.2012.01.006.
219. Behr ER, January C, Schulze-Bahr E, Grace AA, Kaab S, Fiszman M, Gathers S, Buckman S, Youssef A, Pirmohamed M, Roden D. The international serious adverse events consortium (iSAEC) phenotype standardization project for drug-induced torsades de pointes. Eur Heart J. 2013;34(26):1958–63. https://doi.org/10.1093/eurheartj/ehs172.
220. Drew BJ, Ackerman MJ, Funk M, Gibler WB, Kligfield P, Menon V, Philippides GJ, Roden DM, Zareba W, American Heart Association Acute Cardiac Care Committee of the Council on Clinical Cardiology, the Council on Cardiovascular Nursing, and the American College of Cardiology Foundation. Prevention

of torsades de pointes in hospital settings: a scientific statement from the American Heart Association and the American College of Cardiology Foundation. Circ. 2010;121(8):1047–60. https://doi.org/10.1161/CIRCULATIONAHA.109.192704.

221. Kowey PR, Malik M. The QT interval as it relates to the safety of non-cardiac drugs. Eur Heart J Suppl. 2007;9(Suppl G):G3–8. https://doi.org/10.1093/eurheartj/sum047.
222. Vincent GM. Risk assessment in long QT syndrome: the Achilles heel of appropriate treatment. Heart Rhythm. 2005;2(5):505–6. https://doi.org/10.1016/j.hrthm.2005.03.002.
223. Colman MA, Aslanidi OV, Kharche S, Boyett MR, Garratt C, Hancox JC, Zhang H. Pro-arrhythmogenic effects of atrial fibrillation-induced electrical remodelling: insights from the three-dimensional virtual human atria. J Physiol. 2013;591(Pt 17):4249–72. https://doi.org/10.1113/jphysiol.2013.254987.
224. Nattel S, Maguy A, Le Bouter S, Yeh YH. Arrhythmogenic ion-channel remodeling in the heart: heart failure, myocardial infarction, and atrial fibrillation. Physiol Rev. 2007;87(2):425–56. https://doi.org/10.1152/physrev.00014.2006.
225. Shinagawa K. Effects of antiarrhythmic drugs on fibrillation in the remodeled atrium: insights into the mechanism of the superior efficacy of amiodarone. Circ. 2003;107(10):1440–6. https://doi.org/10.1161/01.cir.0000055316.35552.74.
226. Nattel S, Burstein B, Dobrev D. Atrial remodeling and atrial fibrillation: mechanisms and implications. Circ Arrhythm Electrophysiol. 2008;1(1):62–73. https://doi.org/10.1161/CIRCEP.107.754564.
227. Gaspo R, Bosch RF, Bou-Abboud E, Nattel S. Tachycardia-induced changes in Na current in a chronic dog model of atrial fibrillation. Circ Res. 1997;81(6):1045–52. https://doi.org/10.1161/01.res.81.6.1045.
228. Yue L, Melnyk P, Gaspo R, Wang Z, Nattel S. Molecular mechanisms underlying ionic remodeling in a dog model of atrial fibrillation. Circ Res. 1999;84(7):776–84. https://doi.org/10.1161/01.res.84.7.776.
229. Gaborit N, Steenman M, Lamirault G, Le Meur N, Le Bouter S, Lande G, Leger J, Charpentier F, Christ T, Dobrev D, Escande D, Nattel S, Demolombe S. Human atrial ion channel and transporter subunit gene-expression remodeling associated with valvular heart disease and atrial fibrillation. Circ. 2005;112(4):471–81. https://doi.org/10.1161/CIRCULATIONAHA.104.506857.

230. Piccini JP, Pritchett EL, Davison BA, Cotter G, Wiener LE, Koch G, Feld G, Waldo A, van Gelder IC, Camm AJ, Kowey PR, Iwashita J, Dittrich HC. Randomized, double-blind, placebo-controlled study to evaluate the safety and efficacy of a single oral dose of vanoxerine for the conversion of subjects with recent onset atrial fibrillation or flutter to normal sinus rhythm: RESTORE SR. Heart Rhythm. 2016;0:1–7. https://doi.org/10.1016/j.hrthm.2016.04.012.
231. Henry BL, Gabris B, Li Q, Martin B, Giannini M, Parikh A, Patel D, Haney J, Schwartzman DS, Shroff SG, Salama G. Relaxin suppresses atrial fibrillation in aged rats by reversing fibrosis and upregulating Na+ channels. Heart Rhythm. 2016;13(4):983–91. https://doi.org/10.1016/j.hrthm.2015.12.030.
232. Hou JW, Li W, Guo K, Chen XM, Chen YH, Li CY, Zhao BC, Zhao J, Wang H, Wang YP, Li YG. Antiarrhythmic effects and potential mechanism of WenXin KeLi in cardiac Purkinje cells. Heart Rhythm. 2016;13(4):973–82. https://doi.org/10.1016/j.hrthm.2015.12.023.
233. Xiao YF, Ma L, Wang SY, Josephson ME, Wang GK, Morgan JP, Leaf A. Potent block of inactivation-deficient Na+ channels by n-3 polyunsaturated fatty acids. Am J Physiol Cell Physiol. 2006;290(2):C362–70. https://doi.org/10.1152/ajpcell.00296.2005.
234. Xiao YF, Kang JX, Morgan JP, Leaf A. Blocking effects of polyunsaturated fatty acids on Na+ channels of neonatal rat ventricular myocytes. Proc Natl Acad Sci U S A. 1995;92:1100–11004.
235. Leaf A, Albert CM, Josephson M, Steinhaus D, Kluger J, Kang JX, Cox B, Zhang H, Schoenfeld D, Fatty Acid Antiarrhythmia Trial Investigators. Prevention of fatal arrhythmias in high-risk subjects by fish oil n-3 fatty acid intake. Circ. 2005;112(18):2762–8.
236. Raitt MH, Connor WE, Morris C, Kron J, Halperin B, Chugh SS, McClelland J, Cook J, MacMurdy K, Swenson R, Connor SL, Gerhard G, Kraemer DF, Oseran D, Marchant C, Calhoun D, Shnider R, McAnulty J. Fish oil supplementation and risk of ventricular tachycardia and ventricular fibrillation in patients with implantable defibrillators: a randomized controlled trial. JAMA. 2005;293(23):2884–91.
237. Goette A, Schon N, Kirchhof P, Breithardt G, Fetsch T, Hausler KG, Klein HU, Steinbeck G, Wegscheider K, Meinertz T. Angiotensin II-antagonist in paroxysmal atrial fibrillation

(ANTIPAF) trial. Circ Arrhythm Electrophysiol. 2012;5(1):43–51. https://doi.org/10.1161/CIRCEP.111.965178.
238. Schmieder R, Kjeldsen S, Julius S, McInnes G, Zanchetti A, Hua TA. Reduced incidence of new-onset atrial fibrillation with angiotensin II receptor blockade: the VALUE trial. J Hypertens. 2008;26:403–11.
239. GISSI-AF Investigators, Disertori M, Latini R, Barlera S, Franzosi MG, Staszewsky L, Maggioni AP, Lucci D, Di Pasquale G, Tognoni G. Valsartan for prevention of recurrent atrial fibrillation. N Engl J Med. 2009;360:1606–17.
240. Investigators ACTIVEI, Yusuf S, Healey JS, Pogue J, Chrolavicius S, Flather M, Hart RG, Hohnloser SH, Joyner CD, Pfeffer MA, Connolly SJ. Irbesartan in patients with atrial fibrillation. N Engl J Med. 2011;364:928–38.
241. Tayebjee MH, Creta A, Moder S, Hunter RJ, Earley MJ, Dhinoja MB, Schilling RJ. Impact of angiotensin-converting enzyme-inhibitors and angiotensin receptor blockers on long-term outcome of catheter ablation for atrial fibrillation. Europace. 2010;12(11):1537–42. https://doi.org/10.1093/europace/euq284.
242. Ackerman MJ, Priori SG, Willems S, Berul C, Brugada R, Calkins H, Camm AJ, Ellinor PT, Gollob M, Hamilton R, Hershberger RE, Judge DP, Le Marec H, McKenna WJ, Schulze-Bahr E, Semsarian C, Towbin JA, Watkins H, Wilde A, Wolpert C, Zipes DP. HRS/EHRA expert consensus statement on the state of genetic testing for the channelopathies and cardiomyopathies this document was developed as a partnership between the Heart Rhythm Society (HRS) and the European Heart Rhythm Association (EHRA). Heart Rhythm. 2011;8(8):1308–39. https://doi.org/10.1016/j.hrthm.2011.05.020.
243. Verma A, Cairns JA, Mitchell LB, Macle L, Stiell IG, Gladstone D, McMurtry MS, Connolly S, Cox JL, Dorian P, Ivers N, Leblanc K, Nattel S, Healey JS, Committee CCSAFG. 2014 focused update of the Canadian Cardiovascular Society Guidelines for the management of atrial fibrillation. Can J Cardiol. 2014;30(10):1114–30. https://doi.org/10.1016/j.cjca.2014.08.001.
244. Pedersen CT, Kay GN, Kalman J, Borggrefe M, Della-Bella P, Dickfeld T, Dorian P, Huikuri H, Kim YH, Knight B, Marchlinski F, Ross D, Sacher F, Sapp J, Shivkumar K, Soejima K, Tada H, Alexander ME, Triedman JK, Yamada T, Kirchhof P, Document R, Lip GY, Kuck KH, Mont L, Haines D, Indik

J, Dimarco J, Exner D, Iesaka Y, Savelieva I. EHRA/HRS/APHRS expert consensus on ventricular arrhythmias. Europace. 2014;16(9):1257–83. https://doi.org/10.1093/europace/euu194.
245. Nattel S. New ideas about atrial fibrillation 50 years on. Nature. 2002;415:219–26.
246. Bagwe S, Leonardi M, Bissett J. Novel pharmacological therapies for atrial fibrillation. Curr Opin Cardiol. 2007;22:450–7.
247. Van Norman GA. Drugs, devices, and the FDA: part 1. JACC Basic Transl Sci. 2016;1(3):170–9. https://doi.org/10.1016/j.jacbts.2016.03.002.
248. Van Norman GA. Drugs, devices, and the FDA: part 2. JACC Basic Transl Sci. 2016;1(4):277–87. https://doi.org/10.1016/j.jacbts.2016.03.009.
249. Sanguinetti MC, Bennett PB. Antiarrhythmic drug target choices and screening. Circ Res. 2003;93(6):491–9. https://doi.org/10.1161/01.RES.0000091829.63501.A8.
250. Cho HC, Marban E. Biological therapies for cardiac arrhythmias: can genes and cells replace drugs and devices? Circ Res. 2010;106(4):674–85. https://doi.org/10.1161/CIRCRESAHA.109.212936.
251. Wood AJJ. Racial differences in the response to drugs — pointers to genetic differences. N Engl J Med. 2001;344(18):1394–6. https://doi.org/10.1056/NEJM200105033441811.
252. Cambien F, Tiret L. Genetics of cardiovascular diseases: from single mutations to the whole genome. Circ. 2007;116(15):1714–24. https://doi.org/10.1161/CIRCULATIONAHA.106.661751.
253. Roden DM. Cardiovascular pharmacogenomics: current status and future directions. J Hum Genet. 2016;61(1):79–85. https://doi.org/10.1038/jhg.2015.78.
254. Roden DM. Cardiovascular pharmacogenomics. Circ. 2003;108(25):3071–4. https://doi.org/10.1161/01.CIR.0000110626.24310.18.
255. Milan DJ, Lubitz SA, Kaab S, Ellinor PT. Genome-wide association studies in cardiac electrophysiology: recent discoveries and implications for clinical practice. Heart Rhythm. 2010;7(8):1141–8. https://doi.org/10.1016/j.hrthm.2010.04.021.
256. Luo X, Yang B, Nattel S. MicroRNAs and atrial fibrillation: mechanisms and translational potential. Nat Rev Cardiol. 2015;12(2):80–90. https://doi.org/10.1038/nrcardio.2014.178.
257. Yang B, Lin H, Xiao J, Lu Y, Luo X, Li B, Zhang Y, Xu C, Bai Y, Wang H, Chen G, Wang Z. The muscle-specific microRNA miR-1 regulates cardiac arrhythmogenic potential by targeting

GJA1 and KCNJ2. Nat Med. 2007;13(4):486–91. https://doi.org/10.1038/nm1569.
258. Eloff BC, Gilat E, Wan X, Rosenbaum DS. Pharmacological modulation of cardiac gap junctions to enhance cardiac conduction: evidence supporting a novel target for antiarrhythmic therapy. Circ. 2003;108(25):3157–63. https://doi.org/10.1161/01.CIR.0000101926.43759.10.
259. Priori SG. The fifteen years of discoveries that shaped molecular electrophysiology: time for appraisal. Circ Res. 2010;107(4):451–6. https://doi.org/10.1161/CIRCRESAHA.110.226811.
260. Priori SG, Napolitano C. Role of genetic analyses in cardiology: part I: mendelian diseases: cardiac channelopathies. Circ. 2006;113(8):1130–5. https://doi.org/10.1161/CIRCULATIONAHA.105.563205.
261. van Asselt KM, Kok HS, van der Schouw YT, Peeters PH, Pearson PL, Grobbee DE. Role of genetic analyses in cardiology: part II: heritability estimation for gene searching in multifactorial diseases. Circ. 2006;113(8):1136–9. https://doi.org/10.1161/CIRCULATIONAHA.105.563197.
262. Odenstedt J, Linderoth B, Bergfeldt L, Ekre O, Grip L, Mannheimer C, Andrell P. Spinal cord stimulation effects on myocardial ischemia, infarct size, ventricular arrhythmia, and noninvasive electrophysiology in a porcine ischemia-reperfusion model. Heart Rhythm. 2011;8(6):892–8. https://doi.org/10.1016/j.hrthm.2011.01.029.
263. Ackerman JP, Bartos DC, Kapplinger JD, Tester DJ, Delisle BP, Ackerman MJ. The promise and peril of precision medicine: phenotyping still matters most. Mayo Clin Proc. 2016;91(11):1606–16. https://doi.org/10.1016/j.mayocp.2016.08.008.
264. Marsman RF, Bezzina CR, Freiberg F, Verkerk AO, Adriaens ME, Podliesna S, Chen C, Purfurst B, Spallek B, Koopmann TT, Baczko I, Dos Remedios CG, George AL Jr, Bishopric NH, Lodder EM, de Bakker JM, Fischer R, Coronel R, Wilde AA, Gotthardt M, Remme CA. Coxsackie and adenovirus receptor is a modifier of cardiac conduction and arrhythmia vulnerability in the setting of myocardial ischemia. J Am Coll Cardiol. 2014;63(6):549–59. https://doi.org/10.1016/j.jacc.2013.10.062.
265. Denegri M, Bongianino R, Lodola F, Boncompagni S, De Giusti VC, Avelino-Cruz JE, Liu N, Persampieri S, Curcio A, Esposito F, Pietrangelo L, Marty I, Villani L, Moyaho A, Baiardi P, Auricchio A, Protasi F, Napolitano C, Priori SG. Single delivery

of an adeno-associated viral construct to transfer the CASQ2 gene to knock-in mice affected by catecholaminergic polymorphic ventricular tachycardia is able to cure the disease from birth to advanced age. Circ. 2014;129(25):2673–81. https://doi.org/10.1161/CIRCULATIONAHA.113.006901.

266. Fordyce CB, Roe MT, Ahmad T, Libby P, Borer JS, Hiatt WR, Bristow MR, Packer M, Wasserman SM, Braunstein N, Pitt B, DeMets DL, Cooper-Arnold K, Armstrong PW, Berkowitz SD, Scott R, Prats J, Galis ZS, Stockbridge N, Peterson ED, Califf RM. Cardiovascular drug development: is it dead or just hibernating? J Am Coll Cardiol. 2015;65(15):1567–82. https://doi.org/10.1016/j.jacc.2015.03.016.

# Chapter 3
# Class III Antiarrhythmic Drugs

**Juan Tamargo, Ricardo Caballero, and Eva Delpón**

## Introduction

Class III antiarrhythmic drugs (AADs) predominantly block outward-repolarizing potassium currents and prolong cardiac action potential duration (APD) and refractoriness at concentrations at which they do not affect the sodium channels and, therefore, intracardiac conduction velocity is not significantly affected [1]. The prolongation of the APD and refractoriness, combined with the maintenance of normal conduction velocity, leads to an increase in the wavelength of the cardiac impulse, defined as the distance travelled by the depolarization wave

J. Tamargo (✉)
Department of Pharmacology, School of Medicine, Universidad Complutense, CIBERCV, Madrid, Spain
e-mail: jtamargo@med.ucm.es

R. Caballero · E. Delpón
Department of Pharmacology, School of Medicine, Universidad Complutense, Instituto de Investigación Sanitaria Gregorio Marañón, Madrid, Spain

CIBERCV, Madrid, Spain



A. Martínez-Rubio et al. (eds.), *Antiarrhythmic Drugs*, Current Cardiovascular Therapy,
https://doi.org/10.1007/978-3-030-34893-9_3

during the functional refractory period, closes the excitable gap in the reentrant circuit and suppresses reentry (Fig. 3.1). Class III AADs include: amiodarone, dofetilide, dronedarone, ibutilide and sotalol.

However, class III AADs present several disadvantages. First, some of them exhibit reverse-use dependence, i.e. the prolongation of the APD increases at normal or at slower heart

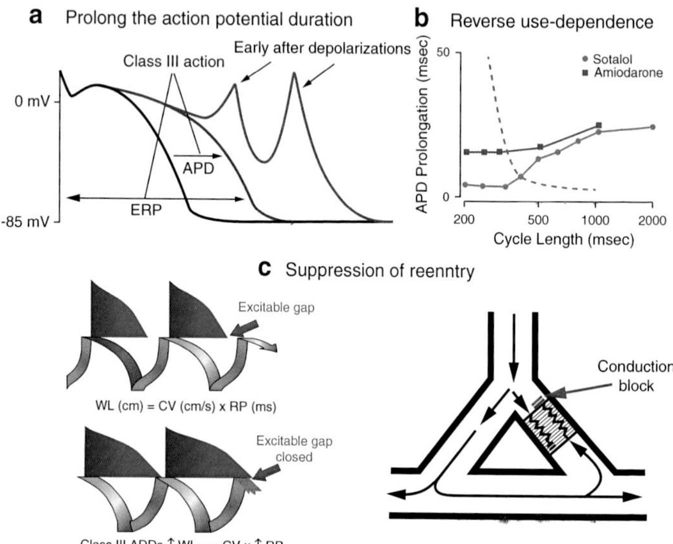


FIGURE 3.1 Class III antiarrhythmic drugs (AADs). (**a**) Class III AADs prolong the cardiac action potential duration (APD) and refractoriness (ERP) and under certain circumstances can induce early depolarizations that induce a polymorphic ventricular tachycardia (torsades de pointes). (**b**) Many class III AADs prolong the APD at slow but not at normal or fast heart rates, i.e., they exhibit reverse use-dependence. (**c**) Class III AADs prolong the APD/ERP, do not modify the conduction velocity (CV) and increase the wavelength of the cardiac impulse (WL), defined as the distance travelled by the depolarization wave during the functional refractory period. As a consequence, they close the excitable gap in the reentrant circuit and they can prevent or abolish reentry. Because the APD/ERP is longer than the conduction time around a reentrant circuit, class III AADs can prevent or abolish impulse reentry

rates (during bradycardia or after a long diastolic interval) but declines as heart rate is increased (i.e., during tachyarrhythmias), which limits their antiarrhythmic efficacy (Fig. 3.1). Second, they produce an excessive and sometimes inhomogeneous prolongation of the ventricular APD (QT interval), which increases the transmural dispersion of cardiac repolarization and can induce early afterdepolarizations (Fig. 3.1) that can trigger the development of polymorphic ventricular tachycardias called torsades de pointes (TdP). The risk of ventricular proarrhythmia is a serious limitation of class III AADs. Third, these drugs produce an acquired long QT syndrome and they should be avoided in combination with other QT-prolonging drugs. Table 3.1 summarizes the main QT-prolonging drugs and the risk factors that predispose to TdP.

TABLE 3.1 (A) Risk factors for QT prolongation, and (B) QT-prolonging drugs [11]

| (A) |
|---|
| • Heart diseases: ischemic heart disease, heart failure, myocarditis, dilated/hypertrophic cardiomyopathy |
| • Age > 65 years |
| • Female gender |
| • High plasma concentrations of QT-prolonging drugs (excessive doses, decreased metabolism and/or excretion) |
| • Electrolyte abnormalities: hypokalemia, hypomagnesemia, hypocalcemia |
| • Cerebrovascular diseases: subarachnoid hemorrhage, ischemic stroke, cerebrovascular accidents |
| • Bradyarrhythmias: bradycardia, AV block, recent cardioversion of AF |
| • Premature complexes leading to short-long-short cycles |
| • Baseline QTc prolongation (>500 ms) |
| • Coadministration of drugs that prolong the QT interval |
| • Genetic polymorphisms (congenital long QT syndrome) |

(continued)

Table 3.1 (continued)

| (B) | |
|---|---|
| Antiarrhythmic drugs | Amiodarone, disopyramide, dofetilide, dronedarone, ibutilide, procainamide (n-acetylprocainamide), quinidine, sotalol |
| Antiemetics | Dolasetron, domperidone, ganisetron, ondansetron |
| Antimicrobials | Azole antifungals (fluconazole, itraconazole, ketoconazole), chloroquine, fluoroquinolones (ciprofloxacin, levofloxacin, moxifloxacin, ofloxacin), macrolides (azithromycin, clarithromycin, erythromycin), pentamidine |
| Psychotropic drugs | Citalopram, clozapine, droperidol, escitalopram, haloperidol, phenothiazines, quetiapine, risperidone, sertindol, thioridazine, tricyclic antidepressants, venlafaxine, ziprasidone |
| Cancer chemotherapy drugs | Amsacrine, anthracyclines (daunorubicin, doxorubicin, epirubicin), arsenic trioxide, 5-fluorouracil, histone deacetylase inhibitors (romidepsin, panobinostat, vorinostat), mitoxantrone, paclitaxel, tamoxifen |
| | Tyrosine kinase inhibitors: carbozantinib, crizotinib, lapatinib, nilotinib, pazopanib, sorafenib, sunitinib, vandetanib, vemurafenib |
| Others | Antihistamines (diphenhydramine, terfenadine, hydroxyzine), bepridil, droperidol, levomethadyl, methadone, octreotide, probucol, protease inhibitors (delavirdine, indinavir, nelfinavir, saquinavir, ritonavir), sumatriptan, thiazides, zolmitriptan |

In this chapter, we review the electrophysiological and pharmacological properties, adverse effects and clinical indications of amiodarone, dofetilide, dronedarone, ibutilide and sotalol. Their pharmacokinetic properties, adverse effects, doses and clinical indications are summarized in Tables 3.2, 3.3, 3.4, 3.5, 3.6, 3.7, and 3.8.

Table 3.2 Pharmacokinetic characteristics of antiarrhythmic drugs

| Drugs | F (%) | $T_{max}$ (h) | PPB (%) | Vd (L/kg) | Metabolism | $t_{½}$ (h) | Renal excretion[a] (%) |
|---|---|---|---|---|---|---|---|
| Amiodarone | 35–65 | 3–8 | 99 | 66 | CYP3A4 and 2C8 | 53 (20–100 days) | 1 |
| Dofetilide | 95 | 2–3 | 65 | 3–4 | CYP3A4 | 7–13 | 80 |
| Dronedarone | 5 | 3–6 | >98 | 20 | CYP3A4 | 13–19 | 15 |
| Ibutilide (IV) | 100 | 1.5 | 40 | 11 | No CYP3A4/2D6 | 6 (2–12) | 7[a] |
| Sotalol | 90–100 | 2.5–4 | 0 | 1.5–2.5 | Not metabolized | 12 (7–18) | 85 |

*F* oral bioavailability, *h* hours, *IV* intravenous, *PPB* protein plasma binding, $t_{1/2}$ drug half-life, $T_{max}$ time to peak plasma levels, *Vd* volume of distribution

[a]Renal excretion without biotransformation

Table 3.3 Adverse effects, contraindications and cautions

| Drug | Adverse effects | Contraindications and cautions |
|---|---|---|
| Amiodarone | 1. Oral Amiodarone:<br>• Cardiovascular: hypotension, bradycardia, AVB, QT prolongation, TdP (rare), slows VT below programmed ICD detection rate, increases defibrillation threshold<br>• Extracardiac: gastrointestinal (nausea, emesis, constipation), ocular (corneal microdeposits, optic neuritis), thyroid abnormalities (hyper- or hypothyroidism), pulmonar (fibrosis, pneumonitis) cutaneous (photosensitivity, blue-gray skin), neurological (ataxia, dizziness, peripheral neuropathy, tremor), hepatotoxicity (increase in transaminases, hepatitis, cirrhosis). Postoperative adult respiratory distress syndrome (rare)<br>2. IV Amiodarone: hypotension, bradycardia, phlebitis at site of administration. QT prolongation, torsades de pointes (rare) | 1. Contraindications: Sinus bradycardia, severe sinus node dysfunction, and 2nd- or 3rd-degree heart block (unless a pacemaker is present). Infranodal conduction disease, cardiogenic shock, severe lung disease, history of thyroid dysfunction or hypersensitivity to amiodarone or to iodine. Hepatic dysfunction.<br>• Baseline QTc >470 ms, conditions and drugs that prolong the QT interval prolongation.<br>2. Cautions: in patients with hypokalemia and/or hypomagnesaemia, congenital or acquired LQTS, taking QT-prolonging drugs.<br>• Delayed conversion to sinus rhythm (up to 8–12 hours)<br>• IV amiodarone contains benzyl alcohol, which may cause fatal "gasping syndrome" in infants and children up to 3 years old |

| | | |
|---|---|---|
| Dofetilide | • QT prolongation, VT and TdP<br>• Headache, dizziness, nausea, chest pain, insomnia | • Contraindications: CrCl <20 mL/min, congenital or acquired long QT syndrome (baseline QTc >440 ms; >500 ms in patients with ventricular conduction problems), previous TdP or known hypersensitivity to dofetilide. Discontinue dofetilide if at any time after a second dose QTc >500 ms (550 ms with ventricular conduction abnormalities). Avoid other QT-prolonging drugs<br>• Cautions: patients with AVB, bradycardia, hypokalemia, hypomagnesemia, diuretic therapy, moderate baseline QT interval prolongation, proarrhythmic events, liver or renal impairment. QT-prolonging drugs.<br>• Avoid the combination with cimetidine, hydrochlorothiazide, ketoconazole, trimethoprim, prochlorperazine or megestrol. |

(continued)

Table 3.3 (continued)

| Drug | Adverse effects | Contraindications and cautions |
|---|---|---|
| Dronedarone | Diarrhea, nausea, vomiting, rash, photosensitivity. It does not affect thyroid or pulmonar functions. Increases serum creatinine levels | 1. Contraindications: bradycardia (<50 bpm), 2nd- or 3rd-degree AVB, complete bundle branch block, distal block, sinus node dysfunction, atrial conduction defects, or sick sinus syndrome, unless a pacemaker is present. Patients with LV systolic dysfunction or current or previous HF, permanent AF, unstable hemodynamic conditions, baseline QTc ≥500 ms, severe hepatic or renal impairment (CrCl <30 mL/min) or liver and lung toxicity related to previous use of amiodarone. Potent CYP3A4 inhibitors and QT prolonging drugs should be avoided<br>2. Interactions. Dronedarone is metabolized by CYP3A: caution with inhibitors (eg., diltiazem, ketoconazole, macrolide antibiotics, protease inhibitors, verapamil, grapefruit juice) and inducers (eg., phenobarbital, phenytoin, rifampin). It inhibits CYP3A4, CYP2D6, P-glycoprotein: increases the exposure to some beta blockers, digoxin, sirolimus, statins, tacrolimus. Monitor the INR. |

| | | |
|---|---|---|
| Ibutilide (IV) | QT prolongation, TdP (3–4% of patients). Slows ventricular rate | 1. Contraindications: baseline QTc >440 ms, advanced or unstable heart disease, congenital or acquired long syndrome, uncorrected hypokalemia or hypomagnesemia, history of polymorphic VT or proarrhythmia, bradycardia or sick sinus syndrome<br>2. Cautions: patients with HF, liver disease or recent MI. |
| Sotalol | • Cardiovascular: bradycardia, AVB, hypotension, HF, syncope, QT prolongation, TdP<br>• Others: fatigue, dizziness, weakness, lightheadedness, dyspnea, bronchitis, nausea, diarrhea, fainting, anxiety, depression | 1. Contraindications: Sinus bradycardia, sick sinus syndrome, or 2nd- and 3rd-degree AVB (unless a pacemaker is present); congenital or acquired LQTS; cardiogenic shock, decompensated systolic HF, Prinzmetal's angina, Raynaud's phenomenon and severe peripheral circulatory disturbances, renal failure (CrCl <40 mL/ min), asthma or related bronchospastic conditions. Avoid other QT-prolonging drugs.<br>2. Cautions: patients with bradycardia, hypotension. Drugs with SA and/or AV–nodal blocking properties. Hypokalemia and diuretic therapy increase QT prolongation |

*AAD* antiarrhythmic drugs, *AF* atrial fibrillation, *AV* atrio-ventricular, *AVB* atrio-ventricular block, *CrCl* creatinine clearance, *HF* heart failure, *ICD* implantable cardiac defibrillator, *INR* international normalized ratio, *IV* intravenous, *LQTS* long *QT* syndrome, *LV* left ventricular, *MI* myocardial infarction, *SA* sinoatrial, *TdP* torsades de pointes, *VT* ventricular tachycardia

TABLE 3.4 Drug interactions of amiodarone

| Drug | Pharmacodynamic/pharmacokinetic | Implications |
|---|---|---|
| Agalsidase alfa or beta | | Avoid the combination |
| Anesthetics, general | Increased risk of bradycardia, hypotension and decreased cardiac output | Patients should be carefully monitored for potential cardiovascular complications |
| Oral anticoagulants: apixaban, dabigatran, edoxaban, rivaroxaban | Amiodarone increases drug exposure and the risk of bleeding | With caution |
| Antihypertensives | Increase the risk of hypotension | Monitor BP when amiodarone is given IV |
| Antiviral drugs: daclasvir, ledipasvir/sofosbuvir, sofosbuvir | Severe bradycardia with this combination | Monitor heart rate during the first 48 h |
| Beta-blockers | Increase the risk of hypotension, bradycardia and AVB | Monitor BP and ECG |
| Bile acid sequestrants (resins) | Reduce the absorption of amiodarone | Administer amiodarone 1 h before or 4 h after the resin |
| Cyclosporine | Amiodarone reduces the clearance and increases the Pc of cyclosporine | Monitor cyclosporine toxicity (renal, hypertension) |
| Cimetidine | Inhibits the metabolism of amiodarone and increases its Pc | Decrease the dose of amiodarone |

| | | |
|---|---|---|
| Class I and III AADs | Amiodarone increases the Pc of class I AADs. Increase the risk of proarrhythmia. Amiodarone inhibits the clearance and increases the Pc of flecainide | Avoid the combination. Monitor the ECG for excessive QT prolongation and proarrhythmia. Reduce (30–50%) the dose of flecainide |
| Class IV AADs: diltiazem, verapamil | Increase the risk of bradycardia, AVB, hypotension and HF. Amiodarone increases the Pc of diltiazem | Monitor the ECG and BP |
| Clopidogrel | Amiodarone inhibits CYP3A4 and the formation of the active metabolite of clopidogrel | Prescribe an alternative platelet $P2Y_{12}$ receptor inhibitor |
| Digoxin | Amiodarone inhibits P-gp, decreases the clearance and increases the Pc of digoxin and the risk of bradycardia and AVB | Monitor the digoxin plasma levels. Reduce (30–50%) the dose of digoxin and monitor the ECG |
| Dopamine, dobutamine | Amiodarone exhibits β-adrenergic blocking effects | Higher IV doses of dopamine and dobutamine are needed |

(continued)

Table 3.4 (continued)

| Drug | Pharmacodynamic/pharmacokinetic | Implications |
|---|---|---|
| Drugs that cause hypokalemia and/or hypomagnesaemia:<br>• Amphotericin, loop and thiazide diuretics, systemic corticosteroids, tetracosactide, laxatives | Prolong the QT interval | Monitor serum potassium and magnesium levels. Monitor the ECG |
| Fentanyl | Increases the risk of hypotension, bradycardia, and decreases cardiac output | Monitor the hemodynamic response |
| Grapefruit juice | Inhibits CYP3A4 and the metabolism of amiodarone | Avoid drinking grapefruit |
| HIV-Protease inhibitors: indinavir, lopinavir, nelfinavir, ritonavir, saquinavir | Inhibit CYP3A4 and increase the Pc of amiodarone | Monitor the ECG. Avoid if possible |
| Ivabradine | Increases the risk of bradycardia and atrial fibrillation | Monitor the ECG |
| Lidocaine | Increased risk of bradycardia, and seizures | Monitor the ECG. Monitor lidocaine Pc/clinical response |

| | | |
|---|---|---|
| Lithium | Reported cases of hypothyroidism | Monitor thyroid function |
| Methotrexate | Amiodarone decreases the metabolism of methotrexate | Monitor for the adverse effects of methotrexate |
| Phenytoin | Amiodarone inhibits hepatic metabolism of phenytoin; phenytoin increases the metabolism of amiodarone reducing its antiarrhythmic efficacy | Reduce the dose of phenytoin (50%). The interaction can take several weeks to become apparent |
| QTc-prolonging drugs (see Table 3.1) | Increase the risk of proarrhythmia (torsades de pointes) | Avoid the combination |
| Rifampicin | Decreases the serum levels of amiodarone | Monitor the ECG |
| Sotalol | Increases the risk of hypotension, bradycardia and QT prolongation | Monitor the hemodynamic response and the ECG |
| Statins: atorvastatin, rosuvastatin, simvastatin | Increase the risk of myopathy | Doses of lovastatin and simvastatin should not exceed 40 mg/day and 20 mg/day, respectively |

(continued)

TABLE 3.4 (continued)

| Drug | Pharmacodynamic/pharmacokinetic | Implications |
|---|---|---|
| St. John's wort | Decreases the plasma levels of amiodarone | Avoid the combination |
| Theophylline | Amiodarone inhibits its metabolism | Monitor theophylline toxicity (nausea, tremor, tachycardia, nervousness) |
| Warfarin | Amiodarone reduces its metabolism and increases the prothrombin time and the risk of bleeding | Reduce (50%) the dose of warfarin. Monitor the INR |

*AADs* antiarrhythmic drugs, *AV* atrio-ventricular, *AVB* atrio-ventricular block, *BP* blood pressure, *CYP* cytochrome P450 superfamily, *ECG* electrocardiogram, *HIV* human immunodeficiency virus, *HF* heart failure, *INR* international normalized ratio, *IV* intravenously, *Pc* plasma levels, *P-gp* P-glycoprotein

Table 3.5 Doses of class III antiarrhythmics

| Drug | Doses |
|---|---|
| Amiodarone (oral) | • PO loading. Rapid control of an urgent arrhythmia: 800–1600 mg/day (in 2–4 divided doses) for 1–3 weeks; then 400–800 mg/day for 3–4 weeks. In less urgent settings: 600–1200 mg daily for 1–3 weeks and 400 mg/day for the next several weeks. A high-dose oral loading can suppress ventricular arrhythmias within 5 days. Maintenance dose: up to 200 mg o.d. (to minimize long-term adverse effects)<br>• Maintenance of SR in AF. Initially 600 mg daily in divided doses for 4 weeks; 400 mg for 4 weeks; maintenance: 100–200 mg o.d.<br>• Rate control in AF: 100–200 mg o.d<br>• VA. Loading dose: 400 mg every 8–12 h for 1–2 weeks, then 300–400 mg daily; reduce dose to 200 mg daily if possible |
| Amiodarone (IV) | IV amiodarone (diluted in 5% glucose) should be initiated/maintained in hospital under specialist supervision<br>• Loading: 150 mg over 10 min, followed by 360 mg over 6 h; then 540 mg over the remaining 24 h (total of 1050 mg over 24 h. IV maintenance: 0.5–1 mg/min<br>• Cardioversion of AF: 5–7 mg/kg IV for 1–2 h, followed by 50 mg/h to a maximum of 1 g over 24 h<br>• SVT: 150 mg IV over 10 min. Maintenance: 1 mg/min (360 mg) over next 6 h; then 0.5 mg/min (540 mg) over remaining 18 h.<br>• Maintenance of SR in AF: 1 mg/min for 6 h; then 0.5 mg/min for 18 h or change to oral dosing; after 24 h, decrease the dose to 0.25 mg/min<br>• Rate control in AF: 300 mg over 30–60 min (preferably via central venous cannula); then, 900 mg IV over 24 h diluted in 500–1000 mL.<br>• Termination of VT: 150 mg IV over 10 minutes<br>• Incessant VT or frequent VT episodes: 150 mg bolus over 10 min, followed by 1 mg/min over the next 6 h and 0.5 mg/min over the remaining 18 h total 1050 mg over 24 h<br>• VF/pulseless VT arrest: 2.5–5 mg/kg bolus monitoring; another dose of 2.5 mg/kg if the VF persists after a further shock<br>• Stable VT: 150 mg bolus. Then, 1 mg/min for 6 h, then 0.5 mg/min × 18 h |

(continued)

Table 3.5 (continued)

| Drug | Doses |
|---|---|
| Dofetilide | • PO. CrCl >60 mL/min: 500 mcg bid. CrCl 40–60 mL/min: 250 mcg bid. CrCl 20- < 40 mL/min: 125 mcg bid. CrCl <20 mL/min: Dofetilide is contraindicated<br>• If 2–3 h after the first dose the QTc has increased >15% compared to the baseline or the QTc is >500 msec (550 msec in patients with ventricular conduction abnormalities) doses should be readjusted as follows: 500 mcg bid → 250 mscg bid; 250 mcg bid → 125 bid and 125 mcg bid → 125 mcg od. If at any time after the second dose is given the QTc is >500 msec (550 msec in patients with ventricular conduction abnormalities), dofetilide should be discontinued |
| Dronedarone | Rate control in AF: 400 mg bid with food |
| Ibutilide (IV) | 0.01 mg/kg (<60 kg) or 1 mg (>60 kg) over 10 min; repeat after 10 min if the arrhythmia persists |
| Sotalol | 1. SVT/VA. Oral: 40–80 mg bid initially. Increase the dose every 2–3 days to 120–160 mg bid. IV: 75 mg over 5 h every 12 h initially; adjusted if necessary every 3 days. Max dose: 150 mg every 12 h<br>• Maintenance of SR in AF: 40–160 mg bid<br>2. Refractory life-threatening VA. Oral: 80 mg bid initially. Increase the dose as needed every 2–3 days to 160–320 mg/day divided every 8–12 h; up to 480–640 mg/day may be required if benefits outweigh the risk of adverse effects |

*AF* atrial fibrillation, *Af* atrial flutter, *Bid* twice daily, *h* hours, *IV* intravenous, *o.d* once daily, *PO* per os (orally), *SVT* supraventricular tachycardia, *SR* sinus rhythm, *VA* ventricular arrhythmias, *VF* ventricular fibrillation, *VT* ventricular tachycardia

Table 3.6 Recommendations of class III AADs for the management of AF

| *1. Rate control in atrial fibrillation* | *Class* | *Level* |
|---|---|---|
| Amiodarone is reasonable for pharmacological cardioversion of AF [24] | IIa | A |
| Dofetilide and IV ibutilide are useful for cardioversion of AF, provided contraindications are absent [24] | I | A |
| In patients with ischemic and/or structural heart disease, amiodarone is recommended for cardioversion of AF [27] | I | A |
| In the absence of pre-excitation, IV digoxin is recommended to control heart rate acutely in HF patients [24] | I | B |
| Digoxin is effective to control resting heart rate in patients with HF with reduced ejection fraction [24] | I | C |
| IV amiodarone can be useful for rate control in critically ill patients without pre-excitation [24] | IIa | B |
| A combination of digoxin and a β-blocker (or a nondihydropyridine calcium channel antagonist for patients with HFpEF) is reasonable to control resting and exercise HR in patients with AF [24] | IIa | B |
| In patients with hemodynamic instability or severely depressed LVEF, amiodarone may be considered for acute control of HR | IIb | B |
| Oral amiodarone may be useful for ventricular rate control when other measures are unsuccessful or contraindicated [24] | IIb | C |

(continued)

Table 3.6 (continued)

| | | |
|---|---|---|
| In HF patients, IV amiodarone can be useful to control HR when other measures are unsuccessful or contraindicated [24] | IIa | C |
| Amiodarone may be considered when resting and exercise HR cannot be adequately controlled using a β-blocker (or a nondihydropyridine calcium channel antagonist in patients with HFpEF) or digoxin, alone or in combination [24] | IIb | C |
| Amiodarone or digoxin may be considered to slow RVR with ACS and AF and severe LV dysfunction and HF or hemodynamic instability [24] | IIb | C |
| In patients with pre-excitation and AF, digoxin or IV amiodarone should not be administered as they may increase the ventricular response and may result in ventricular fibrillation [24, 27] | III | B |
| Dronedarone should not be used to control ventricular rate with permanent AF as it increases the risk of the combined endpoint of stroke, myocardial infarction, systemic embolism, or cardiovascular death [24] | III | B |
| Dofetilide should not be initiated out of hospital because of the risk of excessive QT prolongation that can cause TdP [24] | III | B |
| Dronedarone should not be administered to patients with decompensated HF [24, 27] | III | B |
| *2. Postoperative atrial fibrillation* | | |
| Preoperative amiodarone reduces AF with cardiac surgery and is reasonable as prophylactic therapy for patients at high risk of postoperative AF [24, 27] | IIa | A |

| | | |
|---|---|---|
| It is reasonable to restore SR pharmacologically with ibutilide in patients with postoperative AF [24] | IIa | B |
| IV vernakalant may be considered for cardioversion of postoperative AF in patients without severe HF, hypotension, or severe structural heart disease (especially aortic stenosis) [27] | IIa | B |
| Prophylactic sotalol may be considered for patients with AF risk after cardiac surgery [24] | IIb | B |
| *3. Pharmacological Cardioversion of atrial fibrillation* | | |
| Dofetilide and IV ibutilide are useful for cardioversion of AF, provided there are no contraindications [24] | I | A |
| In patients with no history of ischemic or structural heart disease, vernakalant is recommended for pharmacological cardioversion of new-onset AF [27] | I | A |
| In patients with ischemic and/or structural heart disease, amiodarone is recommended for cardioversion of AF [27] | I | A |
| Because of its potential toxicities, amiodarone should only be used after consideration of risks and when other agents have failed or are contraindicated [24] | I | C |
| IV ibutilide to restore SR or slow the ventricular rate is recommended for patients with pre-excited AF and rapid ventricular response who are not hemodynamically compromised [24] | I | C |
| Oral amiodarone is reasonable for pharmacological cardioversion of AF [24] | IIa | A |
| Pre-treatment with amiodarone or ibutilide should be considered to enhance success of electrical cardioversion and prevent recurrent AF [27] | IIa | B |

(continued)

TABLE 3.6 (continued)

| | | |
|---|---|---|
| In patients with no history of ischemic or structural heart disease, ibutilide should be considered for pharmacological conversion of AF [27] | IIa | B |
| Vernakalant may be considered as an alternative to amiodarone for pharmacological conversion of AF in patients without hypotension, severe HF or severe structural heart disease (especially aortic stenosis) [27] | IIb | B |
| IV amiodarone can be useful to control heart rate with AF when other measures are unsuccessful or contraindicated [24] | IIb | C |
| Dofetilide should not be initiated out of hospital because of the risk of excessive QT prolongation that can cause TdP [24] | III | B |
| *4. Rhythm control therapy in atrial fibrillation* | | |
| Amiodarone, dofetilide, dronedarone or sotalol are recommended in patients with AF to maintain SR, depending on underlying heart disease and comorbidities [24] | *I* | *A* |
| Dronedarone or sotalol are recommended for prevention of recurrent symptomatic AF in patients with normal LV function and without pathological LV hypertrophy [27] | I | A |
| Dronedarone is recommended for prevention of recurrent symptomatic AF in patients with stable coronary artery disease, and without HF [27] | I | A |
| Amiodarone is recommended for prevention of recurrent symptomatic AF in patients with HF [27] | I | B |

| | | |
|---|---|---|
| Amiodarone is more effective in preventing AF recurrences than other AAD, but extracardiac toxic effects are common and increase with time. For this reason, other AAD should be considered first [24, 27] | I/II | C |
| Ibutilide should be considered for acute therapy of pre-excited AF [27] | IIa | B |
| Amiodarone combined with a β-blocker or nondihydropyridine calcium channel antagonists can be useful to prevent recurrent AF in patients with HCM | IIa | C |
| Sotalol, dofetilide, and dronedarone may be considered for a rhythm-control strategy in patients with HCM [24] | IIb | C |
| Dronedarone should not be used for treatment of AF in patients with NYHA class III and IV HF or patients who have had an episode of decompensated HF in the past 4 weeks [24] | III | B |
| AADs for rhythm control should not be continued when AF becomes permanent [24, 27] | III | B |
| IV amiodarone is potentially harmful in patients with pre-excited AF [24, 27] | III | B |
| AAD therapy is not recommended in patients with prolonged QT interval (>0.5 s) or those with significant sinoatrial node disease or AV node dysfunction who do not have a functioning permanent pacemaker [27] | III | C |

*AAD* antiarrhythmic drug, *ACS* acute coronary syndromes, *AF* atrial fibrillation, *Af* atrial flutter, *AV* atrioventricular, *HCM* hypertrophic cardiomyopathy, *HF* heart failure, *HFpEF* heart failure with preserved ejection fraction, *HR* heart rate, *IV* intravenous, *LV* left ventricular, *LVEF* left ventricular ejection fraction, *SR* sinus rhythm, *RVR* rapid ventricular response, *TdP* torsades de pointes

TABLE 3.7 Recommendations of class III AADs for the management of supraventricular arrhythmias

| Recommendations | Class/Level ACC/AHA/HRS [26] | Class/Level ESC [29] |
|---|---|---|
| **1. Supraventricular tachycardia of unknown mechanism** | | |
| *Ongoing Treatment* | | |
| Sotalol may be reasonable for ongoing management in patients with symptomatic SVT who are not candidates for, or prefer not to undergo, catheter ablation | IIb, B | |
| Dofetilide may be reasonable for ongoing management in patients with symptomatic SVT who are not candidates for, or prefer not to undergo, catheter ablation and in whom β-blockers, diltiazem, flecainide, propafenone, or verapamil are ineffective or contraindicated | IIb, B | |
| Oral amiodarone may be considered for ongoing management in patients with symptomatic SVT who are not candidates for, or prefer not to undergo, catheter ablation and in whom β-blockers, diltiazem, dofetilide, flecainide, propafenone, sotalol, or verapamil are ineffective or contraindicated | IIb, C | |
| Oral digoxin may be reasonable for ongoing management in patients with symptomatic SVT without pre-excitation who are not candidates for, or prefer not to undergo, catheter ablation | IIb, C | |

| | | |
|---|---|---|
| **2. Acute treatment of wide QRS tachycardia in the absence of an established diagnosis** | | |
| IV amiodarone may be considered if vagal manoeuvres and adenosine fail in the acute management of wide QRS tachycardia in the absence of an established diagnosis | | IIb, B |
| **3. Focal atrial tachycardia** | | |
| *a) Acute Treatment* | | |
| IV amiodarone may be reasonable in the acute setting to either restore SR or slow the ventricular rate in hemodynamically stable patients with focal AT | IIb, C | IIb, C |
| IV ibutilide may be reasonable in the acute setting to restore SR in hemodynamically stable patients with focal AT | IIb, C | IIb, C |
| *b) Ongoing Treatment* | | |
| Oral sotalol or amiodarone may be reasonable for ongoing management in patients with focal AT | IIb, C | |
| Amiodarone may be considered if other measures fail | | IIb, C |

(continued)

Table 3.7 (continued)

| **Recommendations** | **Class/Level ACC/ AHA/HRS** [26] | **Class/Level ESC** [29] |
|---|---|---|
| **4. Atrial flutter/macro-reentrant tachycardia** | | |
| *a) Acute Treatment* | | |
| Oral dofetilide or IV ibutilide, under close monitoring due to proarrhythmic risk, are useful for acute cardioversion in patients with Af | I, A | |
| IV ibutilide or IV or oral (in-hospital) dofetilide are recommended for conversion to in the absence of QTc interval prolongation | | I, B |
| IV amiodarone may be tried if other measures are not available or desirable | | IIb, C |
| IV amiodarone can be useful for acute control of the ventricular rate (in the absence of pre-excitation) in patients with Af and systolic HF when β-blockers are contraindicated or ineffective | IIa, B | |
| *b) Ongoing Treatment* | | |
| Amiodarone, dofetilide or sotalol can be useful to maintain SR in patients with symptomatic, recurrent Af; drug choice depends on underlying heart disease and comorbidities | IIa, B | |
| Amiodarone may be considered to maintain SR if other measures fail | | IIb, C |

| | | |
|---|---|---|
| **5. Treatment of AVNRT** | | |
| *a) Acute Treatment* | | |
| IV amiodarone may be considered for acute treatment in hemodynamically stable patients with AVNRT when other therapies are ineffective or contraindicated | IIb, C | |
| *b) Ongoing Treatment* | | |
| Oral sotalol or dofetilide may be reasonable for ongoing management in patients with AVNRT who are not candidates for, or prefer not to undergo, catheter ablation | IIb, B | |
| Oral digoxin or amiodarone may be reasonable for ongoing treatment of AVNRT in patients who are not candidates for, or prefer not to undergo, catheter ablation | IIb, B | |
| **6. Therapy of AVRT due to manifest or concealed accessory pathways** | | |
| *a) Acute Treatment* | | |
| IV ibutilide is beneficial for acute treatment in patients with pre-excited AF (orthodromic AVRT) who are hemodynamically stable | I, C | IIa, B |

(continued)

TABLE 3.7 (continued)

| **Recommendations** | **Class/Level ACC/ AHA/HRS** [26] | **Class/Level ESC** [29] |
|---|---|---|
| *b) Ongoing Treatment* | | |
| Oral amiodarone may be considered in patients with AVRT and/or pre-excited AF who are not candidates for, or prefer not to undergo, catheter ablation and in whom other AADs are ineffective or contraindicated | IIb, C | |
| Oral dofetilide or sotalol may be reasonable for ongoing management in patients with AVRT and/or pre-excited AF who are not candidates for, or prefer not to undergo, catheter ablation | IIb, B | |
| Amiodarone is not recommended and potentially harmful for acute treatment in patients with pre-excited AF | III, C | III, B |
| **7. SVT in ACHD patients** | | |
| *a) Acute Treatment* | | |
| IV ibutilide can be effective for acute treatment in ACHD patients and atrial flutter who are hemodynamically stable | IIa, B | |
| Oral dofetilide or sotalol may be reasonable for acute treatment in ACHD patients and AT and/or Af who are hemodynamically stable | IIb, B | |

| | | |
|---|---|---|
| *b) Ongoing Treatment* | | |
| Amiodarone may be reasonable for prevention of recurrent AT or Af in ACHD patients for whom other medications and catheter ablation are ineffective or contraindicated | IIb, B | IIb, C |
| Oral sotalol therapy can be useful for prevention of recurrent AT or Af in ACHD patients | IIa, B | |
| Oral dofetilide may be reasonable for prevention of recurrent AT or Af in ACHD patients | IIb, B | |
| Sotalol is not recommended as a first-line AAD as it is related to an increased risk of pro-arrhythmias and mortality | | III, C |
| **8. SVT during pregnancy** | | |
| *a) Acute Treatment* | | |
| IV amiodarone may be considered for acute treatment in pregnant patients with potentially life-threatening SVT when other therapies are ineffective or contraindicated | IIb, C | |
| IV ibutilide may be considered for termination of atrial flutter | | IIb, C |

(continued)

TABLE 3.7 (continued)

| **Recommendations** | **Class/Level ACC/AHA/HRS** [26] | **Class/Level ESC** [29] |
|---|---|---|
| *b) Ongoing Treatment* | | |
| Oral amiodarone may be considered for ongoing management in pregnant patients when treatment of highly symptomatic, recurrent SVT is required and other therapies are ineffective or contraindicated | IIb, C | |
| Sotalol can be effective for ongoing management in pregnant patients with highly symptomatic SVT | IIa, C | |
| Amiodarone is not recommended in pregnant women | | III, C |

*AADs* antiarrhythmic drugs, *ACHD* adult congenital heart disease, *Af* atrial flutter, *AT* atrial tachycardia, *AVNRT* atrioventricular nodal reentrant tachycardia, *AVRT* atrioventricular reentrant tachycardia, *IV* intravenous, *SR* sinus rhythm, *SVT* supraventricular tachycardia

TABLE 3.8 Recommendations of class III AADs for the management of ventricular arrhythmias

| Recommendations | Class | Level |
|---|---|---|
| *Acute management of specific VA* | | |
| In patients with hemodynamically unstable VA that persist or recur after a maximal energy shock, IV amiodarone should be administered to attempt to achieve a stable rhythm after further defibrillation [28] | I | A |
| In patients with hemodynamically stable VT, administration of IV amiodarone or sotalol may be considered to attempt to terminate VT [28] | IIb | B |
| In patients with suspected acute MI, prophylactic administration of lidocaine or high-dose amiodarone for the prevention of VT is potentially harmful [28] | III | B |
| *Management of Cardiac Arrest* | | |
| In patients with hemodynamically unstable VA that persist or recur after a maximal energy shock, IV amiodarone should be administered to attempt to achieve a stable rhythm after further defibrillation [28] | I | A |
| In patients with hemodynamically stable VT, administration of IV amiodarone or sotalol may be considered to attempt to terminate VT [28] | IIb | B |
| In patients with suspected acute MI, prophylactic administration of high-dose amiodarone for the prevention of VT is potentially harmful [28] | III | B |

(continued)

Table 3.8 (continued)

| Recommendations | Class | Level |
|---|---|---|
| *Prevention and management of SCD associated with acute coronary syndromes: in-hospital phase* | | |
| IV amiodarone is recommended for the treatment of polymorphic VT [25] | I | C |
| *Stable coronary artery disease after MI with preserved ejection fraction* | | |
| Amiodarone may be considered for relief of symptoms from VAs in survivors of a MI but it has no effect on mortality [25] | IIb | B |
| *Treatment of PVC in patients with structural heart disease/left ventricular dysfunction* | | |
| In patients with frequent symptomatic PVC or NSVT amiodarone should be considered [25] | IIa | B |
| *Treatment of patients with LV dysfunction and sustained recurrent monomorphic VT* | | |
| Amiodarone treatment should be considered to prevent VT in patients with or without an ICD [25] | IIa | C |
| *Prevention of VT recurrences in patients with LV dysfunction and sustained VT* | | |
| Amiodarone is recommended in patients with recurrent ICD shocks due to sustained VT [25] | I | B |
| Amiodarone should be considered after a first episode of sustained VT in patients with an ICD [25] | IIa | B |
| *Treatment and prevention of Recurrent VA in Patients With Ischemic Heart Disease* | | |

| | | |
|---|---|---|
| In patients with ischemic heart disease and recurrent VA, with significant symptoms or ICD shocks despite optimal device programming and ongoing treatment with a β-blocker, amiodarone or sotalol is useful to suppress recurrent VA [28] | I | B |
| *Secondary Prevention of SCD in Patients With NICM* | | |
| In patients with NICM who survive a cardiac arrest, have sustained VT, or have symptomatic VA who are ineligible for an ICD (due to a limited life-expectancy and/or functional status or lack of access to an ICD), amiodarone may be considered for prevention of SCD [28] | IIb | B |
| *Treatment of Recurrent VA in Patients With NICM* | | |
| In patients with NICM and an ICD who experience spontaneous VA or recurrent appropriate shocks despite optimal device programming treatment with amiodarone or sotalol can be beneficial [28] | IIa | B |
| *Treatment of PVC-induced cardiomyopathy* | | |
| Amiodarone is reasonable to reduce recurrent arrhythmias, and improve symptoms and LV function [28] | IIa | B |
| *Treatment of patients with hypertrophic cardiomyopathy* | | |
| In patients with HCM and a history of sustained VT or VF, amiodarone may be considered when an ICD is not feasible or not preferred by the patient [28] | IIb | C |

(continued)

Table 3.8 (continued)

| Recommendations | Class | Level |
|---|---|---|
| *Treatment of patients with dilated cardiomyopathy* | | |
| Amiodarone should be considered in patients with an ICD that experience recurrent appropriate shocks in spite of optimal device programming [25] | IIa | C |
| Amiodarone is not recommended for the treatment of asymptomatic NSVT in patients with DCM [25] | III | A |
| *Arrhythmogenic right ventricular cardiomyopathy* | | |
| Amiodarone should be considered to improve symptoms in patients with frequent PVC or NSVT who are intolerant of or have contraindications to β-blockers [25] | IIa | C |
| *Short QT Syndrome* | | |
| Sotalol may be considered in asymptomatic patients with a diagnosis of SQTS and a family history of SCD [25] | IIb | C |
| *Management of arrhythmias during pregnancy* | | |
| Sotalol should be considered for acute conversion of hemodynamically stable monomorphic sustained VT [25] | IIa | C |

| | | |
|---|---|---|
| IV amiodarone should be considered for acute conversion of sustained, monomorphic VT when hemodynamically unstable, refractory to electrical cardioversion or not responding to other drugs [25] | IIa | C |
| *Adult Congenital Heart Disease* | | |
| Prophylactic treatment with anti-arrhythmic drugs (other than β-blockers) is not recommended [25] | III | B |
| In patients with ACHD who have asymptomatic VA, prophylactic therapy with amiodarone is potentially harmful [25, 28] | III | B |
| Prophylactic anti-arrhythmic therapy is not recommended for asymptomatic infrequent PVC in patients with CHD and stable ventricular function [25] | III | C |

*ACHD* adult congenital heart disease, *CHD* coronary heart disease, *DCM* dilated cardiomyopathy, *HCM* hypertrophic cardiomyopathy, *ICD* implantable cardioverter defibrillator, *IV* intravenous, *LV* left ventricular, *MI* myocardial infarction, *NICM* non-ischemic cardiomyopathy, *NSVT* non-sustained ventricular tachycardia, *PVC* premature ventricular complexes, *SCD* sudden cardiac death, *SQTS* short QT syndrome, *VA* ventricular arrhythmia, *VT* ventricular tachycardia

# Amiodarone

Amiodarone is a iodinated benzofuran derivative that exhibits a "wide-spectrum" of antiarrhythmic properties. It blocks inwardly depolarizing $Na^+$ ($I_{Na}$) and L-type $Ca^{2+}$ ($I_{CaL}$) currents and several outward repolarizing $K^+$ currents, including the transient ($I_{to}$), the inward rectifier ($I_{K1}$), the ultrarapid ($I_{Kur}$), rapid ($I_{Kr}$), and slow ($I_{Ks}$) components of the delayed rectifier and the acetylcholine-activated ($I_{KAch}$) [2–5]. Amiodarone inhibits the $I_{Na}$ by blocking the inactivated state of sodium channels with a fast diastolic recovery from block. This effect is accentuated in depolarized tissues (voltage-dependent block) and at fast rates (rate-dependent block), but it is almost nonexistent at slow heart rates. In fact, amiodarone reduces cardiac excitability and conduction velocity and prolongs the QRS and H-V intervals at fast rates. Additionally, amiodarone noncompetitively antagonizes α- and β-adrenoceptors (class II effect) [2–6], inhibits both the conversion of thyroxine (T4) to triiodothyronine (T3) and the entry of T3 and T4 into cells [7], and produces a vasodilator effect mediated via the blockade of $I_{CaL}$ and β-adrenergic receptors. The blockade of $I_{CaL}$ and β-adrenergic receptors explains why amiodarone produces bradycardia and atrio-ventricular (AV) block. Thus, amiodarone exhibits class I, III and IV antiarrhythmic actions of the Vaughan Williams classification.

**Electrophysiological Actions** The acute and chronic electrophysiological effects of amiodarone in humans are very different [2, 5, 6, 8, 9]. After *intravenous administration*, the main effect is the lengthening of AV nodal refractoriness and intranodal conduction (with prolongation of the PR and A-H intervals) possibly related to the blockade of $I_{CaL}$ and the non-competitive β-adrenergic antagonism. However, the drug produces minimal effects on the APD and refractoriness of the atrial and ventricular muscle, by pass tracts, or His-Purkinje system and there is almost no effect on the QRS, H-V and QTc intervals or the monophasic action potentials [1–3, 5, 6]. Thus, the class III action of the drug is not observed.

However, *long-term treatment* with oral amiodarone prolongs the APD and refractoriness in all cardiac tissues, including bypass tracts, without affecting the resting membrane potential. Interestingly, amiodarone lengthens the APD preferentially in cardiac tissues with the shortest APD (His bundle, atrial muscle and ventricular epicardium and endocardium), with lesser effects, or even a shortening at slow rates, in Purkinje fibres and M cells [1–3, 5, 6]. Thus, in contrast to other class I and III AADs, amiodarone produces a homogeneous prolongation of the APD (QT interval) and reduces transmural dispersion of repolarization across the ventricular wall and the possible re-entry of cardiac impulses. Additionally, amiodarone prolongs the APD at all driving rates, i.e., it does not produce reverse use-dependence. Furthermore, despite amiodarone prolongs the ventricular APD, the risk of TdP is less than with other AADs, possibly because it blocks both the $I_{CaL}$ and β-adrenoceptors, does not produce reverse use-dependence and produces a more homogenous recovery of ventricular repolarization reducing the transmural dispersion of repolarization. In chronic treatments and at fast driving rates, amiodarone blocks the $I_{Na}$ (prolongs the QRS complex) and decreases cardiac excitability and conduction velocity and increases the VF threshold. Desethylamiodarone (DEA), the main active metabolite, has relatively greater effects on the $I_{Na}$ and contributes to the antiarrhythmic efficacy of amiodarone [3]. On the ECG, amiodarone prolongs the RR, PR, A-H, H-V, QRS, JT and QT intervals (occasionally it can produce U waves). Oral amiodarone was more effective than IV amiodarone in lengthening the anterograde effective refractory period of the accessory AV pathway.

In the sinoatrial node and other cardiac pacemaker cells, amiodarone decreases the slope of phase 4 depolarization (pacemaker potential) and the rate of spontaneous excitation and suppresses the slow action potentials (abnormal automaticity) elicited in abnormally depolarized cardiac cells as well as the early afterdepolarizations generated in Purkinje fibres and M cells [2–5]. In the AV node, amiodarone slows intranodal conduction and increases refractoriness and, therefore, reduces the ventricular rate in patients with supraventirulcar arrhythmias. In patients with AF, amiodarone prolongs the refractory periods both in the atria and in the pulmonary veins, slows AV nodal conduction and, in experimental models, it prevents atrial remodelling [10]. The effects of oral amiodarone on sinoatrial and AV nodal function are maximal within 2 weeks, whereas the effects on VT and ventricular refractoriness appear gradually, becoming maximal at ≥10 weeks.

**Hemodynamic Effects** Amiodarone is a peripheral and coronary vasodilator. After oral administration, amiodarone slows sinus rate (15–20%) and prolongs the PR and QT intervals but does not depress the left ventricular ejection fraction (LVEF). Indeed, the LVEF may increase slightly even in patients with reduced LVEF, possibly because its vasodilator effect reduces LV afterload. However, after IV administration amiodarone decreases heart rate, systemic vascular resistances, blood pressure and contractile force; thus, it should be given cautiously to patients with depressed LVEF because of the risk of bradycardia and hypotension [5, 6].

**Pharmacokinetics** (Table 3.2) After oral administration, amiodarone presents a slow, variable and incomplete absorption (bioavailability of 35–65%) and peak plasma levels are reached after 3–8 h [11]. Food increases its oral bioavailability and reduces gastrointestinal adverse effects [12]. The onset of action after oral administration occurs after 2–3 days (1–2 h after IV administration) [9]. Amiodarone is highly protein bound (99%) and extensively distributed (Vd 70 L/kg). It accumulates in the heart (cardiac levels are 10–50 times higher than in plasma), adipose tissue, liver, lungs and skin, crosses the placenta and is found in breast milk. This wide tissular distribution explains why even when the onset of drug action occurs after 2–3 days, steady-state plasma levels are reached after several months unless large loading doses are used, and why the drug effects persist for weeks or months after drug discontinuation [9, 11]. Amiodarone is extensively metabolized in the liver by CYP450 3A4 and 2C8, leading to various active metabolites. DEA also accumulates in almost all tissues and exhibits electrophysiologic effects quite similar to those of amiodarone. Both amiodarone and DEA are excreted primarily via the hepatic-biliary route undergoing some enterohepatic recirculation, so that doses do not need to be reduced in patients with renal disease. Amiodarone is eliminated very slowly. There is an initial 50% reduction in plasma levels 3–10 days after drug discontinuation which probably represents drug elimination from well-perfused tissues, followed by a terminal elimination half-life (t) of 53 days (range 26–107 days). The therapeutic plasma levels are between 1.0 and 2.5 mg/mL [6]. Amiodarone and DEA are not dialyzable.

**Adverse Effects** (Table 3.3) They are reported in up to 75% of patients treated with amiodarone for more than 2 years, leading to drug discontinuation in 18–37% of patients. Some side effects may be potentially fatal [9, 13, 14]. Adverse effects are more common on chronic therapy and at high doses, but they still occur even at dosages ≤200 mg/day. Cardiac side effects include symptomatic bradycardia (especially in the elderly), AV block, conduction disturbances, worsening heart failure (HF) and QT prolongation [9, 13, 14]. However, the risk of TdP is very uncommon (<0.5%) [15], probably because of its class II and IV properties, but may occur in patients with hypokalemia or bradycardia, or those receiving QT-prolonging drugs. Phlebitis and hypotension are observed when administered IV.

Adverse extracardiac effects are gastrointestinal (nausea, vomiting, constipation, anorexia), ocular (almost all patients develop asymptomatic corneal microdeposits; rare: optic neuritis and atrophy with visual loss), neurological (proximal muscle weakness, fatigue, peripheral neuropathy, headache, ataxia, tremors, impaired memory, sleep disturbances), cutaneous (rash, photosensitivity, alopecia, blue-gray skin discoloration), hyperthyroidism or hypothyroidism and hepatotoxicity (elevated transaminase levels, hepatitis, cirrhosis and fatal hepatic necrosis) [6, 9, 13–17]. Amiodarone can increase creatinine plasma levels due to partial inhibition of the tubular organic cationic transporter system, rather than a decline in renal function. In fact, the drug does not affect the glomerular filtration rate (GFR), renal blood flow, and $Na^+$ or $K^+$ excretion. Most of these adverse effects are reversible after dose reduction or drug discontinuation, but because of its long half-life, some of them may persist for many months (skin discoloration slowly reverses after 18 months but may not disappear). Neurological and gastrointestinal adverse effects are common during loading doses and usually improve with lower maintenance doses.

Pulmonary toxicity (interstitial pneumonitis, pulmonary fibrosis) occurs in 1–15% of patients receiving doses ≥400 mg/day. Pulmonary function tests show a restrictive pattern with reduced forced vital capacity and diffusing capacity, and chest computed tomography can reveal evidence of fibrosis and diffuse ground glass confluent opacities. Advanced age, high cumulative dose (>400 mg/day), duration of therapy (>6 months), reduced predrug diffusion capacity and preexisting pulmonary disease are risk factors for the development of pulmonary toxicity [14, 18, 19]. Pulmonary toxicity can be fatal in about 10% of patients [13]. Treatment includes drug discontinuation and administration of glucocorticoids [9].

Amiodarone inhibits the peripheral conversion of T4 to T3, producing a slight increase in T4, reverse T3 and thyroid-stimulating hormone (TSH), and a slight decrease in T3 levels. Hypothyroidism appears in 2–6% during the first year of treatment (TSH >10 mU/L) particularly in areas with high dietary iodine intake [7, 20]. Drug discontinuation and/or levothyroxine are the main treatments for amiodarone-induced hypothyroidism. Hyperthyroidism (TSH < 0.35 mU/L) appears in 0.9% of patients and predominates in areas with iodine deficiency [21]. Because it may precipitate cardiac arrhythmias, hyperthyroidism should be excluded if recurrence of arrhythmias appears during amiodarone therapy [7]. Even if amiodarone is discontinued, thyrotoxicosis persists for up to 8 months. Type 1 amiodarone-induced thyrotoxicosis (AIT) occurs in patients with an underlying thyroid pathology and is treated with high doses of thionamides (eg, methimazole or propylthiouracil) to block thyroid hormone synthesis, adding potassium perchlorate to block iodide uptake by the thyroid and deplete intrathyroidal iodine stores. Type 2 AIT is a result of a destructive thyroiditis that results in excess release of preformed T4 and T3 into the circulation and is treated with glucocorticoids. Total thyroidectomy is the only measure that consistently allows continued use of amiodarone. Therefore, thyroid function tests should be performed every 3 months for the first year and every 6–12 months unless thyroid dysfunction appeared.

Because adverse effects are usually dose-related their incidence can be reduced by using very low doses (100–200 mg daily) [9, 14]. Additionally, it is recommended to examine before and periodically during treatment the ECG, chest x-ray, skin, peripheral nerves, thyroid, hepatic, visual and pulmonary function (including carbon monoxide diffusion capacity testing) [9].

Amiodarone and DEA cross the placenta and are detected in breast milk. Amiodarone is associated with severe adverse fetal effects (neurodevelopmental abnormalities, preterm birth, fetal growth restriction and fetal neonatal hypo-/hyperthyroidism and bradycardia) [22, 23]. Therefore, amiodarone is not recommended in women who are, or may become, pregnant (Pregnancy category X) and in nursing mothers [11]. Oral amiodarone may be considered for ongoing management in pregnant patients when treatment of highly symptomatic patients is required and other therapies are ineffective or contraindicated [24–29].

**Drug Interactions** Amiodarone and DEA inhibit CYP450 isoenzymes (CYP1A1/2, 3A4, 2C9 y 2D6) and some transporters [P-glycoprotein (P-gp) and organic cation transporter 2 (OCT2)]. Additionally, amiodarone is a substrate for CYP3A4 [11]. Therefore, amiodarone has the potential for multiple interactions with other drugs that are summarized in Table 3.4.

**Contraindications and Cautions** See Table 3.3.

**Dosage and Administration** See Table 3.5.

**Indications** Amiodarone is indicated for a wide spectrum of supraventricular [atrial fibrillation (AF) or flutter (Af), atrial tachycardia, AV nodal reentrant tachycardia and AV reentrant tachycardia] and ventricular tachyarrhythmias [ventricular tachycardia (VT) and fibrillation (VF)] in patients with structural heart disease (coronary artery disease, LV hypertrophy, HF or LV dysfunction, hypertrophic cardiomyopathy), being the drug of choice when other AADs are ineffective, not tolerated or contraindicated [24–29]. Furthermore, because amiodarone produces less negative inotropic effects or hypotension than β-blockers, diltiazem or verapamil, it is preferred in critically ill patients or in those with hemodynamic instability. However, amiodarone presents several disadvantages, including its slow onset of action after oral administration, so that it should be administered IV or at loading doses to achieve effects rapidly, its long half-life, and its poor safety profile and multiple drug interactions. Because of long-term amiodarone therapy is associated with cardiac and extracardiac adverse effects, it remains as a second-line treatment in patients who are suitable for other AADs or in young patients [9, 24–29].

1. *Atrial fibrillation/flutter* (Table 3.6). Amiodarone is used for the maintenance of sinus rhythm (SR) conversion of AF/Af to SR and ventricular rate control. Amiodarone is the most effective drug for the maintenance of SR in patients with recurrent symptomatic AF/Af [15, 30–33]. It is superior to class I AADs and sotalol and the drug of choice in patients with structural heart disease and the

only AAD recommended in patients with congestive HF or significant aortic stenosis [24, 27, 30, 34, 35]. Amiodarone is superior to sotalol or propafenone for maintenance of SR after cardioversion [30] and in a substudy of the AFFIRM trial, amiodarone was superior to both sotalol and a mixture of class I drugs. In the SAFE-T trial, amiodarone was superior to sotalol, but both drugs had similar efficacy in the subgroup of patients with ischemic heart disease [35].

Amiodarone is also effective for the conversion of AF/Af to SR. However, most data derived from use in patients with AF, while few data are available for patients with Af [24, 27]. Although it has the disadvantage that conversion is often delayed beyond 6 h, amiodarone also slows ventricular rates and it has no risk of postconversion ventricular arrhythmias. For the acute conversion of AF, IV amiodarone is as effective as IV propafenone [36] and both amiodarone and flecainide appear more effective than sotalol in restoring SR [37–39]. Pretreatment with amiodarone can facilitate DC cardioversion and prevent AF recurrences; in relapses to AF after successful cardioversion, repeating DC cardioversion after prophylactic amiodarone can improve the efficacy of DC cardioversion to maintain the SR and prevent the recurrences [37, 40]. Furthermore, amiodarone should be considered to achieve rhythm control and maintain SR in patients with hypertrophic cardiomyopathy and recurrent symptomatic AF [24, 27, 41].

Short-term oral amiodarone treatment following ablation for paroxysmal or persistent AF did not reduce the recurrence of AF/Af at the 6-month follow-up but prolonged time to first documented recurrence and more than halved arrhythmia-related hospitalization and cardioversion rates within the blanking period [42]. Administered before cardiothoracic surgery or postoperatively, amiodarone (alone or in combination with β-blockers) decreased the incidence of post-operative AF (POAF) and hospital stay compared to β-blocker therapy [43–46] and was effective in converting POAF to SR [47, 48].

Amiodarone can be useful for rate control in patients whose heart rate cannot be controlled with combination therapy (e.g. β-blockers or verapamil/diltiazem combined with digoxin) or when these drugs are contraindicated or poorly tolerated [24, 27]. Intravenous amiodarone slows the ventricular rate (10–12 bpm after 8–12 h) [34, 49].

Amiodarone prolongs the anterograde refractory period of the accessory pathway and can be used both for rate control and to achieve conversion in patients with pre-excitation and AF, although urgent electrical cardioversion is often necessary. IV amiodarone is not recommended in these patients, because case reports of accelerated ventricular rhythms and VF [50].

2. *Supraventricular tachycardias* (SVT) (Table 3.7). Evidence for amiodarone for the ongoing management of SVT is limited [26, 29]. IV amiodarone may be considered for acute treatment in hemodynamically stable patients and for ongoing treatment, but because of its safety profile, oral amiodarone is a second-line agent recommended when catheter ablation or other AADs are ineffective or contraindicated (i.e. in patients with structural heart disease) [26, 29].
3. *Ventricular arrhythmias* (Table 3.8). Amiodarone is recommended for the treatment and prophylaxis of life-threatening recurrent ventricular arrhythmias (VT and/or VF) and life-threatening recurrent hemodynamically unstable VT not responding to other AADs, particularly in patients with structural heart disease (i.e. HF, myocardial infarction-MI, hypertension, or cardiomyopathies) or after cardiac surgery when other AADs are not tolerated or contraindicated [25, 28, 51–53]. However, there is modest evidence from randomized controlled trials supporting its use and nowadays it has been replaced by the implantable cardioverter-defibrillator (ICD) therapy. Doses of amiodarone should be as low as possible and restricted to selected patients with refractory ventricular arrhythmias and in young patients it should be reserved as a bridge to more definitive treatment options such as catheter ablation.

Amiodarone is more effective than sotalol and presents a lower risk of ventricular proarrhythmia, but chronic therapy (18–24 months) and high doses of amiodarone (>400 mg/day) increase the risk of adverse effects that require drug discontinuation [9, 51, 54]. Therefore, doses of amiodarone should be as low as possible and restricted to selected patients with refractory ventricular arrhythmias. Chronic treatment in young patients should be reserved as a bridge to more definitive treatment options such as catheter ablation [28].

Several studies compared IV amiodarone with other AADs (lidocaine, procainamide or bretylium) for the prophylaxis and treatment of VF and recurrent, hemodynamically destabilizing VT when they can no longer be controlled by successive electrical cardioversion or defibrillation [28, 55–59]. Administered during incessant VT, amiodarone produced a gradual slowing of the VT cycle length, with eventual termination of the arrhythmia [60]. However, these trials showed that IV amiodarone was moderately effective during a 24–48 h period against VT and VF and the arrhythmia frequently recurred. Furthermore, in a retrospective study, IV amiodarone produced an acute termination of sustained monomorphic VT only in 29% of patients [61]. Very recently the PROCAMIO study compared for the first time in a randomized design IV procainamide and amiodarone for the treatment of the acute episode of sustained monomorphic well-tolerated VT. Procainamide therapy was associated with less major cardiac adverse events and a higher proportion of tachycardia termination within 40 min [62].

In patients with sustained VT or VF and cardiac arrest several placebo-controlled trials and meta-analysis found that amiodarone decreased the recurrences and improved symptoms and survival, but when compared with ICD therapy there was a significant reduction (28%) in the relative risk of death with the ICD that was due almost entirely to a 50% reduction in arrhythmic death [63–66]. Therefore, in these patients amiodarone has been replaced by

ICD. However, in the ICD era amiodarone (plus β-blockade) may still be used in ICD-treated patients to decrease the frequency of shocks from VT/VF episodes or to control supraventricular tachyarrhythmias elicited by device therapy [64, 66]. When amiodarone is added to an ICD, the defibrillation threshold is usually increased and reprogramming prior to discharge from hospital may be necessary. Amiodarone is also indicated to improve symptoms in patients with DCM with an ICD who experience recurrent appropriate shocks in spite of optimal device programming and in patients with arrhythmogenic right ventricular cardiomyopathy and presenting frequent premature ventricular beats (PVBs) or non-sustained VT who are intolerant or have contraindications to β-blockers [25, 28].

The ARREST and ALIVE trials, analyzed the effects of IV amiodarone in hemodynamically destabilizing refractory VT/VF, VT when they can no longer be controlled by successive electrical cardioversion or defibrillation. In patients with out-of-hospital cardiac arrest due to refractory VT or VF after 3 direct-current shocks, those who received amiodarone were more likely than those who received placebo or lidocaine to have a return of spontaneous circulation and to survive to be admitted to the hospital [55, 57]. However, neither amiodarone nor lidocaine result in a significantly higher rate of survival to hospital discharge or favourable neurologic outcome at discharge. Thus, amiodarone may be useful for resuscitating some cardiac arrest victims.

A meta-analysis evaluated the effectiveness of amiodarone for primary or secondary prevention in sudden cardiac death (SCD) compared with placebo, no intervention or any other AAD in patients at high risk (primary prevention) or who have recovered from a cardiac arrest or a syncope due to VT and/or VF (secondary prevention) [51, 67]. There was low-to-moderate quality evidence that amiodarone reduced SCD, cardiac and all-cause mortality when compared to placebo or no intervention for primary prevention, but its effects were superior to other AADs. However, it was uncertain if amiodarone reduced or increased SCD and mortality for secondary prevention because the quality of the evidence was very low.

The CASCADE study evaluated AAD therapy in survivors of out-of-hospital VF not associated with a Q-wave MI who were at especially high-risk of recurrence of VF. All patients received an ICD in addition to randomized therapy [68]. The risk of the primary outcome, a composite of cardiac death, sustained VT/VF, or syncopal ICD shock, was significantly reduced by amiodarone. Patients on amiodarone were less likely to receive ICD shocks and syncope followed by a shock from a defibrillator was less common in patients treated with amiodarone. These results suggested a benefit of amiodarone over class I AADs. However, it is uncertain whether the observed benefit is due to the harmful effect of conventional AAD therapy and/or a beneficial effect of amiodarone, or most likely, their combination.

Intravenous amiodarone is the preferred AAD for incessant VT or frequent symptomatic VT episodes and severe LV dysfunction because in contrast to many other AADs it does not increase mortality. Two placebo-controlled studies analyzed the effects of amiodarone on the risk of resuscitated VF or arrhythmic death among survivors of MI treated with β-blockers at baseline reaching contradictory results. In the EMIAT trial, amiodarone did not modify all-cause mortality and cardiac mortality as compared with placebo [69]. Conversely, in the CAMIAT trial, amiodarone reduced the incidence of VF or arrhythmic death among survivors of acute MI with frequent or repetitive frequent or repetitive ventricular premature depolarisations. Similarly, several major trials in patients with a history of HF and LV dysfunction, arrived at conflicting results [70]. The GESICA trial suggested low-dose amiodarone improved survival, decreased hospital admissions for congestive HF, and improved functional class in patients with HF independently of the presence of complex ventricular arrhythmias [71]. However, in the STAT-CHF trial recruiting patients with HF (LVEF ≤40%) and ≥ 10 PVBs/h, amiodarone as compared to placebo was effective in suppressing ventricular arrhythmias, slowed heart rate and increased LVEF by 42% at 2 years, but it did not reduce the incidence of SCD or prolong survival among patients with HF, except for a trend toward reduced mortality among those with nonischemic cardiomyopathy [72]. In the SCD-HeFT study, recruiting patients with New York Heart Association (NYHA) class II-III (LVEF≤35%), amiodarone had no favorable effect on survival, whereas ICD therapy reduced overall mortality by 23% [73]. In a meta-analysis of 13 trials recruiting patients with recent MI or congestive HF, prophylactic amiodarone reduced the rate of arrhythmic/sudden death (29%), but it only displayed a modest reduction (13%) on total mortality [53]. The treatment benefit was uniform across the congestive HF and post–MI trial patients and was independent of major prognostic variables, such as LV function. Furthermore, a contemporary study in patients with post-acute MI with HF and/or LV systolic dysfunction from VALIANT trial, amiodarone use was associated with an excess in early and late all-cause and cardiovascular mortality [74]. Thus, further studies are needed to define the role of amiodarone in post-MI patients with HF and/or LV systolic dysfunction.

## Dofetilide

Dofetilide is a methanesulfonamide drug not available in Europe. It selectively blocks the $I_{Kr}$ and unlike most other AADs has minimal effects on other ion channels [75]. As a consequence, dofetilide prolongs dose-dependently the APD and refractoriness of atrial and ventricular myocardium (but the effect is more prominent in the atria) and accessory pathways, without slowing intracardiac conduction. Like ibutilide and sotalol, dofetilide exhibits the phenomenon of reverse use-dependence, so that the prolongation of APD and refractoriness diminished as the heart rate increases, while at slow heart rates the prolongation of the APD and the risk of early afterdepolarizations (proarrhythmia) increases [75]. It prolongs the QT and JT intervals but has no effect on heart rate, intracardiac conduction (no changes in the PR, QRS, A-H and H-V intervals) or significant hemodynamic effects and appears to be hemodynamically safe in patients with HF or a prior MI. Drug potency is affected by extracellular potassium concentration, and hypokalemia and hyperkalemia increases and decreases drug potency, respectively [76].

**Pharmacokinetics** (Table 3.2) Dofetilide is well absorbed (bioavailability 92–95%) and peak plasma levels are reached within 2–3 h. It binds to plasma proteins (60–70%) and 80% of the dose is excreted in urine (80% as unchanged dofetilide) and the remaining 20% as inactive or minimally active metabolites. Its $t_{½}$ is 7–13 hours [11, 75, 77].

**Adverse Effects** (Table 3.3) The most significant adverse effect of dofetilide is QT prolongation–related TdP. Rates of TdP ranged from 1% to ~3% in the DIAMOND trials [78]. The risk of TdP is highest at the time of drug initiation (80% within the first 3 days of therapy), in women, patients with severe HF, recent MI, hypokalemia, prolonged baseline QT or after conversion from AF to SR. The risk can be reduced maintaining normal serum potassium and magnesium levels, and following the manufacturer's algorithm in patients with renal disease, bradycardia, or baseline QT interval. To minimize the risk of proarrhythmia, patients initiated or re-initiated on dofetilide should be placed for a minimum of 3 days in a facility that can provide calculations of creatinine clearance, continuous ECG monitoring, and cardiac resuscitation. Other adverse effects include headache, chest pain, dizziness, respiratory tract infection, dyspnea, insomnia, rash, flu-like syndrome, nausea and diarrhea. There are no well-controlled studies that have been done in pregnant women (Pregnancy Category: C).

**Drug Interactions** Dofetilide does not inhibit or induce any CYP450 enzyme isoforms. Avoid its combinations with drugs that prolong the QT interval, other antiarrhythmic agents or potent CYP3A4 inhibitors (cimetidine, dolutegravir, grapefruit juice, HIV protease inhibitors, macrolide antibiotics, verapamil, prochlorperazine) that increase its plasma levels [11, 77].

**Contraindications and Cautions** See Table 3.3.

**Dosage and Administration** See Table 3.5.

Dofetilide therapy should be initiated in-hospital under continuous ECG monitoring because of the risk of excessive QT prolongation, periodic calculation of creatinine clearance (CrCl) and expert personnel for the treatment of ventricular arrhythmias [24, 26, 28]. Dosage adjustments are determined by QTc changes and CrCl. Renal function and QTc should be monitored every 3 months. The drug is contraindicated if the baseline QTc >440 m or the CrCl <20 mL/min. If 2–3 h after the first dose of dofetilide the QTc increased by >15% compared with baseline or the QTc is >500 ms (550 ms in patients with ventricular conduction abnormalities), subsequent dosing should be reduced by 50%. At 2–3 h after each subsequent dose, determine QTc and if at any time after the second dose the QTc is >500 ms (550 ms in patients with ventricular conduction abnormalities), dofetilide should be discontinued [24, 26, 28].

**Indications** Dofetilide is indicated for the acute conversion of recent-onset AF/Af (≤7 days) and the maintenance of SR (Table 3.6) [24, 27, 79, 80]. Dofetilide can be used in patients with structural heart disease or coronary artery disease. In the SAFIRE-D study, 70% of the pharmacological conversions occurred within 24 h and 91% within 36 h [80]. Furthermore, dofetilide appears safe and effective in preventing AF in patients refractory to other AADs undergoing catheter ablation [81]. Between 40% and 60% of patients on dofetilide remained in SR at 1 year (25% on placebo). Dofetilide is not associated with an increased mortality risk in patients with AF/Af [32].

Dofetilide restores and maintains SR in patients with congestive heart failure or recent MI and left ventricular dysfunction [82–84]. In patients with AF/Af and significant LV dysfunction, the DIAMOND studies showed that dofetilide was superior to placebo for the restoration and maintenance of SR and even when it had no effect on all-cause mortality, restoration and maintenance of SR was associated with significant reduction in mortality. Additionally, dofetilide reduced the risk for either all-cause or HF rehospitalization. Thus, dofetilide is an alternative to amiodarone in patients with AF/Af and LV dysfunction. In patients with AF/Af, severe LV dysfunction and recent MI, dofetilide did not affect all-cause or cardiac mortality, or total arrhythmic deaths. Thus, unlike flecainide and propafenone, dofetilide can be used in patients with structural heart disease or coronary artery disease.

Oral dofetilide may be reasonable in: (a) patients with AVRT and/or pre-excited AF who are not candidates for, or prefer not to undergo, catheter ablation [26]. In patients with paroxysmal supraventricular tachycardia (PSVT) dofetilide and propafenone were equally effective in preventing recurrences or decreasing the frequency of PSVT compared with placebo [85]. (b) For prevention of recurrent atrial tachycardia or Af in adult congenital heart disease patients, the long-term efficacy of the drug (defined by either complete suppression or partial improvement of symptoms) ranges from 70% to 85% [86, 87].

Dofetilide decreases the VF threshold in patients undergoing defibrillation testing prior to ICD implantation, suppresses the inducibility of VT and decreases the frequency of ICD shocks. It is as effective as sotalol in preventing the induction of sustained VT, but is significantly better tolerated during the acute phase [88] and in patients with an ICD and ventricular arrhythmias, dofetilide decreases the frequency of VT/VF and ICD shocks even when other ADDs, including amiodarone, are ineffective [89].

However, dofetilide is not frequently used because therapy must be started in an inpatient setting for 3 days and the risk of proarrhythmia. Thus, it should be reserved under ECG monitoring for highly symptomatic patients, in patients with depressed LVEF, who are not candidates for catheter ablation and/or when other AADs are ineffective or contraindicated.

## Dronedarone

Dronedarone is a noniodinated benzofuran derivative with a structure similar to that of amiodarone. The lack of the iodine moiety minimizes the risk of thyroid toxicity, and the addition of a methyl-sulfonyl group decreases its lipophilicity and tissular distribution which is expected to reduce organ toxicity due to tissular accumulation and to shorten its half-life [90]. Like amiodarone, dronedarone blocks $Na^+$, $Ca^{2+}$ ($I_{CaL}$) and several $K^+$ currents ($I_{to}$, $I_{Kur}$, $I_{Kr}$, $I_{Ks}$, $I_{K1}$ and $I_{KAch}$) and produces a non- competitive inhibition of α- and β-adrenergic receptors and a vasodilator effect mediated via the $I_{CaL}$ blockade and activation of the NO pathway [90–93]. Dronedarone and amiodarone exhibit similar effects on the $I_{CaL}$, $I_{Kr}$ and $I_{Ks}$, but dronedarone is a more potent blocker of $I_{Na}$ and $I_{KAch}$ and exhibits more potent non-competitive antiadrenergic effects than amiodarone.

**Electrophysiological Actions** Dronedarone prolongs the APD and refractoriness in all cardiac tissues, an effect independent of the rate of stimulation, and reduces transmural dispersion of repolarization. It slows heart rate and AV nodal conduction and prolongs the RR, PR, QT, JT and A-H intervals on the ECG with no change in H-V and QRS intervals [91, 92]. Dronedarone decreases blood pressure, myocardial contractility and slightly increases the defibrillation threshold. Dronedarone has little effect on cardiac performance except in patients with compromised LVEF and should not be used in those with clinical signs of HF.

**Pharmacokinetics** (Table 3.2) Dronedarone is rapidly and well absorbed after oral administration (70–90%), but it undergoes extensive first-pass metabolism, so that oral bioavailability is ~5% (15% when administered with a high-fat meal) [11, 90]. Dronedarone is extensively metabolized in the liver via CYP3A4 (and CYP2D6) to an active N-debutyl metabolite. Peak plasma levels of dronedarone and its metabolite are reached within 3–6 h and steady-state plasma levels within 4–8 days. Dronedarone and its active metabolite bind to plasma proteins (>98%) and are widely distributed (Vd 20 L/kg), crossing the blood–brain and placental barriers. Dronedarone presents a lower Vd (tissular accumulation) and a shorter a $t_{1/2}$ (13–19 h) than amiodarone and 85% of the drug being excreted in feces. Dronedarone and its metabolite are completely eliminated from the body within 2 weeks after the end of treatment. Drug pharmacokinetics is not influenced by age, gender, weight, or renal function, but dose adjustments are recommended in patients with severe hepatic dysfunction [11, 90].

**Adverse Effects** (Table 3.3) The most frequent are gastrointestinal (diarrhea, nausea, abdominal pain, vomiting, dyspepsia), abnormal liver function tests, asthenia, bradycardia, and QT prolongation. Uncommon adverse effects include: headache, rash and photosensitivity. Dronedarone increases serum creatinine levels due to partial inhibition of the tubular organic cationic transporter system, but the drug does not affect the GFR [94]. Sinus bradycardia is less frequent than with amiodarone and TdP have not been reported.

The ANDROMEDA trial which randomized patients with LV systolic dysfunction (LVEF 35%) and NYHA class III or IV symptoms within the prior month was prematurely discontinued because of increased mortality in the dronedarone group related to the worsening of HF [95]. In the PALLAS trial, dronedarone also increased rates of HF, stroke, and death from cardiovascular causes in patients with permanent AF who were at risk for major vascular events [96]. Thus, dronedarone should not be used in patients with recently decompensated HF or with permanent AF.

Dronedarone may cause fetal harm and it is contraindicated in women who are, or may become, pregnant (Pregnancy category X); it is not known whether dronedarone is excreted in human milk.

**Drug Interactions** Dronedarone is a moderate inhibitor of CYP3A4 and CYP2D6, and a potent inhibitor of P-gp and is metabolized by CYP3A4, so that it can present many drug interactions [11].

Coadministration of dronedarone with β-blockers, verapamil, or diltiazem increases their depressant effects on sinoatrial and AV nodes. Because diltiazem and verapamil are weak CYP3A4 inhibitors, in patients treated with dronedarone, diltiazem and verapamil should be initiated at low doses and dose uptitration should be done after ECG assessment. Class I or III antiarrhythmics increase the risk of proarrhythmia and should be discontinued before the administration of dronedarone. Dronedarone increases the plasma levels of digoxin (a P-gp substrate) and the risk of bradycardia and AV block. In the PALLAS trial, the use of digoxin was associated with an increased risk of arrhythmia or sudden death in dronedarone-treated patients [96]. Thus, the dose of digoxin should be halved and ECG and digoxin plasma levels carefully monitored.

Dronedarone is primarily metabolized by CYP3A4. Potent CYP3A4 inhibitors [azole antifungals (itraconazole, pozaconazole, voriconazole), cimetidine, cyclosporine, macrolides (clarithromycin, telithromycin), nefazodone, ritonavir, grapefruit juice] and inducers (carbamazepine, phenobarbital, phenytoin, rifampin, St John's Wort) significantly increase and decrease, respectively, exposure of dronedarone and should be administered with caution or avoided [90, 92]. Reduce the dose of dronedarone when coadministered with moderate CYP3A4 inhibitors (diltiazem, erythromycin, verapamil). Dronedarone can increase the exposure of statins that are substrates of CYP3A4 and/or P-gp (atorvastatin, lovastatin, simvastatin) and the risk of myopathy; thus, the dose of lovastatin and simvastatin should be limited to 20 mg/day and 10 mg/day, respectively. Dronedarone may increase the plasma levels of immunosupressants (tacrolimus, sirolimus, everolimus, cyclosporine); monitor their plasma concentrations, and adjust doses as appropriate [11]. Unlike amiodarone, dronedarone does not modify the INR, but it increases the exposure of dabigatran and this combination should be avoided. Avoid the combination of dronedarone with QT-prolonging drugs.

**Contraindications and Cautions** See Table 3.3.

**Dosage and Administration** See Table 3.5.

**Indications** Dronedarone is approved for the maintenance of SR after successful cardioversion in clinically stable adult patients with paroxysmal or persistent AF [97–99], but it is less effective than amiodarone [32, 100, 101]. In patients with paroxysmal or persistent AF or Af with additional risk factors for death, the ATHENA trial showed that dronedarone significantly reduced the composite outcome of first hospitalization due to cardiovascular events or death as compared with placebo [102]. Additionally, dronedarone decreased the mean ventricular rate during the recurrence of AF [98, 99]. In a short-term study, amiodarone was significantly more effective than dronedarone at preventing recurrence of AF, but was associated with significantly more adverse thyroid, neurological, ocular, and dermatological adverse effects [103].

## Ibutilide

Ibutilide is a methanesulfonamide derivative that prolongs cardiac repolarization through the inhibition of the $I_{Kr}$ and the activation of the late inward sodium current ($I_{NaL}$) during the plateau phase of the cardiac action potential [104].

**Electrophysiologic Actions** Like other class III agents, ibutilide prolongs APD and refractoriness of the atrial and ventricular myocardium, AV node, His-Purkinje system, and accessory pathways, prolongs the QT and JT intervals and produces a mild slowing of the sinus rate, but it has no effect on the PR, A-H, QRS and H-V intervals [105–107]. The prolongation of QT interval is related to the dose, rate of infusion and heart rate. Indeed, the prolongation of APD and refractoriness becomes less pronounced at higher tachycardia rates, i.e. ibutilide exhibits reverse use dependence. Ibutilide has no significant hemodynamic effects or negative inotropic effects and can be used safely in patients with structural heart disease and prior MI. It can lower the energy threshold required for VF.

**Pharmacokinetics** (Table 3.2) Ibutilide is administered IV. It binds to plasma proteins (40%), presents a large Vd (11 L/kg) and is extensively metabolized in the liver; one hydroxy metabolite has weak class III effects. Ibutilide is renally excreted and its $t_{½}$ presents a marked interpatient variability (2–12 h) [107]. The pharmacokinetics of ibutilide is independent of dose, age and LV function.

**Adverse Effects** (Table 3.3) The most serious adverse effect is a dose-dependent QT prolongation that returns to normal values 2–4 h after stopping the IV infusion [104–106]. TdP can occur in up to 4% of patients during or shortly after the infusion period (within the first 4–6 h of dosing) and the risk increases in patients with LVEF <20% [108]. Non-sustained monomorphic VT may occur in ~5% and proarrhythmia requiring cardioversion occurred in ~2% of treated patients [109, 110]. To reduce the risk of proarrhythmia, high doses of ibutilide and rapid infusion rates should be avoided; IV pretreatment with magnesium sulfate reduces the incidence of ventricular arrhythmias, including TdP [111, 112]. Therefore, patients receiving ibutilide should undergo continuous ECG monitoring during administration and for at least 4 hours after completion of dosing. Other noncardiac adverse effects are headache, bradycardia, hypotension, palpitations and nausea [11, 109]. The safety of ibutilide during pregnancy has not been well studied, and its use during pregnancy should be restricted to patients in whom no safer alternative exists (pregnancy category: C).

**Drug Interactions** (Table 3.4) Class I or class III AADs should not be given concurrently with ibutilide (or within 4 h after infusion); other antiarrhythmics should be withheld prior to conversion with ibutilide.

**Contraindications and Cautions** See Table 3.3.

**Dosage and Administration** See Table 3.5.

Because of the risk for ventricular proarrhythmia, ibutilide should be initiated in-hospital on continuous ECG monitoring by personnel trained in identification and treatment of ventricular arrhythmias during the drug administration and for 6–8 h thereafter and with resuscitation facilities available. The infusion should be stopped if the QTc is >500 ms or conversion to SR occurs. Although dose adjustment is not necessary in patients with hepatic or renal impairment, patients with liver disease may metabolize ibutilide more slowly and require longer postinfusion monitoring [107].

**Indications** Intravenous ibutilide is indicated for the rapid conversion of recent-onset AF/Af (≤ 7 days) to SR, but it is more effective for the conversion of Af (Table 3.6) [105–107, 110, 113–115]. In AF or Af, a single dose of ibutilide successfully converted 53% patients; an additional 22% patients is converted with the second dose, which resulted in an overall conversion rate of 75% [116]. The mean termination time was 27 min after the start of the infusion. Ibutilide was more effective than amiodarone, procainamide or sotalol in converting recent-onset Af to SR; however, ibutilide and amiodarone are equally effective in converting recent-onset AF to SR [33, 105, 106, 108, 113, 117]. In patients with persistent AF/Af the efficacy was 44% and 49%, respectively. Ibutilide is safe and effective for the rapid conversion of AF and Af after cardiac surgery (conversion rate 57% at the dose of 1 mg) [115]. Ibutilide also facilitates electrical cardioversion in patients with AF refractory to prior electrical cardioversions and prevent recurrent AF [24, 27]. All 50 patients receiving ibutilide before electrical cardioversion achieved SR while only 36 of 50 who did not receive the drug. The 14 patients who did not respond to electrical cardioversion were successfully cardioverted when a second attempt was made after ibutilide pretreatment [108]. However, because of the risk of proarrhythmia, ibutilide should not be used in patients with frequent short episodes of paroxysmal AF because even if the drug is effective to terminate the arrhythmia it is not useful for long-term prevention. The effectiveness of ibutilide for treatment of focal AT is unclear [26, 105, 106].

Furthermore, ibutilide prolongs accessory pathway refractoriness and can temporarily slow ventricular rate during pre-excited AF and may be used for the pharmacologic cardioversion of micro-reentrant AT [118] and AV reentrant tachycardia [119].

## Sotalol

Sotalol is a non-selective β1-adrenoceptor blocker without intrinsic sympathomimetic activity that, in addition, inhibits the $K^+$ current $I_{Kr}$, i.e., it is a mixed class II and class III AAD [11, 120, 121].

**Electrophysiological Actions** Sotalol is a racemic mixture of dextro- and levo-isomers. Both isomers have comparable class III activity, but *l*-sotalol is responsible for the β-blocking activity

[121, 122]. The β-blocking effects appear at low oral doses (half-maximal at 80 mg/day), while the class III effects are observed at doses >160 mg/day. Sotalol dose-dependently prolongs atrial and ventricular APD and refractoriness, slows heart rate, decreases AV nodal conduction, increases AV nodal refractoriness and prolongs the RR, PR, A-H and QT intervals of the ECG, but does not modify the QRS and H-V intervals. It also slows conduction along any bypass tract in both directions. The prolongation of the APD is greater at slower rates (reverse use-dependence) and under these conditions, sotalol may cause early afterdepolarizations triggering TdP. Unlike amiodarone, sotalol appears to reduce the defibrillation threshold [26].

*Hemodynamics*. Sotalol exerts a direct negative inotropic effect through its β-blocker activity, but it may indirectly increase $Ca^{2+}$ entry and cardiac contractility by prolonging repolarization, particularly at slow heart rates. However, in patients with reduced LVEF, sotalol can decrease the cardiac index, increase filling pressures and precipitate overt HF [120, 121]. Therefore, it must be used cautiously in patients with LV dysfunction or HF and should be avoided in patients with LVEF <20%, although is well tolerated in those with normal cardiac function. In 415 patients with AF/Af and PSVT, new or worsening HF occurred in 1.2% of patients, but in these studies patients with NYHA classes III-IV were excluded.

**Pharmacokinetics** (Table 3.2) Sotalol is completely absorbed (oral bioavalability 90–100%), reaching peak plasma concentrations within 2.5–4 h and steady-sate plasma levels in 2–3 days. It does not bind to plasma proteins, is not metabolized in the liver and is excreted unchanged primarily by the kidneys. Its $t_{1/2}$ is 7–18 h. The dose must be reduced in the elderly and in patients with renal impairment [11, 120].

**Adverse Effects** (Table 3.3) They are those commonly seen with other β-blockers, including bradycardia and AV block, asthenia, fatigue, hypotension, dizziness and cardiac ischemia after abrupt discontinuation. Proarrhythmia is the most serious adverse effect. TdP appears in 0.3% of patients treated with ≤240 mg/day, in 4.4% of those treated with 480 mg/day, in ~1.3% of patients when the QTc <500 ms and in 3.4–5.6% when the QTc is between 500–550 ms. In the PAFAC trial TdP appear in 1% of patients [123]. Proarrhytmia was probably the cause of the increased mortality observed with d-sotalol in patients with LV dysfunction post-MI [32, 124]. The risk of TdP increases in females, at high doses (>320 mg/day) and in patients with bradycardia, baseline QTc intervals >450 ms, electrolyte disturbances (hypokalemia and hypomagnesaemia), severe LV failure, treated with QT-prolonging drugs or with congenital long-QT syndrome.

Sotalol crosses the placenta and is present in breast milk (Pregnancy category B). β-blockers are commonly used in pregnant women with cardiovascular conditions and are associated with intrauterine growth retardation [23].

**Drug interactions** (Table 3.4) Sotalol should be used with caution or avoided in patients treated with QT-prolonging drugs and additive effects are expected if co-administered with other β-blockers. Class IA, IC and III AADs are not recommended as concomitant therapy with sotalol. Coadministration with digoxin can increase the risk of bradycardia and AVB and coadministration with diltiazem or verapamil may increase the risk of hypotension, bradycardia, or AVB. In diabetic patients sotalol may mask symptoms of hypoglycemia (tachycardia, tremor) or worsen hyperglycemia; so, the doses of insulin or antidiabetic drugs may require adjustment. β2-receptor agonists should be administered at higher dosages in patients treated with sotalol. Antacids containing aluminum hydroxide and magnesium hydroxide given 2 h or less before sotalol may reduce its bioavailability.

**Contraindications and Cautions** See Table 3.3.

**Dosage and Administration** See Table 3.5.

Patients initiated or reinitiated on sotalol should be placed in a facility that can provide cardiac resuscitation and continuous electrocardiographic monitoring for a minimum of 3 days [24–28]. The starting oral dose is 80 mg bid in patients with a QT <450 ms and a CrCl >60 mL/min. Doses may be increased in increments of 80 mg/day every 2–3 days to reach steady-state levels (maximum dose of 160 mg bid) provided the QTc interval <500 ms. Higher doses (480–640 mg/day) are used in patients with refractory life-threatening ventricular arrhythmias. Because sotalol can cause TdP or severe bradycardia, it may be considered to initiate the treatment in-hospital, particularly in patients in whom sinus bradycardia may cause syncope or when the conversion of AF/Af to SR prolong the QT interval. The use of high doses of sotalol requires careful ECG monitoring, especially in patients with impaired renal function.

In patients with ventricular arrhythmias and a CrCl between 30 and 59 mL/min sotalol must be administered od; with a CrCl between 10 and 29 mL/min the dose should be administered every 36–48 h, and with a CrCl <10 mL/min the dose should be individualized.

In patients with AF/Af and renal impairment (CrCl <60 mL/min) sotalol should be administered bid; if the CrCl is between 40 and 59 mL/min sotalol should be administered od; if the CrCl <40 mL/min sotalol is contraindicated.

#### Indications

Sotalol is approved for the:

1. *Maintenance of SR following cardioversion of recurrent AF/Af* (Table 3.6). For the maintenance of SR sotalol is as effective as flecainide or propafenone, but it can be administered to patients with structural heart disease or coronary artery disease where class IC drugs are contraindicated and without an additional agent to slow AV-nodal conduction [26, 33]. However, sotalol is less effective than amiodarone. In patients with persistent AF amiodarone and sotalol were equally efficacious in converting AF to SR but amiodarone was superior for maintaining SR; however, both drugs had similar efficacy in patients with ischemic heart disease [125]. Furthermore, in the CTAF trial,

after a mean of 16 months of follow-up 65% of patients treated with amiodarone and 37% of patients treated with sotalol or propafanone remained free of AF recurrence [30]. Similarly, in a large meta-analysis, efficacy of sotalol is similar to that of most AADs other than amiodarone [32]. Thus, sotalol can replace amiodarone when adverse effects are expected.

Pretreatment with sotalol can facilitate DC cardioversion and prevent recurrent AF and in relapses to AF after successful cardioversion, repeating DC cardioversion after sotalol facilitates the successful cardioversion (Table 3.6). Sotalol is also effective to decrease the incidence of POAF and to control ventricular rate during AF/Af [43, 126].

2. *Supraventricular tachycardias.* Sotalol may be reasonable for ongoing management in patients with SVT who are not candidates for, or prefer not to undergo, catheter ablation (Table 3.7) [26, 127]. Additionally, sotalol slows the ventricular response to atrial tachyarrhythmias and offers an effective alternative to DC cardioversion in adults and adolescents with congenital heart disease and hemodynamically stable atrial tachyarrhythmias [128]. One study randomized patients with reentrant SVT (AVNRT or AVRT) or other atrial tachyarrhythmias (eg, AF, Af, AT) to sotalol (80–160 mg bid) or placebo and found significant reductions in recurrence risk, including for patients with reentrant SVT, with no proarrhythmic adverse effects [127]. However, because of the potential for proarrhythmia, sotalol should be reserved for patients with SVT who are not candidates for, or prefer not to undergo, catheter ablation and for whom other AADs are ineffective or cannot be prescribed.
3. *Treatment of life-threatening sustained ventricular arrhythmias and acute conversion of hemodynamically stable monomorphic sustained VT* (Table 3.8). In patients with hemodynamically stable VT, sotalol was superior to lidocaine for the acute termination of sustained VT [129]. In patients with life-threatening arrhythmias (sustained VT/VF) which were also inducible by programmed electrical

stimulation (PES), the ESVEM trial showed that sotalol was significantly more efficacious at decreasing death and ventricular arrhythmias than other six class I AADs [130]. In patients who had received an ICD for secondary prevention of serious malignant ventricular arrhythmias, the combination of amiodarone with a β-blocker prevented shocks better than the β-blocker alone, although sotalol alone tended to reduce ICD shocks [131]. However, in another placebo-controlled study in patients with ICD, sotalol reduced the risk of death from any cause or the delivery of a first shock for any reason by 48% whether or not ventricular function was depressed. Sotalol also prevented the occurrence of shocks in response to supraventricular arrhythmias [132]. Two studies that compared the efficacy of metoprolol and sotalol yielded contradictory results. In one trial, sotalol was less effective than metoprolol for reducing recurrence of ventricular arrhythmia events; however, this study did not include inappropriate shocks that were a prominent feature in the previous studies [133]. In another trial, metoprolol was as efficacious as sotalol in preventing VT/VF recurrences in patients with an ICD [134]. In patients with sustained VT/VF and a ICD, sotalol reduced the recurrences in comparison to no AAD treatment and the frequency of ICD discharges, but it did not improve survival [135].

Because of its proarrhythmic risk, the use of sotalol is not recommended in patients with less severe arrhythmias (non-sustained VT or supraventricular tachyarrhythmias), even if symptomatic. Sotalol can be used safely in patients with coronary artery disease, but it should also be avoided in patients with severe HF (NYHA functional class III or IV). Although specific studies in treating atrial arrhythmias after MI have not been conducted, the administration of sotalol started 5–15 days after the MI did not increase rate after a 12 month follow-up [136].

**Acknowledgments** This work was supported by grants from the Institute of Health Carlos III (PI16/00398 and CB16/11/00303), MINECO (SAF2017-88116-P) and Comunidad de Madrid [ITACA-CM (S2017/BMD-3738)].

## References


1. Tamargo J, Delpón E. Pharmacologic bases of antiarrhythmic therapy. Chapter 54. In: Zipes DP, Jalife J, Stevenson WG, editors. Cardiac electrophysiology. 8th ed. Estados Unidos: Elsevier; 2017. p. 513–24.
2. Singh BN. Antiarrhythmic actions of amiodarone: a profile of a paradoxical agent. Am J Cardiol. 1996;78:41–53.
3. Kodama I, Kamiya K, Toyama J. Cellular electropharmacology of amiodarone. Cardiovasc Res. 1997;35:13–29.
4. Tamargo J. Happy 50th anniversary of amiodarone (1969–2019). Int J Cardiol. 2019;293:115–6.
5. Vamos M, Hohnloser SH. Amiodarone and dronedarone: an update. Trends Cardiovasc Med. 2016;26:597–602.
6. Connolly SJ. Evidence-based analysis of amiodarone efficacy and safety. Circulation. 1999;100:2025–34.
7. Harjai KJ, Licata AA. Effects of amiodarone on thyroid function. Ann Intern Med. 1997;126:63–73.
8. Wellens HJJ, Brugada P, Abdollah H, Dassen WR. A comparison of the electrophysiologic effects of intravenous and oral amiodarone in the same patient. Circulation. 1984;69:120–4.
9. Epstein AE, Olshansky B, Naccarelli GV, Kennedy JI Jr, Murphy EJ, Goldschlager N. Practical management guide for clinicians who treat patients with amiodarone. Am J Med. 2016;129:468–75.
10. Shinagawa K, Shiroshita-Takeshita A, Schram G, Nattel S. Effects of antiarrhythmic drugs on fibrillation in the remodeled atrium: insights into the mechanism of the superior efficacy of amiodarone. Circulation. 2003;107:1440–6.
11. Tamargo J, Caballero R, Delpón E. Chapter 8.1: Cardiovascular drugs—from A to Z. In: Kaski JC, Kjeldsen K, editors. The ESC handbook on cardiovascular pharmacotherapy. 2nd ed. Oxford: Oxford University Press; 2019. p. 413–812.
12. Meng X, Mojaverian P, Doedee M, Lin E, Weinryb I, Chiang ST, et al. Bioavailability of amiodarone tablets administered with and without food in healthy subjects. Am J Cardiol. 2001;87:432–5.
13. Vorperian VR, Havighurst TC, Miller S, January CT. Adverse effects of low dose amiodarone: a meta-analysis. J Am Coll Cardiol. 1997;30:791–8.
14. Ruzieh M, Moroi MK, Aboujamous NM, Ghahramani M, Naccarelli GV, Mandrola J, et al. Meta-analysis comparing the

relative risk of adverse events for amiodarone versus placebo. Am J Cardiol. 2019. pii: S0002-9149(19)31046-X.
15. Zimetbaum P. Amiodarone for atrial fibrillation. N Engl J Med. 2007;356:935–41.
16. Passman RS, Bennett CL, Purpura JM, Kapur R, Johnson LN, Raisch DW, et al. Amiodarone-associated optic neuropathy: a critical review. Am J Med. 2012;125:447–53.
17. Orr CF, Ahlskog JE. Frequency, characteristics, and risk factors for amiodarone neurotoxicity. Arch Neurol. 2009;66:865–9.
18. Papiris SA, Triantafillidou C, Kolilekas L, Markoulaki D, Manali ED. Amiodarone: review of pulmonary effects and toxicity. Drug Saf. 2010;33:539–58.
19. Colby R, Geyer H. Amiodarone-induced pulmonary toxicity. JAAPA. 2017;30:23–6.
20. Elnaggar MN, Jbeili K, Nik-Hussin N, Kozhippally M, Pappachan JM. Amiodarone-induced thyroid dysfunction: a clinical update. Exp Clin Endocrinol Diabetes. 2018;126:333–41.
21. Cohen-Lehman J, Dahl P, Danzi S, Klein I. Effects of amiodarone therapy on thyroid function. Nat Rev Endocrinol. 2010;6:34.
22. Bartalena L, Bogazzi F, Braverman LE, Braverman LE. Effects of amiodarone administration during pregnancy on neonatal thyroid function and subsequent neurodevelopment. J Endocrinol Investig. 2001;24:116–30.
23. Regitz-Zagrosek V, Roos-Hesselink JW, Bauersachs J, Blomström-Lundqvist C, Cıfkova R, De Bonis M, et al. ESC Scientific Document Group. 2018 ESC Guidelines for the management of cardiovascular diseases during pregnancy. Eur Heart J. 2018;39:3165–241.
24. January CT, Wann LS, Alpert JS, Calkins H, Cigarroa JE, Cleveland JC Jr, et al. ACC/AHA Task Force Members. 2014 AHA/ACC/HRS Guideline for the management of patients with atrial fibrillation: Executive Summary. A Report of the American College of Cardiology/American Heart Association Task Force on Practice Guidelines and the Heart Rhythm Society. Circulation. 2014;130:2071–4.
25. Priori S, Blomström-Lundqvist C, Mazzanti A, Blom N, Borggrefe M, Camm J, et al. 2015 ESC Guidelines for the management of patients with ventricular arrhythmias and the prevention of sudden cardiac death. Eur Heart J. 2015;36:2793–867.
26. Page RL, Joglar JA, Caldwell MA, Calkins H, Conti JB, Deal BJ, et al. 2015 ACC/AHA/HRS Guideline for the management

of adult patients with supraventricular tachycardia: Executive Summary: A Report of the American College of Cardiology/American Heart Association Task Force on Clinical Practice Guidelines and the Heart Rhythm Society. J Am Coll Cardiol. 2016;67:1575–623.
27. Kirchhof P, Benussi S, Kotecha D, Ahlsson A, Atar D, Casadei B, et al. 2016 ESC guidelines for the management of atrial fibrillation developed in collaboration with EACTS: The Task Force for the management of atrial fibrillation of the European Society of Cardiology (ESC) Developed with the special contribution of the European Heart Rhythm Association (EHRA) of the ESC Endorsed by the European Stroke Organisation (ESO). Eur Heart J. 2016;37:2893–962.
28. Al-Khatib SM, Stevenson WG, Ackerman MJ, Bryant WJ, Callans DJ, Curtis AB, et al. 2017 AHA/ACC/HRS guideline for management of patients with ventricular arrhythmias and the prevention of sudden cardiac death. Heart Rhythm. 2018;15:e773-e189.
29. Brugada J, Katritsis DG, Arbelo E, Arribas F, Bax JJ, Blomström-Lundqvist C, et al.; ESC Scientific Document Group. 2019 ESC Guidelines for the management of patients with supraventricular tachycardia. The Task Force for the management of patients with supraventricular tachycardia of the European Society of Cardiology (ESC). Eur Heart J. 2019. pii: ehz467. https://doi.org/10.1093/eurheartj/ehz467.
30. Roy D, Talajic M, Dorian P, Connolly S, Eisenberg MJ, Green M, et al. Amiodarone to prevent recurrence of atrial fibrillation. Canadian Trial of Atrial Fibrillation Investigators. N Engl J Med. 2000;342:913–20.
31. AFFIRM First Antiarrhythmic Drug Substudy Investigators. Maintenance of sinus rhythm in patients with atrial fibrillation: an AFFIRM substudy of the first antiarrhythmic drug. J Am Coll Cardiol. 2003;42(1):20–9.
32. Lafuente-Lafuente C, Valembois L, Bergmann JF, Belmin J. Antiarrhythmics for maintaining sinus rhythm after cardioversion of atrial fibrillation. Cochrane Database Syst Rev. 2015;3:CD005049.
33. Miller MR, McNamara RL, Segal JB, Kim N, Robinson KA, Goodman SN, et al. Efficacy of agents for pharmacologic conversion of atrial fibrillation and subsequent maintenance of sinus rhythm: a meta-analysis of clinical trials. J Fam Pract. 2000;49:1033–46.

34. Chevalier P, Durand-Dubief A, Burri H, Cucherat M, Kirkorian G, Touboul P. Amiodarone versus placebo and class Ic drugs for cardioversion of recent-onset atrial fibrillation: a meta-analysis. J Am Coll Cardiol. 2003;41:255–62.
35. Singh SN, Tang XC, Reda D, Singh BN. Systematic electrocardioversion for atrial fibrillation and role of antiarrhythmic drugs: a substudy of the SAFE-T trial. Heart Rhythm. 2009;6:152–5.
36. Kochiadakis GE, Igoumenidis NE, Parthenakis FI, Chlouverakis GI, Vardas PE. Amiodarone versus propafenone for conversion of chronic atrial fibrillation: results of a randomized, controlled study. J Am Coll Cardiol. 1999;33:966–71.
37. Singh BN, Singh SN, Reda DJ, Tang XC, Lopez B, Harris CL, et al. Amiodarone versus sotalol for atrial fibrillation. N Engl J Med. 2005;352:1861–72.
38. Vijayalakshmi K, Whittaker VJ, Sutton A, Campbell P, Wright RA, Hall JA, et al. A randomized trial of prophylactic antiarrhythmic agents (amiodarone and sotalol) in patients with atrial fibrillation for whom direct current cardioversion is planned. Am Heart J. 2006;151:863.e1–6.
39. Reisinger J, Gatterer E, Heinze G, Wiesinger K, Zeindlhofer E, Gattermeier M, et al. Prospective comparison of flecainide versus sotalol for immediate cardioversion of atrial fibrillation. Am J Cardiol. 1998;81:1450–4.
40. Channer KS, Birchall A, Steeds RP, Walters SJ, Yeo WW, West JN, et al. A randomized placebo-controlled trial of pretreatment and short- or long-term maintenance therapy with amiodarone supporting DC cardioversion for persistent atrial fibrillation. Eur Heart J. 2004;25:144–50.
41. Elliott PM, Anastasakis A, Borger MA, Borggrefe M, Cecchi F, Charron P, et al. 2014 ESC Guidelines on diagnosis and management of hypertrophic cardiomyopathy: the Task Force for the Diagnosis and Management of Hypertrophic Cardiomyopathy of the European Society of Cardiology (ESC). Eur Heart J. 2014;35:2733–79.
42. Darkner S, Chen X, Hansen J, Pehrson S, Johannessen A, Nielsen JB, et al. Recurrence of arrhythmia following short-term oral AMIOdarone after CATheter ablation for atrial fibrillation: a double-blind, randomized, placebo-controlled study (AMIO-CAT trial). Eur Heart J. 2014;35:3356–64.
43. Arsenault KA, Yusuf AM, Crystal E, Healey JS, Morillo CA, Nair GM, et al. Interventions for preventing post-oper-

ative atrial fibrillation in patients undergoing heart surgery. Cochrane Database Syst Rev. 2013;1:CD003611.

44. Burgess DC, Kilborn MJ, Keech AC. Interventions for prevention of postoperative atrial fibrillation and its complications after cardiac surgery: a meta-analysis. Eur Heart J. 2006;27:2846–57.
45. Zhu J, Wang C, Gao D, Zhang C, Zhang Y, Lu Y, Gao Y. Meta-analysis of amiodarone versus beta-blocker as a prophylactic therapy against atrial fibrillation following cardiac surgery. Intern Med J. 2012;42:1078–87.
46. Chatterjee S, Sardar P, Mukherjee D, Lichstein E, Aikat S. Timing and route of amiodarone for prevention of postoperative atrial fibrillation after cardiac surgery: a network regression meta-analysis. Pacing Clin Electrophysiol. 2013;36:1017–23.
47. Kowey PR, Levine JH, Herre JM, Pacifico A, Lindsay BD, Plumb VJ, et al. Randomized double-blind comparison of intravenous amiodarone and bretylium in the treatment of patients with recurrent, hemodynamically destabilizing ventricular tachycardia or fibrillation. The Intravenous Amiodarone Multicenter Investigators Group. Circulation. 1995;92:3255–63.
48. Heldal M, Atar D. Pharmacological conversion of recent-onset atrial fibrillation: a systematic review. Scand Cardiovasc J Suppl. 2013;47:2–10.
49. Letelier LM, Udol K, Ena J, Weaver B, Guyatt GH. Effectiveness of amiodarone for conversion of atrial fibrillation to sinus rhythm: a meta-analysis. Arch Intern Med. 2003;163:777–85.
50. Simonian SM, Lotfipour S, Wall C, Langdorf MI. Challenging the superiority of amiodarone for rate control in Wolff-Parkinson-White and atrial fibrillation. Intern Emerg Med. 2010;5:421–6.
51. Claro JC, Candia R, Rada G, Baraona F, Larrondo F, Letelier LM. Amiodarone versus other pharmacological interventions for prevention of sudden cardiac death. Cochrane Database Syst Rev. 2015;12:CD008093.
52. Bunch TJ, Mahapatra S, Murdock D, Molden J, Weiss JP, May HT, et al. Ranolazine reduces ventricular tachycardia burden and ICD shocks in patients with drug-refractory ICD shocks. Pacing Clin Electrophysiol. 2011;34:1600–6.
53. Amiodarone Trials Meta-Analysis Investigators (ATMAI). The effect of prophylactic amiodarone on mortality after acute myocardial infarction and in congestive heart failure: meta-analysis of individual data from 6500 patients in randomized trials. Lancet. 1997;350:1417–24.

54. Connolly SJ, Dorian P, Roberts RS, Gent M, Bailin S, Fain ES, et al. Comparison of beta-blockers, amiodarone plus beta-blockers, or sotalol for prevention of shocks from implantable cardioverter defibrillators: the OPTIC Study: a randomized trial. JAMA. 2006;295:165–71.
55. Kudenchuk PJ, Cobb LA, Copass MK, Cummins RO, Doherty AM, Fahrenbruch CE, et al. Amiodarone for resuscitation after out-of-hospital cardiac arrest due to ventricular fibrillation. N Engl J Med. 1999;341:871–8.
56. Kudenchuk PJ, Brown SP, Daya M, Rea T, Nichol G, Morrison LJ, et al. Amiodarone, lidocaine, or placebo in out-of-hospital cardiac arrest. N Engl J Med. 2016;374:1711–22.
57. Dorian P, Cass D, Schwartz B, Cooper R, Gelaznikas R, Barr A. Amiodarone as compared with lidocaine for shock-resistant ventricular fibrillation. N Engl J Med. 2002;346:884–90.
58. Levine JH, Massumi A, Scheinman MM, Winkle RA, Platia EV, Chilson DA, et al. Intravenous amiodarone for recurrent sustained hypotensive ventricular tachyarrhythmias. Intravenous Amiodarone Multicenter Trial Group. J Am Coll Cardiol. 1996;27:67–75.
59. Somberg JC, Bailin SJ, Haffajee CI, Paladino WP, Kerin NZ, Bridges D, et al. Intravenous lidocaine versus intravenous amiodarone (in a new aqueous formulation) for incessant ventricular tachycardia. Am J Cardiol. 2002;90:853–9.
60. Scheinman MM, Levine JH, Cannom DS, Friehling T, Kopelman HA, Chilson DA, et al. Dose-ranging study of intravenous amiodarone in patients with life-threatening ventricular tachyarrhythmias. The Intravenous Amiodarone Multicenter Investigators Group. Circulation. 1995;92:3264–72.
61. Marill KA, deSouza IS, Nishijima DK, Stair TO, Setnik GS, Ruskin JN. Amiodarone is poorly effective for the acute termination of ventricular tachycardia. Ann Emerg Med. 2006;47:217–24.
62. Ortiz M, Martin A, Arribas F, Coll-Vinent B, Del Arco C, Peinado R, et al. Randomized comparison of intravenous procainamide vs. intravenous amiodarone for the acute treatment of tolerated wide QRS tachycardia: the PROCAMIO study. Eur Heart J. 2017;38:1329–35.
63. AVID Investigators. A comparison of antiarrhythmic-drug therapy with implantable defibrillators in patients resuscitated from near-fatal ventricular arrhythmias. N Engl J Med. 1997;337:1576–83.

64. Connolly SJ, Hallstrom AP, Cappato R, Schron EB, Kuck KH, Zipes DP, et al. Meta-analysis of the implantable cardioverter defibrillator secondary prevention trials. AVID, CASH and CIDS studies. Antiarrhythmics vs Implantable Defibrillator study. Cardiac Arrest Study Hamburg. Canadian Implantable Defibrillator Study. Eur Heart J. 2000;21:2071–8.
65. Bokhari F, Newman D, Greene M, Korley V, Mangat I, Dorian P. Long-term comparison of the implantable cardioverter defibrillator versus amiodarone: eleven-year follow-up of a subset of patients in the Canadian Implantable Defibrillator Study (CIDS). Circulation. 2004;110:112–6.
66. Steinberg JS, Martins J, Sadanandan S, Goldner B, Menchavez E, Domanski M, et al. Antiarrhythmic drug use in the implantable defibrillator arm of the Antiarrhythmics Versus Implantable Defibrillators (AVID) Study. Am Heart J. 2001;142:520–9.
67. Farre J, Romero J, Rubio JM, Ayala R, Castro-Dorticós J. Amiodarone and "primary" prevention of sudden death: critical review of a decade of clinical trials. Am J Cardiol. 1999;83:55D–63D.
68. CASCADE Investigators. Cardiac arrest in Seattle: conventional versus amiodarone drug evaluation. Am J Cardiol. 1991;67:578–84.
69. Julian DG, Camm AJ, Frangin G, Julian DG, Frangin GA, Schwartz PJ. Randomized trial of effect of amiodarone on mortality in patients with left ventricular dysfunction after recent myocardial infarction (EMIAT). Lancet. 1997;347:667–74.
70. Cairns JA, Connolly SJ, Roberts R, Gent M. Randomised trial of outcome after myocardial infarction in patients with frequent or repetitive ventricular premature depolarisations: CAMIAT. Canadian Amiodarone Myocardial Infarction Arrhythmia Trial Investigators. Lancet. 1997;349:675–82.
71. Doval HC, Nul DR, Grancelli HO, Perrone SV, Bortman GR, Curiel R. Randomised trial of low-dose amiodarone in severe congestive heart failure. Grupo de Estudio de la Sobrevida en la Insuficiencia Cardiaca en Argentina (GESICA). Lancet. 1994;344:493–8.
72. Singh SN, Fletcher RD, Fisher SG, Singh BN, Lewis HD, Deedwania PC, et al. Amiodarone in patients with congestive heart failure and asymptomatic ventricular arrhythmia. Survival Trial of Antiarrhythmic Therapy in Congestive Heart Failure. N Engl J Med. 1995;333:77–82.

73. Bardy GH, Lee KL, Mark DB, Poole JE, Packer DL, Boineau R, et al. Amiodarone or an implantable cardioverter-defibrillator for congestive heart failure. N Engl J Med. 2005;352:225–37.
74. Thomas KL, Al-Khatib SM, Lokhnygina Y, Solomon SD, Kober L, McMurray JJ, et al. Amiodarone use after acute myocardial infarction complicated by heart failure and/or left ventricular dysfunction may be associated with excess mortality. Am Heart J. 2008;155:87–93.
75. Mounsey JP, DiMarco JP. Cardiovascular drugs. Dofetilide. Circulation. 2000;102:2665–270.
76. Yang T, Roden DM. Extracellular potassium modulation of drug block of IKr. Implications for torsade de pointes and reverse usedependence. Circulation. 1996;93:407–11.
77. McClellan KJ, Markham A. Dofetilide: a review of its use in atrial fibrillation and atrial flutter. Drugs. 1999;58:1043–59.
78. Pedersen HS, Elming H, Seibaek M, Burchardt H, Brendorp B, Torp-Pedersen C, et al. Risk factors and predictors of torsade de pointes ventricular tachycardia in patients with left ventricular systolic dysfunction receiving dofetilide. Am J Cardiol. 2007;100:876–80.
79. Falk RH, Pollak A, Singh SN, Friedrich T. Intravenous dofetilide, a class III antiarrhythmic agent, for the termination of sustained atrial fibrillation or flutter. Intravenous Dofetilide Investigators. J Am Coll Cardiol. 1997;29:385–90.
80. Singh S, Zoble RG, Yellen L, Brodsky MA, Feld GK, Berk M, et al. Efficacy and safety of oral dofetilide in converting to and maintaining sinus rhythm in patients with chronic atrial fibrillation or atrial flutter: the symptomatic atrial fibrillation investigative research on dofetilide (SAFIRE-D) study. Circulation. 2000;102:2385–90.
81. Shamiss Y, Khaykin Y, Oosthuizen R, Tunney D, Sarak B, Beardsall M, et al. Dofetilide is safe and effective in preventing atrial fibrillation recurrences in patients accepted for catheter ablation. Europace. 2009;11:1448–55.
82. Torp-Pedersen C, Moller M, Bloch-Thomsen PE, Køber L, Sandøe E, Egstrup K, et al. Dofetilide in patients with congestive heart failure and left ventricular dysfunction. Danish Investigations of Arrhythmia and Mortality on Dofetilide Study Group. N Engl J Med. 1999;341:857–65.
83. Kober L, Bloch Thomsen PE, Moller M, Torp-Pedersen C, Carlsen J, Sandøe E, et al. Effect of dofetilide in patients with

recent myocardial infarction and left ventricular dysfunction: a randomised trial. Lancet. 2000;356:2052–8.

84. Pedersen OD, Bagger H, Keller N, Marchant B, Køber L, Torp-Pedersen C. Efficacy of dofetilide in the treatment of atrial fibrillation-flutter in patients with reduced left ventricular function: a Danish investigations of arrhythmia and mortality on dofetilide (diamond) substudy. Circulation. 2001;104:292–6.
85. Tendera M, Wnuk-Wojnar AM, Kulakowski P, Malolepszy J, Kozlowski JW, Krzeminska-Pakula M, et al. Efficacy and safety of dofetilide in the prevention of symptomatic episodes of paroxysmal supraventricular tachycardia: a 6-month double-blind comparison with propafenone and placebo. Am Heart J. 2001;142:93–8.
86. Wells R, Khairy P, Harris L, Anderson CC, Balaji S. Dofetilide for atrial arrhythmias in congenital heart disease: a multicenter study. Pacing Clin Electrophysiol. 2009;32:1313–8.
87. Tanel RE, Walsh EP, Lulu JA, Saul JP. Sotalol for refractory arrhythmias in pediatric and young adult patients: initial efficacy and long-term outcome. Am Heart J. 1995;130:791–7.
88. Boriani G, Lubinski A, Capucci A, Niederle R, Kornacewicz-Jack Z, Wnuk-Wojnar AM, et al. Ventricular Arrhythmias Dofetilide Investigators. A multicentre, double-blind randomized crossover comparative study on the efficacy and safety of dofetilide vs sotalol in patients with inducible sustained ventricular tachycardia and ischaemic heart disease. Eur Heart J. 2001;22:2180–91.
89. Baquero GA, Banchs JE, Depalma S, Young SK, Penny-Peterson ED, Samii SM, et al. Dofetilide reduces the frequency of ventricular arrhythmias and implantable cardioverter defibrillator therapies. J Cardiovasc Electrophysiol. 2012;23:296–301.
90. Schweizer PA, Becker R, Katus HA, Thomas D. Dronedarone: current evidence for its safety and efficacy in the management of atrial fibrillation. Drug Des Devel Ther. 2011;5:27–39.
91. Patel C, Yan GX, Kowey PR. Dronedarone. Circulation. 2009;120:636–44.
92. Tamargo J, López-Farré A, Caballero R, Delpón E. Dronedarone. Drugs Today (Barc). 2011;47:109–33.
93. Kathofer S, Thomas D, Karle CA. The novel antiarrhythmic drug dronedarone: comparison with amiodarone. Cardiovasc Drug Rev. 2005;23:217–30.
94. Tschuppert Y, Buclin T, Rothuizen LE, Decosterd LA, Galleyrand J, Gaud C, Biollaz J. Effect of dronedarone on

renal function in healthy subjects. Br J Clin Pharmacol. 2007;64:785–91.

95. Køber L, Torp-Pedersen C, McMurray JJ, Gøtzsche O, Lévy S, Crijns H, et al. Dronedarone Study Group. Increased mortality after dronedarone therapy for severe heart failure. N Engl J Med. 2008;358:2678–87.
96. Connolly SJ, Camm AJ, Halperin JL, Joyner C, Alings M, Amerena J, et al. Dronedarone in high-risk permanent atrial fibrillation. N Engl J Med. 2011;365:2268–76.
97. Davy JM, Herold M, Hoglund C, Timmermans A, Alings A, Radzik D, et al. Dronedarone for the control of ventricular rate in permanent atrial fibrillation: the Efficacy and safety of dRonedArone for the cOntrol of ventricular rate during atrial fibrillation (ERATO) study. Am Heart J. 2008;156:527.e1–9.
98. Singh BN, Connolly SJ, Crijns HJ, Roy D, Kowey PR, Capucci A, et al. Dronedarone for maintenance of sinus rhythm in atrial fibrillation or flutter. N Engl J Med. 2007;357:987–99.
99. Khan MH, Rochlani Y, Aronow WS. Efficacy and safety of dronedarone in the treatment of patients with atrial fibrillation. Expert Opin Drug Saf. 2017;16:1407–12.
100. Piccini JP, Hasselblad V, Peterson ED, Washam JB, Califf RM, Kong DF. Comparative efficacy of dronedarone and amiodarone for the maintenance of sinus rhythm in patients with atrial fibrillation. J Am Coll Cardiol. 2009;54:1089–95.
101. Vamos M, Hohnloser SH. Amiodarone and dronedarone: an update. Trends Cardiovasc Med. 2016;26:597–602.
102. Hohnloser SH, Crijns HJ, van Eickels M, Gaudin C, Page RL, Torp-Pedersen C, et al. Effect of dronedarone on cardiovascular events in atrial fibrillation. N Engl J Med. 2009;360:668–78.
103. Le Heuzey JY, De Ferrari GM, Radzik D, Santini M, Zhu J, Davy JM. A short-term, randomized, double-blind, parallel-group study to evaluate the efficacy and safety of dronedarone versus amiodarone in patients with persistent atrial fibrillation: the DIONYSOS study. J Cardiovasc Electrophysiol. 2010;21:597–605.
104. Naccarelli GV, Lee KS, Gibson JK, VanderLugt J. Electrophysiology and pharmacology of ibutilide. Am J Cardiol. 1996;78:12–6.
105. Stambler BS, Beckman KJ, Kadish AH, Camm JA, Ellenbogen KA, Perry KT, et al. Acute hemodynamic effects of intravenous ibutilide in patients with or without reduced left ventricular function. Am J Cardiol. 1997;80:458–63.

106. Stambler BS, Wood MA, Ellenbogen KA. Antiarrhythmic actions of intravenous ibutilide compared with procainamide during human atrial flutter and fibrillation: electrophysiological determinants of enhanced conversion efficacy. Circulation. 1997;96:4298–306.
107. Murray KT. Ibutilide. Circulation. 1998;97:493–7.
108. Oral H, Souza JJ, Michaud GF, Knight BP, Goyal R, Strickberger SA, et al. Facilitating transthoracic cardioversion of atrial fibrillation with ibutilide pretreatment. N Engl J Med. 1999;340:1849–54.
109. Kowey PR, VanderLugt JT, Luderer JT. Safety and risk/benefit analysis of ibutilide for acute conversion of atrial fibrillation/flutter. Am J Cardiol. 1996;78:46–52.
110. Nair M, George LK, Koshy SK. Safety and efficacy of ibutilide in cardioversion of atrial flutter and fibrillation. J Am Board Fam Med. 2011;24:86–92.
111. Patsilinakos S, Christou A, Kafkas N, Nikolaou N, Antonatos D, Katsanos S, et al. Effect of high doses of magnesium on converting ibutilide to a safe and more effective agent. Am J Cardiol. 2010;106:673–6.
112. Tercius AJ, Kluger J, Coleman CI, White CM. Intravenous magnesium sulfate enhances the ability of intravenous ibutilide to successfully convert atrial fibrillation or flutter. Pacing Clin Electrophysiol. 2007;30:1331–5.
113. Kafkas NV, Patsilinakos SP, Mertzanos GA, Papageorgiou KI, Chaveles JI, Dagadaki OK, et al. Conversion efficacy of intravenous ibutilide compared with intravenous amiodarone in patients with recent-onset atrial fibrillation and atrial flutter. Int J Cardiol. 2007;118:321–5.
114. Volgman AS, Carberry PA, Stambler B, Lewis WR, Dunn GH, Perry KT, et al. Conversion efficacy and safety of intravenous ibutilide compared with intravenous procainamide in patients with atrial flutter or fibrillation. J Am Coll Cardiol. 1998;31:1414–9.
115. VanderLugt JT, Mattioni T, Denker S, Torchiana D, Ahern T, Wakefield LK, et al. Efficacy and safety of ibutilide fumarate for the conversion of atrial arrhythmias after cardiac surgery. Circulation. 1999;100:369–75.
116. Andò G, Di Rosa S, Rizzo F, Carerj S, Bramanti O, Giannetto M, et al. Ibutilide for cardioversion of atrial flutter: efficacy of a single dose in recent-onset arrhythmias. Minerva Cardioangiol. 2004;52:37–42.

117. Bernard EO, Schmid ER, Schmidlin D, Scharf C, Candinas R, Germann R. Ibutilide versus amiodarone in atrial fibrillation: a double-blinded, randomized study. Crit Care Med. 2003;31:1031–4.
118. Eidher U, Freihoff F, Kaltenbrunner W, Steinbach K. Efficacy and safety of ibutilide for the conversion of monomorphic atrial tachycardia. Pacing Clin Electrophysiol. 2006;29:358–62.
119. Glatter KA, Dorostkar PC, Yang Y, Lee RJ, Van Hare GF, Keung E, et al. Electrophysiological effects of ibutilide in patients with accessory pathways. Circulation. 2001;104:1933–9.
120. Hohnloser SH, Woosley RL. Sotalol. N Engl J Med. 1994;331:31–8.
121. Manoach M, Tribulova N. Sotalol: the mechanism of its antiarrhythmic-defibrillating effect. Cardiovasc Drug Rev. 2001;19:172–82.
122. Kato R, Ikeda N, Yabek SM, Kannan R, Singh BN. Electrophysiologic effects of the levo- and dextrorotatory isomers of sotalol in isolated cardiac muscle and their in vivo pharmacokinetics. J Am Coll Cardiol. 1986;7:116–25.
123. Fetsch T, Bauer P, Engberding R, Koch HP, Lukl J, Meinertz T, et al. Prevention of atrial fibrillation after cardioversion: results of the PAFAC trial. Eur Heart J. 2004;25:1385–94.
124. Waldo AL, Camm AJ, deRuyter H, Friedman PL, MacNeil DJ, Pauls JF, et al. Effect of d-sotalol on mortality in patients with left ventricular dysfunction after recent and remote myocardial infarction. The SWORD Investigators. Survival with oral d-sotalol. Lancet. 1996;348:7–12.
125. Singh BN, Singh SN, Reda DJ, Tang XC, Lopez B, Harris CL, et al. Amiodarone versus sotalol for atrial fibrillation. N Engl J Med. 2005;352:1861–72.
126. Kerin NZ, Jacob S. The efficacy of sotalol in preventing postoperative atrial fibrillation: a meta-analysis. Am J Med. 2011;124:875.e1–9.
127. Wanless RS, Anderson K, Joy M, Joseph SP. Multicenter comparative study of the efficacy and safety of sotalol in the prophylactic treatment of patients with paroxysmal supraventricular tachyarrhythmias. Am Heart J. 1997;133:441–6.
128. Rao SO, Boramanand NK, Burton DA, Perry JC. Atrial tachycardias in young adults and adolescents with congenital heart disease: conversion using single dose oral sotalol. Int J Cardiol. 2009;136:253–7.

129. Ho DS, Zecchin RP, Richards DA, Uther JB, Ross DL. Double-blind trial of lignocaine versus sotalol for acute termination of spontaneous sustained ventricular tachycardia. Lancet. 1994;344:18–23.
130. Mason JW. A comparison of seven antiarrhythmic drugs in patients with ventricular tachyarrhythmias. Electrophysiologic Study versus Electrocardiographic Monitoring Investigators. N Engl J Med. 1993;329:452–8.
131. Connolly SJ, Dorian P, Roberts RS, Gent M, Bailin S, Fain ES, et al. Comparison of beta-blockers, amiodarone plus beta-blockers, or sotalol for prevention of shocks from implantable cardioverter defibrillators: the OPTIC Study: a randomized trial. JAMA. 2006;295:165–71.
132. Pacifico A, Hohnloser SH, Williams JH, Tao B, Saksena S, Henry PD, et al. Prevention of implantable defibrillator shocks by treatment with sotalol. d,l-Sotalol Implantable Cardioverter-Defibrillator Study Group. N Engl J Med. 1999;340:1855–62.
133. Seidl K, Hauer B, Schwick NG, Zahn R, Senges J. Comparison of metoprolol and sotalol in preventing ventricular tachyarrhythmias after the implantation of a cardioverter/defibrillator. Am J Cardiol. 1998;82:744–8.
134. Kettering K, Mewis C, Dornberger V, Vonthein R, Bosch RF, Seipel L, et al. Efficacy of metoprolol and sotalol in the prevention of recurrences of sustained ventricular tachyarrhythmias in patients with an implantable cardioverter defibrillator. Pacing Clin Electrophysiol. 2002;25:1571–6.
135. Kühlkamp V, Mewis C, Mermi J, Bosch RF, Seipel L. Suppression of sustained ventricular tachyarrhythmias: a comparison of d,l-sotalol with no antiarrhythmic drug treatment. J Am Coll Cardiol. 1999;33:46–52.
136. Julian DG, Prescott RJ, Jackson FS, Szekely P. Controlled trial of sotalol for one year after myocardial infarction. Lancet. 1982;1:1142–7.

# Chapter 4
# Beta-blockers as Antiarrhythmic Agents

**Catalin Adrian Buzea, Anca Rodica Dan, and Gheorghe-Andrei Dan**

C. A. Buzea (✉)
Carol Davila University of Medicine and Pharmacy, Bucharest, Romania

Department of Cardiology, Clinical Hospital Colentina, Bucharest, Romania

A. R. Dan
Department of Cardiology, Clinical Hospital Colentina, Bucharest, Romania

G.-A. Dan
"Carol Davila" University of Medicine, Colentina University Hospital, Bucharest, Romania



A. Martínez-Rubio et al. (eds.), *Antiarrhythmic Drugs*, Current Cardiovascular Therapy,
https://doi.org/10.1007/978-3-030-34893-9_4

# Cardiac Beta-Adrenergic Receptors and Remodeling in Myocardial Infarction and Heart Failure

## *Autonomic Innervation of the Heart*

### Intrinsic and Extrinsic Nervous System

The normal autonomic innervation of the heart consists of extrinsic and intrinsic components. The extrinsic innervation comprises sympathetic and parasympathetic components. The sympathetic fibers originate from the cervical ganglia (communicating with nerves C1–C3, and less with C4), cervicothoracic ganglia (communicating with nerves C7–C8 and T1–T2), and thoracic ganglia (with T4 being the lowest) [1]. The fibers from these ganglia form the *superior, middle* and *inferior* cardiac nerves that reach the surface of the heart following the carotid, subclavian and brachiocephalic arteries, whereas the *thoracic* cardiac nerve has a more complicated trajectory alongside the thoracic vertebrae and intercostal arteries [1]. The sympathetic fibers penetrate then the myocardium and end as terminal fibers at the endocardium. Despite the throughout distribution of these fibers, there is a different density between chambers and cardiac layers and between conduction system and working myocardium [2–4]. The parasympathetic fibers originate from the medulla and are carried *via* vagus nerve branches: *superior*, *inferior* and *thoracic* cardiac branches [1]. The vagal branches converge to a distinct fat pad, namely third fat pad, from where the parasympathetic fibers are more heterogeneously distributed compared to the sympathetic terminals [5]. The sinoatrial node (SAN) and atrioventricular node (AVN) are well innervated and to a lesser degree the superior and posterior arias of the atria. The ventricles parasympathetic innervation is sparse [3, 4, 6].

The intrinsic innervation of the heart consists of a network of ganglia organized into ganglionic plexi (GP) which may act as integration centers [7, 8]. The parasympathetic fibers synapse in these cardiac ganglia as well as the preganglionic sympathetic fibers. Multiple locations of GPs where identified: dorsal surface of atria, inferior vena cava, inferior atrial and pulmonary vein, left atrium junctions, and the anterior surface of the ventricles, primarily at the emerge of major vessels [1, 7, 9].

## Effects of Sympathetic/Parasympathetic Activity

The sympathetic response is mediated by the norepinephrine, which acts on the adrenergic receptors (AR). They are classified by their response to agonists into α and β types, which are further divided into subtypes: α1 and α2-AR and β1, β2 and β3-AR. The β1-AR is the most represented in the heart [10, 11], with a β1/β2 ratio of 1.5:1 in the atria and 4:1 in the ventricles [12]. Endogenous norepinephrine exerts its positive inotropic and chronotropic effects through β1-AR stimulation [13]. After binding the receptor, a complex intracellular signaling system is activated which ultimately ends with the phosphorylation of multiple proteins involved in ion channel and contractile function (Fig. 4.1, adapted from [6]).

The global effects of β1-AR stimulation consist in increased contractility, increased inward $Na^+$ current and pacemaker current, and shortening of action potential duration (APD) and of the refractory period, which consecutively reflects in the increased of heart rate and the conduction velocity [6, 14].

The β2-AR are less well represented in the heart, but they are denser in the SAN suggesting they have a role in the regulation of heart rate [15]. Nevertheless, the stimulation of β2-AR increases the heart rate to the same degree as β1-AR [12].

The parasympathetic response is mediated by acetylcholine, activating muscarinic and nicotinic receptors. At the heart level, the effects of parasympathetic stimulation are mediated by M2 muscarinic receptors (see Fig. 4.1) which are denser in atrial and nodal tissues and less in the ventricles [16].

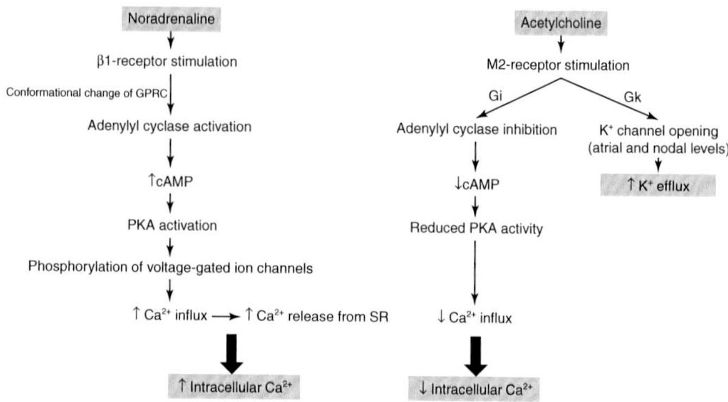


FIGURE 4.1 Cellular effects of sympathetic and parasympathetic stimulation. *cAMP* cyclic adenosine monophosphate, *GPCR* G protein-coupled receptor, *Gi,Gk* guanine nucleotide binding proteins, *PKA* protein kinase A, *SR* sarcoplasmic reticulum

The effect of muscarinic receptor activation is different on atrial compared to ventricular myocytes. In both, M2- receptor activation leads to reduced activity of adenylate cyclase and subsequently to a decrease of intracellular $Ca^{2+}$ and contractility. On the other hand, on atrial tissue and SAN and AVN, there is a supplementary effect consisting in the activation of a $K^+$ channel ($I_{Ach}$) which leads to lowering of heart rate and slower conduction [17].

## *Sympathetic Remodeling*

It is widely accepted that many arrhythmias are related to the imbalance of the autonomic nervous system, meaning an excess of sympathetic stimulation and reduced parasympathetic activity [14]. The cardiac sympathetic remodeling represents structural and functional modifications as a response to different conditions affecting the heart. To the date, there are four types of remodeling: hyperinnervation, denervation, altered neurotransmitter production and neuronal hyperexcitability [18].

## Hyperinnervation

An increased density of nerve fibers was demonstrated in many conditions like myocardial infarction (MI) or heart failure (HF) [19–22]. The neuronal regrowth is related to the neurotrophic factors, of which the nerve growth factor (NGF) implication is well demonstrated. NGF promotes sympathetic differentiation and peripheral axonal growth and its levels are increased following a MI [22–25]. Also, the neural growth is regulated by several factors, like ephrins and semaphorins, and these could be involved in sympathetic remodeling. Sema3A is a class 3 secreted semaphorin and a potent neural chemorepellent with a negative impact on cardiac sympathetic innervation [26]. The overexpression of sema3A in the border zone after MI seems to reduce the sympathetic hyperinnervation and the vulnerability for arrhythmias [27].

## Denervation and Axon Degeneration

The lack of sympathetic stimulation could also contribute to electrical instability. Denervation and reduced sympathetic activation was demonstrated in patients with MI or HF [28, 29] and there are multiple factors contributing to sympathetic denervation, like increased level of pro-NGF (a precursor protein of NGF) [30] or chondroitin sulfate proteoglycans [31]. This denervation, alongside hyperinnervation previously mentioned, seems to be an important factor in the development of arrhythmias [32, 33].

## Altered Neurotransmitter Production

Besides neural density alterations, other factors like modifications in neurotransmitter or neuropeptides production could participate to the arrhythmic substrate [14, 18]. For example, after MI there is an increased concentration of neuropeptide Y secondary to sympathetic overdrive, which inhibits acetylcholine release and produces vasoconstriction with negative consequences on the cardiac substrate [14, 34].

### Increased Neuronal Excitability

In the territories with adrenergic denervation, an exaggerated response to sympathetic stimulation was observed, so-called denervation supersensitivity [35, 36]. Loss of postsynaptic norepinephrine reuptake and increase of the β-receptors number and of adenylate cyclase activity are among the factors involved in this phenomenon [36]. Nevertheless, the superexcitability to adrenergic stimulation seems to play a role in the vulnerability to arrhythmias [14, 37].

## *Role of Autonomic Nervous Activity in Arrhythmias*

### Atrial Tachyarrhythmias

Coumel et al. described for first time the role of autonomic nervous system imbalance in atrial fibrillation (AF) development [38] and both sympathetic and parasympathetic stimulation could lead to this arrhythmia based on cardiac substrate; whereas vagal activity is demonstrated to be related to nocturnal AF and normal cardiac substrate, the adrenergic stimulation represents the trigger for AF related to organic heart disease [39–45]. A research done on dogs stated that the acetylcholine-mediated AF was facilitated by the isoproterenol, suggesting both components of ANS have a role in AF genesis [46]. Also, a study with implanted radio-transmitters demonstrated both sympathetic and parasympathetic activity preceding AF onset [47, 48].

The abnormal intracellular $Ca^{2+}$ transient and shortened APD determined by adrenergic stimulation and the shortening of the atrial effective refractory period (ERP) secondary to vagal activity seems to generate an inward sodium-calcium exchange current and subsequently early afterdepolarizations (EAD) [49].

### Ventricular Tachyarrhythmias

Based on the available evidence, the relationship between increased adrenergic stimulation and ventricular arrhythmias and sudden cardiac death is widely accepted [19, 50–53].

The susceptibility for ventricular arrhythmias is increased in the presence of ischemia [54–56] and any factor which elicits an increase in sympathetic activity, including exercise or psychological stress, could be the precipitating factor [57–61]. A study of explanted hearts showed marked nerve sprouting around diseased myocardium, especially in patients with a history of ventricular arrhythmias [19]. Direct electrical stimulation of sympathetic nerves increases the level of nerve sprouting and decreases the threshold for ventricular fibrillation [55, 62, 63]. Also, there is evidence of increased adrenergic activity right before the onset of ventricular arrhythmias [64, 65].

## Pharmacologic Properties of Beta-Adrenergic Blockers (BB)

### *General Considerations*

The beta-blockers (BB) represent a heterogeneous class of drugs that competitively antagonize the β adrenergic receptors. The differences between the representants of this class are based on multiple characteristics like selectivity for the subtype of the receptor, presence of intrinsic sympathomimetic activity (ISA), concomitant α-blockade, vasodilation capacity, and pharmacokinetic properties. A classification of BB is provided in Table 4.1.

*The first generation* of non-selective BB, of which the main prototype remains propranolol, is characterized by an affinity for both β1 and β2 receptors. The *second generation* like metoprolol or atenolol blocks predominantly the β1 receptors at low doses which confers a cardioselectivity for these drugs. Though this selectivity is relative as they may block β2 receptors at high doses [68]. This is important especially for patients with bronchospastic pulmonary diseases. The *third generation* of BB includes both non-selective and β1-selective drugs which have additional properties. For example, carvedilol and labetalol have α1-blocking properties thus facilitating peripheral vasodilation and reduced vascular resistance [69]. Nebivolol also facilitates vasodilation mediated by nitric oxide (NO) release. There is some evidence carvedilol may favor NO production as well [70]. Other BB like pindolol, acebutolol or labetalol have some ISA

TABLE 4.1 Classification of beta-receptor blockers (adapted after [66, 67])

| Type of beta receptor antagonist | Drug | β1-blockade potency | β1-selectivity |
|---|---|---|---|
| Non-selective (first generation) | Nadolol | 1.0 | 0 |
| | Penbutolol | 1.0 | 0 |
| | Pindolol | 6.0 | 0 |
| | Propranolol | 1.0 | 0 |
| | Timolol | 6.0 | 0 |
| | Sotalol | 0.3 | 0 |
| | Levobunolol | not available | 0 |
| | Metipranolol | not available | 0 |
| β1-selective (second generation) | Acebutolol | 0.3 | + |
| | Atenolol | 1.0 | ++ |
| | Bisoprolol | 10.0 | ++ |
| | Esmolol | 0.02 | ++ |
| | Metoprolol | 1.0 | ++ |
| Non-selective with ancillary properties (third generation) | Carteolol | 10.0 | 0 |
| | Carvedilol | 10.0 | 0 |
| | Bucindolol | 1.0 | 0 |
| | Labetalol | 0.3 | ++ |
| β1-selective with ancillary properties (third generation) | Betaxolol | 1.0 | ++ |
| | Celiprolol | 1.0 | ++ |
| | Nebivolol | 10.0 | ++ |

properties, meaning they may prevent the profound beta-blockade effects at rest. Some BB as carvedilol demonstrated antioxidant effects either by protection against reactive oxygen species or by increasing NO levels [71, 72]. An overview of these extra mechanisms of different BB is shown in Table 4.2.

TABLE 4.2 Additional mechanisms of some β-adrenoceptor antagonists (adapted after [67]

| Drug | Intrinsic agonist activity | α1 receptor blocking | Membrane stabilizing activity | Nitric oxide production | Antioxidant activity |
|---|---|---|---|---|---|
| Penbutolol | + | | | | |
| Pindolol | +++ | | + | | |
| Propranolol | | | ++ | | |
| Acebutolol | + | | | | |
| Metoprolol | | | +[a] | | |
| Carteolol | ++ | | | + | |
| Carvedilol | | + | ++ | | + |
| Labetalol | + | + | + | | |
| Betaxolol | + | | + | | |
| Celiprolol | | | | + | |
| Nebivolol | | | | + | |

[a]Only at very high doses

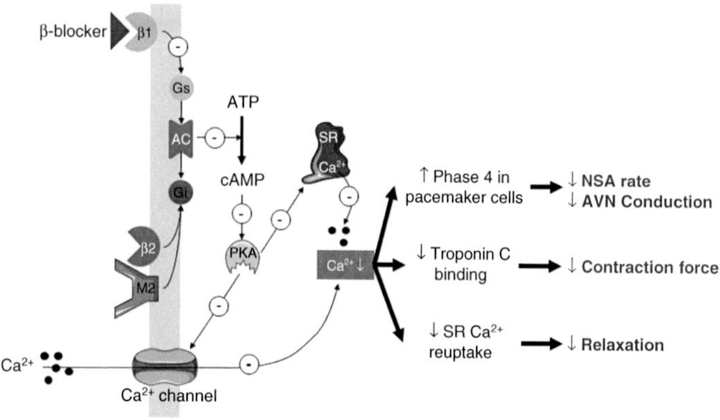


FIGURE 4.2 The main mechanism of BB and cardiovascular effects. *β1,2* beta-adrenergic receptors, *M2* muscarinic receptor type 2, *Gs* stimulating G-protein, *Gi* inhibitory G-protein, *ATP* adenosine triphosphate, *cAMP* cyclic adenosine monophosphate, *PKA* phosphokinase A, *SR* sarcoplasmic reticulum, *NSA* node sino-atrial, *AVN* atrioventricular node

The major pharmacological effects of BB are exerted on the cardiovascular system and they are mainly related to the blockade of β1 receptors which is the dominant adrenergic receptor in the heart. The potency and selectivity of β1-blockade are different among the representants of this class as shown in Table 4.1. Through the competitive blocking of β1-AR BB drugs reduce the inotropic and chronotropic effects of catecholamines and decrease the NSA rate, the conduction in atria and AVN and the automaticity (see Fig. 4.2, adapted from [73]). These pharmacological effects are visible when there is a high level of adrenergic activity, like during exercise, and they are present to a lesser degree at rest.

## *Pharmacokinetics*

The differences in pharmacokinetic properties of BB (see Table 4.3) influence not only the dosage of the drug but also the extent of their beneficial and potentially harmful effects.

TABLE 4.3 Pharmacokinetics properties of the β-blockers (adapted after [67, 73])

| Drug | Lipid solubility | Oral availability | Plasma half-life (H) | Protein binding (%) | Elimination |
|---|---|---|---|---|---|
| Nadolol | 0 | 30–50 | 20–24 | 30 | Kidney |
| Penbutolol | +++ | ~100 | ~5 | 80–98 | Liver |
| Pindolol | + | ~100 | 3–4 | 40 | Liver, kidney |
| Propranolol | +++ | 30 | 3–5 | 90 | Liver |
| Timolol | + | 75 | 4 | <10 | Liver, kidney |
| Sotalol | 0 | 90–100 | 7–18 | 5 | Kidney |
| Acebutolol | 0 | 20–60 | 3–4 | 26 | Kidney partially |
| Atenolol | 0 | 50–60 | 6–7 | 6–16 | Kidney |
| Bisoprolol | + | 80 | 9–12 | ~30 | Liver, kidney |
| Esmolol | + | NA | 0.15 | 55 | Kidney |
| Metoprolol | Moderate /+ | 40–50 | 3–7 | 12 | Liver |
| Carteolol | + | 85 | 6 | 23–30 | Kidney |
| Carvedilol | + | ~30 | 7–10 | 98 | Liver |

(continued)

TABLE 4.3 (continued)

| Drug | Lipid solubility | Oral availability | Plasma half-life (H) | Protein binding (%) | Elimination |
|---|---|---|---|---|---|
| Labetalol | Low/+++ | ~33 | 3–4 | ~50 | Liver>>kidney |
| Betaxolol | ++ | ~80 | 15 | 50 | Liver, then kidney |
| Celiprolol | + | 30–70 | 5 | 4–5 | NA |
| Nebivolol | Low/+++ | NA | 11–30 | 98 | Liver, kidney |

*NA* not available

## Absorption

Most of BB are orally administrated but their availability differs because of the first-pass liver effect. Lipophilic BB have a higher first-pass metabolism which confers a lower plasma half-life. The lipid solubility dictates the capacity to pass the blood-brain barrier and the main elimination route. Agents with high lipophilic profile, like propranolol, are more able to determine the central nervous system (CNS) effects whereas BB with low lipid solubility have a low penetration to this level. There are also a few BB drugs that may be administered intravenously. Currently, propranolol, metoprolol, labetalol, and esmolol have approved parenteral formulation. Of particular interest is esmolol which has an ultra-short half-time of 9 min, being converted to inactive metabolites by red cells esterase. Its beta-blocking effect disappears in ~30 min which promotes esmolol as a candidate of choice in acute settings where a rapid β-blockade is desirable but the hemodynamic stability of patient is uncertain.

## Distribution

Propranolol, carvedilol or labetalol have a high protein-binding capacity. This could lead to a higher plasmatic level in the case of hypoproteinemia and thus a dose modification could be necessary.

## Biotransformation

Plasma half-life time influences the mode of administration of BB. The shortest half-life is seen in the case of esmolol, which could be preferred in patients with potential hemodynamic instability. The drugs with longer half-life like nebivolol, sotalol, carvedilol or metoprolol succinate have better trough-to-peak ratios and therefore could be administrated once daily. This could be a better option for chronic diseases and for improving patient's adherence to therapy.

### Elimination

The route of elimination varies greatly among BB drugs. Lipid soluble agents as propranolol, labetalol and carvedilol are metabolized by the liver. High hydrophilic drugs like atenolol or sotalol are excreted by the kidney. Nebivolol and bisoprolol are eliminated by both liver and kidney routes. Therefore, in patients with severe liver or kidney diseases choosing the BB and the dosage according to these pharmacokinetic properties is advisable.

## Electrophysiologic Mechanism of Beta-Adrenergic Blockers

### *General Considerations*

Adrenergic stimulation has a major impact on cardiac electrophysiology due to a complex combination of ion currents modifications. By blocking sympathetic stimulation on cardiac cells, BB have an opposing effect, which results mainly in the lengthening of the action potential duration (APD), and therefore antiarrhythmic properties. As antiarrhythmics, BB have an impact on different mechanisms like reentry, automaticity or early and delayed afterdepolarizations (EAD, DAD). An overview of electrophysiological (EP) effects of BB and their consequences is shown in Fig. 4.3 (adapted from [74]).

### *Effects on $I_{Ks}$ and $I_{Kr}$*

Adrenergic stimulation increases $I_{Ks}$ and this seems to prevent the excessive prolongation of APD during the $I_{Ca}$ increase [75]. In congenital long QT syndromes (LQTS) characterized by a loss-of-function mutation in KCNH2 (LQTS type 2) or KCNQ1/ KCNE1 (LQTS type 1/type 5), there is a reduction of $I_{Kr}$ and, respectively, $I_{Ks}$ currents and consequently a higher risk of EAD and ventricular tachycardias

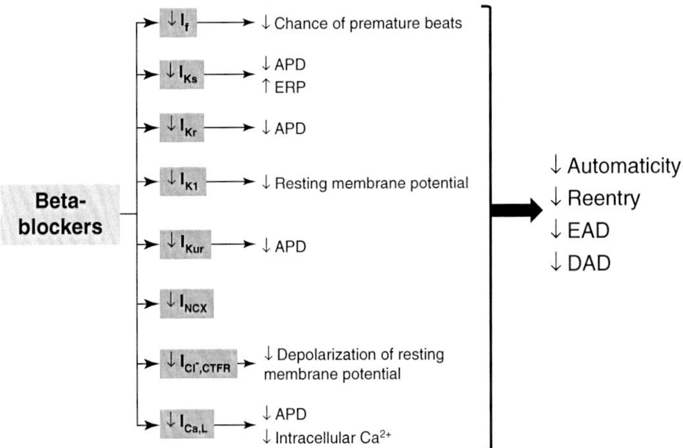


FIGURE 4.3 Ion currents affected by beta blockers and the effect on action potential and arrhythmic mechanisms. *APD* action potential duration, *ERP* effective refractory period, *EAD* early afterdepolarization, *DAD* delayed afterdepolarization, *ic* intracellular

(VT) during adrenergic stimulation. Downregulation of these two currents was in electrical remodeling secondary to heart failure [76, 77]. Thus, BB could be useful in such cases.

The ultra-rapid delayed rectifier current ($I_{Kur}$) is expressed only in atrial myocardium and is upregulated during AF [78]. Its composition consists of Kv1.5 α-subunits and is affected by adrenergic stimulation via PKA phosphorylation and consequently could be modulated by BB therapy [79]. An interesting finding related to the BB effect on $I_{Kur}$ is that the effect seems to be different between left and right atria. Whereas pure beta-blockers had a stronger effect on left atrium ERP, sotalol showed a more pronounced effect on the right atrium [80].

## Effects on $I_{K1}$

Sympathetic stimulation of cardiomyocytes leads to a dose-dependent modulation of the inward rectifier current ($I_{K1}$) and this is significantly reduced in the presence of heart failure [81, 82]. Also, in Andersen syndrome characterized by mutations in Kir2.1 channels was demonstrated a reduced $I_{K1}$ current density which contributes to the prolongation of QT (LQTS7) and ventricular arrhythmias [83]. An increased $I_{K1}$ density was seen in AF [84, 85]. In a study based on mathematical modeling chronic therapy with BB resulted in prolongation of APD and ERP and a positive shifting in membrane resting potential in atrial cells as a consequence of decreasing $I_{K1}$ current, alongside $I_{to}$ current [86].

## *Effects on $I_f$ (funny)*

The funny current ($I_f$) represents the major determinant of the diastolic depolarization and pacemaker activity. It has unusual properties like permeability for both $Na^+$ and $K^+$ ions, activation by hyperpolarization and slow kinetics [87]. It is expressed predominantly in the NSA, but also in other regions with pacemaker capabilities like AVN and Purkinje cells. By inhibiting adrenergic augmentation of $I_f$ current BB may have beneficial effects on enhanced pacemaker activity, especially in situations with a high sympathetic drive.

## *Effects on $I_{NCX}$*

The cardiac sodium-calcium exchanger ($I_{NCX}$) is responsible for the regulation of the intracellular $Ca^{2+}$. When its activity is amplified, like in heart failure, it may contribute to the generation of DAD and ventricular arrhythmias [88]. BB may increase sarcoplasmic reticulum $Ca^{2+}$ ATPase pump (SERCA) expression and decrease the $I_{NCX}$ and therefore lowering the risk of VT [89].

## *Effects on $I_{CTFR}$*

Norepinephrine seems to determine a cAMP-activated chloride current ($I_{Cl^-,CTFR}$) *via* a cardiac variant of the cystic fibrosis transmembrane conductance regulator protein (CTFR) [90, 91]. The major effect of $I_{Cl^-,CTFR}$ is represented by the shortening of APD and this could facilitate reentrant arrhythmias [92], but the role of this current on arrhythmogenesis and the potential role of BB therapy is unknown.

BB reduce the $Ca^{2+}$ influx determined by the sympathetic increase of the $I_{Ca.L}$ current (see Fig. 4.2) and consequently the proarrhythmic effect of intracellular $Ca^{2+}$ overload [93].

### *Effects in Heart Failure*

The mechanisms behind the beneficial effect of BB in HF are complex and include improving of β-adrenergic signaling, the resensitization of the β-receptor, reducing the cytosolic $Ca^{2+}$ overload via bradycardia and normalization of ryanodine receptors (see Fig. 4.4) [94–96].

## Beta-Adrenergic Blockers for Clinical Arrhythmias

### *General Considerations*

BB agents are of great value in clinical practice in a plethora of arrhythmias, both supraventricular and ventricular (Table 4.4) [78, 97, 98]. Because of their heterogeneity in properties, the clinical benefit may differ significantly in various clinical settings. This may be useful for the clinician in order to choose the appropriate drug for a specific situation.

### *Sinus Tachycardia*

Sinus tachycardia usually is determined by physiological adaptation. Therefore this condition does not impose a treatment but in the presence of symptoms related to the fast heart rate treatment with beta-blockers could be useful [99].

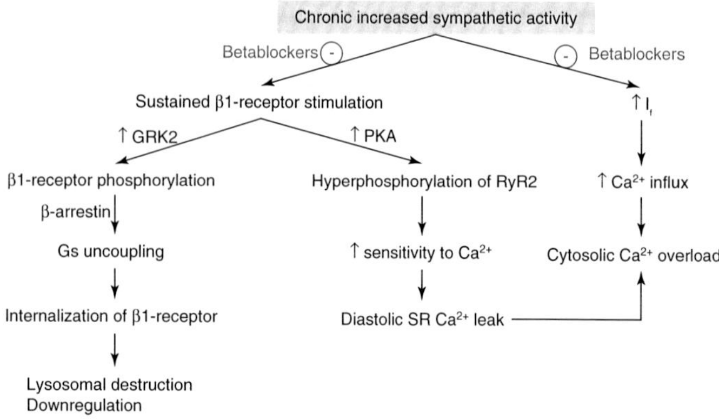


FIGURE 4.4 Proposed mechanisms of beneficial action of beta-blockers in heart failure. *GRK2* G protein-coupled receptor kinase, *PKA* protein kinase A, *SR* sarcoplasmic reticulum, *RyR2* ryanodine receptor, *Gs* stimulating G-protein

TABLE 4.4 Use of beta blockers in arrhythmias

| Arrhythmias/clinical settings |
|---|
| Supraventricular arrhythmias |
| Sinus tachycardia |
| Ectopic atrial tachycardia (for cardioversion or prevention) |
| Atrioventricular nodal reciprocating tachycardia |
| Focal junctional tachycardia |
| Non-paroxysmal junctional tachycardia |
| WPW with symptomatic arrhythmias |
| Atrial flutter (rate control) |
| Atrial fibrillation |
| Prevention (post-conversion, post-AMI, HF, post-surgery) |
| Conversion to sinus rhythm |
| Rate control |
| Ventricular arrhythmias |
| Control of arrhythmias after AMI |
| Prevention of SCD in HF and post-AMI |
| Prevention in inherited cardiac arrhythmias |

Inappropriate sinus tachycardia represents a persistently increased heart rate at rest unrelated to the level of physical, emotional or pathological stress. It should be differentiated from other atrial tachycardias or postural orthostatic tachycardia syndrome (POTS) and usually is an exclusion diagnosis. Patients with this condition may benefit occasionally from betablockade, however, this treatment is often ineffective and may be accompanied by hypotension [97, 100].

Postural orthostatic tachycardia syndrome (POTS) represents an excessive increase of heart rate during orthostatic posture associated with diverse symptoms like palpitations, fatigability, exercise intolerance, lightheadedness but not with orthostatic hypotension. The mechanisms underlying POTS are not fully understood. A genetic mutation in norepinephrine transporter (NET) was identified and its presence resulted in increased plasmatic and urine levels and decreased reuptake of norepinephrine [101]. Recent researches demonstrated the involvement of α1, β1 and β2 receptors autoantibodies which may be responsible for the pathophysiological manifestations of POTS [102, 103] In some reports of POTS cases, a benefit was obtained with propranolol or bisoprolol [104, 105]. A beta blocker with α1-blocking properties, like labetalol, may be more appropriate in case of patients with POTS who develop hypertension in a standing position [106].

## *Focal Atrial Tachycardias*

Focal atrial tachycardias (AT) is defined by regular atrial activity from atrial areas outside of sinus node with centrifugal spread and atrial rates ranged from 100 to 250 bpm, rarely 300 bpm [99]. The underlying mechanism of this group of arrhythmias consists of automatic, triggered or micro-reentry activity [107]. The incidence of focal ATs is <1% in symptomatic patients but increases with age [108, 109]. In children focal AT is seen in up to 23% in patients with normal heart, but more frequently in those with congenital heart disease [110]. The non-sustained focal AT are benign and rarely symptomatic, therefore they usually do not impose a treatment. The incessant form of focal AT could lead to tachycardia-induced cardiomyopathy [111].

There is limited data regarded the efficacy of BB therapy in focal AT and no randomized studies are available. In the acute setting intravenous BB may be used for either terminate the arrhythmia, which is rare, or for controlling the ventricular rate through increasing AVN block [97, 99]. For long-term management, BB may be used in symptomatic patients for prevention of recurrences or controlling the heart rate, especially if focal AT are related to the increased sympathetic tonus, like perioperative [78, 99, 112].

BB have limited utility in multifocal atrial tachycardia (MAT) because of underlying pulmonary condition, usually severe. In the absence of bronchospasm or acute decompensation of respiratory disease, BB may be used both in acute or chronic settings for rate control or for conversion to sinus rhythm [97]. Regarding the agent of choice, there is limited data on the efficacy and safety of beta-selective metoprolol in patients with pulmonary disease [113, 114]. For acute rate control in selected patients, a dose of 2–3 mg of metoprolol iv. may be given every 2–3 min up to a total of 15 mg ([115].). Also, there is a case report of successful termination of MAT in a patient with a severe chronic obstructive pulmonary disease using esmolol iv [116].

## *Atrioventricular Nodal Reentrant Tachycardia*

Atrioventricular nodal reentrant tachycardia (AVNRT) is a typical reentrant arrhythmia based on the dual pathway electrophysiology of AVN. It appears more frequent in women and usually is not associated with structural cardiac disease.

BB may be used for acute termination of AVNRT in hemodynamically stable patients, but usually is not recommended at first-line therapy unless there are contraindications or lack of efficacy to adenosine or calcium-channel blockers [78, 97, 99]. There is little evidence regarding the efficacy of BB in the acute treatment of AVNRT and some of the trials demonstrated rather a low rate of success [117]. An open study comparing esmolol and propranolol in patients with AVNRT showed a conversion rate as low as 14% for esmolol and 16% for propranolol [118]. Also, a randomized trial comparing the efficacy of diltiazem and esmolol in the acute treatment of AVNRT was stopped prematurely because of a clear superiority of calcium blocker [119].

For the prevention of AVNRT, the most successful choice is represented by catheter ablation, while the pharmacological approach is available for the patients who are not willing to perform the ablation. In this regard beta blockers, as drugs with impact on AVN conduction, may be a viable choice. There are no large randomized trials to reveal the efficacy of BB therapy in chronic management of AVNRT but generally, the drug efficacy ranged from 30 to 50% [120].

### *Atrioventricular Reentrant Tachycardia with Accessory Pathways*

In patients with accessory pathways, 95% of the occurring tachyarrhythmias are represented by atrioventricular reentrant tachycardia (AVRT). The ECG expression differs as to the conduction through AVN during the tachycardia is orthodromic or antidromic.

The use of BB for acute treatment of AVRT is not recommended because of the risk of enhancing the conduction over the accessory pathway if atrial fibrillation occurs [78, 97]. There is no trial examining the efficacy and safety of chronic BB therapy in patients with preexcitation syndrome. Nevertheless, the current guidelines suggest that BB may be used in patients in which electrophysiological testing demonstrated that the bypass tract is incapable of rapid anterograde conduction [99].

### *Atrial Flutter*

Atrial flutter (AFL) is the most representative form of macroreentrant tachyarrhythmias and accounts for about 15% of supraventricular tachyarrhythmias, frequently preceding or coexisting with atrial fibrillation (AF) [120]. Male gender, elderly, and the presence of heart failure or chronic obstructive pulmonary disease are the factors associated with the highest risk of developing AFL. Also, 60% of patients developed AFL in relation to a predisposing acute event, like surgery or exacerbation of pulmonary disease [121].

BB have a role in controlling heart rate both in acute and recurrent AFL, but not for conversion to nor for maintaining sinus rhythm. It is generally accepted that rate control of AFL is more difficult compared to AF, possibly because of slower and regular atrial rate. It is difficult to analyze the evidence regarding the efficacy of treatment in AFL because most trials included both AFL and AF. For acute rate control, the preferred BB is esmolol because of the rapid onset of effect [122, 123]. The dosage of intravenous BB approved for acute rate control in AFL/AF is detailed in Table 4.5.

For chronic treatment, BB are useful for rate control in AFL if catheter ablation is not performed, especially in patients with

Table 4.5 BB commonly used for acute rate control in atrial flutter and atrial fibrillation (adapted from [124, 125]

| Drug | Initial bolus | Repeated dosing |
|---|---|---|
| Esmolol | 500 mcg over 1–5 min then 50 mcg/kg/min infusion over 4 min | *If fails*<br>Repeated loading dose then 100 mcg/kg/min infusion over 4 min<br>*If it fails*<br>Repeat loading dose then titrate upward the infusion with increments of 50 mcg/kg/min over 4 min<br>Maximum dose: 300 mcg/kg/min |
| Metoprolol tartrate | 2.5–5 mg over 2 min | Repeat at 5 min as needed up to a maximum dose of 15 mg |
| Propranolol | 1 mg over 1 min | Repeat at 2 min as needed up to a maximum dose of 3 mg |

chronic heart failure, without a preference for a specific agent. BB are not recommended in patients with preexcitation [78, 97].

## Atrial Fibrillation

Atrial fibrillation (AF) is the most common pathologic tachyarrhythmia in adults with an estimated prevalence of 3% in patients aged 20 years or older [125]. It accounts for a third of hospitalizations for arrhythmias and it is independently associated with increased mortality.

The main strategies in the management of AF are the restoration and maintenance of sinus rhythm or rate control. The choice of strategy and of the pharmacological drug is dependent on multiple factors like symptoms, patient characteristics, and co-morbidities, or left ventricular ejection fraction (LVEF). When restoration of sinus rhythm is considered BB have little utility. There are few trials of cardioversion of AF after administration of esmolol but the magnitude of the effect is small [122, 126]. The current guidelines for the management of AF do not recommend any BB as a therapy for pharmacological cardioversion [125].

When sinus rhythm was restored, and a rhythm control strategy is considered BB may be useful in selected patients for the prevention of recurrences of AF. In a small randomized study, bisoprolol was as effective as sotalol in the prevention of AF with fewer side effects [127]. In a direct comparison, carvedilol and bisoprolol had comparable effectiveness in the prevention of AF, with a rate of recurrences of 46% and, respectively, 32% [128]. However, both studies are based on small populations. A recent meta-analysis concluded that metoprolol showed a significant reduction of AF relapses (OR 0.62, 95% CI 0.44 to 0.88, $P = 0.008$) based on two studies encompassing 562 patients [129]. Despite the little evidence regarding the efficacy of BB in the prevention of AF in a European survey 76% of centers would use BB as first agents due to low risk of adverse reactions [130]. The current guidelines, while not excluding BB as recommended therapy for AF prophylaxis, consider this class less effective and potentially harmful in case of vagally mediated AF [124, 131]

BB therapy has a special place in the treatment of perioperative AF. In the POISE trial, initiation of metoprolol succinate in patients undergoing non-cardiac surgery was associated with a lower rate of postoperative AF, but with the cost of the increased rate of stroke and mortality [132]. Some explanations of this contradictory effect were related to the use of long-acting drug and the initiation of therapy short time before surgery. Post-hoc analysis of the POISE trial revealed that hypotension, bradycardia and stroke rate were the factors determining both higher mortality and sepsis rates. The hypotension could favorize the development of sepsis and the prevention of tachycardia could delay the recognition of this complication. These adverse effects could be related to the initiation of BB on the day of surgery, to the use of long-acting BB and to the lack of titration of dose in order to ensure the tolerability and stability of the patient [133]. Therefore, in non-cardiac surgery, it is recommended to continue BB therapy if the patient is already under treatment and it is reasonable to initiate BB when the preoperative assessment suggests a high risk for developing AF (like the presence of myocardial ischemia or high score of Revised Cardiac Risk Index), but the initiation should be more than 1 day before surgery [133]. In the case of newly postoperative AF controlling the heart rate with BB represents the main recommendation, especially in the presence of underlying coronary artery disease or low LVEF [134]. In cardiac surgery, the incidence of postoperative AF varies according to the type of procedure and it is estimated at 20–40%, with higher values (30–50%) in case of valvular surgery [135]. A Cochrane review performed on 33 trials showed a significant reduction of postoperative AF with BB therapy, predominantly propranolol, compared to placebo (16.3% vs 31.7%) [136]. Also, the withdrawal of BB was associated with the development of postoperative AF [137, 138]. A more recent systematic review regarding the role of perioperative BB therapy included 88 randomized trials with 19,161 patients [139]. Compared to placebo the BB use was associated with a significant lower incidence of postoperative AF and AFL both in cardiac surgery (RR 0.48, 95%CI 0.40 to 0.57, $p < 0.00001$) and non-cardiac surgery (RR 0.73, 95%CI 0.56 to 0.95, $p = 0.019$).

BB are effective and usually preferred agents for heart rate control in AF, both in acute and chronic settings. For acute rate control intravenous metoprolol, esmolol, and propranolol have been used successfully, especially in conditions of increased adrenergic status like postoperative AF or thyrotoxicosis [112, 125]. Esmolol, with a very short half-time, is the preferred agent when there is doubt regarding the hemodynamic stability of the patient. Also, BB is the recommended choice in patients with low LVEF, since non-dihydropyridine calcium blockers are virtually contraindicated in this population.

A recent challenge regarding the treatment of the patients with HF and concomitant AF resulted from some meta-analysis which showed little if no benefit of BB therapy on mortality. In 2013 Rienstra et al. performed an analysis on four trials which enrolled 8680 patients with HF from which 19% had baseline AF. In this subgroup of patients BB therapy had no effect on mortality (OR 0.86, 95%CI 0.66 to 1.13, $p = 0.28$) [140]. Also, Kotecha et al. published another meta-analysis of 11 RCTs in which BB had no effect on mortality in patients with AF and HF (HR: 0.96, 95% CI: 0.81 to 1.12; $p = 0.58$) regardless the heart rate [141]. Contrary to these data in a propensity-matched analyses of a subgroup of patients from AF-CHF (Atrial Fibrillation and Congestive Heart Failure) trial with no BB at baseline, the BB therapy was associated with a lower all-cause mortality (HR: 0.763; 95% CI: 0.562 to 1.037; $p = 0.0838$) irrespective of the type or the burden of AF [142].

## Beta-Adrenergic Blockers and Sudden Cardiac Death (SCD) Prevention

### *Ventricular Tachycardias*

The efficacy of BB therapy in the treatment of VT differs based on the presence or absence of structural heart disease. In patients with idiopathic VT (like adenosine-sensitive VT originating from right ventricle outflow tract, verapamil-sensitive VT originating from left posterior fascicle, or papillary muscle VT) and normal cardiac substrate BB may be used in reducing symptoms and arrhythmic burden, but usually associate a higher rate of recurrence comparing to ablation therapy [78, 98, 143]. In a prospective study performed on a population of 330 patients with ventricular arrhythmias originating from right ventricle outflow tract catheter ablation was superior to medical therapy regarding the rate of recurrences [144].

In the settings of acute coronary syndromes early treatment with BB may be used for prevention or to reduce the rate of recurrences of VT [145, 146]. Also, BB may reduce the risk of death in recurrent VT/VF (electrical storm) refractory to amiodarone and/or lidocaine [78, 143]. In a small study of 49 patients with electrical storm and acute myocardial infarction, the sympathetic blockade with esmolol or propranolol was associated with better survival at 1 week compared to lidocaine and procainamide/bretylium tosylate [147]. In patients who received an implantable defibrillator (ICD), the administration of BB reduces the need for shocks [148]. The same conclusion was demonstrated by a subanalysis of a cohort of patients with ischemic cardiomyopathy and ICD from the MADIT-II trial in which BB therapy was associated with significantly lower mortality and of the risk of VT requiring ICD intervention [149].

In a systematic review of RCTs with patients with myocardial infarction, the treatment with BB is associated with a 23% reduction of risk of death in long-term trials [150]. A *post-hoc* analysis of pooled data from EMIAT (European Myocardial Infarct Amiodarone Trial) and CAMIAT (Canadian Amiodarone Myocardial Infarction Trial) studies demonstrated a clear benefit of adding BB to the amiodarone treatment on arrhythmic death in patients postmyocardial infarction, compared to amiodarone alone [151]. In stable coronary disease, the use of BB is recommended but their efficacy on the prevention of VT and SCD is not clear in the patients with preserved LVEF [98]. A recent meta-analysis showed no benefit on cardiovascular mortality from BB therapy in patients with LVEF ≥50%, but the number of patients included in this category was too low to allow a definite conclusion [152].

In patients with reduced LVEF, the role of BB in the prevention of VT/VF and of SCD is clearly demonstrated. In the U.S. Carvedilol Heart Failure Study treatment with carvedilol was associated with a significantly lower incidence of SCD compared to placebo (1.7% vs 3.8%, $p = 0.03$) [153]. In the Metoprolol CR/XL Randomised Intervention Trial in Congestive Heart Failure (MERIT-HF) metoprolol reduced the risk of SCD (OR 0.59, 95%CI 0.45–0.78, $p = 0.0002$, compared to placebo) [154]. A similar beneficial effect on arrhythmic death was demonstrated for bisoprolol in CIBIS-II trial [155]. A meta-analysis of four large RCTs performed in patients with HF and BB treatment showed a risk reduction of the sudden death of 37% ($p < 0.0001$), demonstrating the main role of BB in the reduction of fatal ventricular arrhythmias in HF [156]. Another large meta-analysis based on 24,779 patients with HF the treatment with BB demonstrated a 32% reduction in the risk of SCD compared to placebo/control [157]. It seems the beneficial role of BB therapy is maintained also in patients with nonischemic cardiomyopathy and HF [158]. The current guidelines do not prefer a specific BB agent (from those accepted in HF) based on the antiarrhythmic properties. However, in the COMET trial which compared two BB agents approved for the treatment of HF the use of carvedilol was associated with a lower incidence of SCD compared to metoprolol tartrate (RR 0.77, CI 0.64 to 0.93, $p = 0.0073$) [159].

## *Inherited Arrhythmias*

### Arrhythmogenic Right Ventricular Cardiomyopathy

Arrhythmogenic right ventricular cardiomyopathy (ARVC) represents a myocardial disease, often with an autosomal-dominant familial transmission, characterized by the replacement of right ventricle myocardium with fibrofatty tissue. The VT in ARVC is usually monomorphic and it occurs during or immediately after exercise, demonstrating a relationship with sympathetic stimulation. Therefore, a beta blocker, preferably without nonvasodilating properties, is usually recommended in patients with ARVC for reducing the burden of ventricular arrhythmias [143, 160]. Though, there is no proof of benefit on SCD and some reports showed no protective effect of BB against VT [161].

## Hypertrophic Cardiomyopathy

Hypertrophic Cardiomyopathy (HCM) is an autosomal-dominant genetic disease characterized by an increase of left ventricle walls thickness not determined by abnormal loading conditions.

BB therapy has no effective role in the prevention of SCD in HCM but instead may reduce the number on non-sustained VT and consequently the number of ICD interventions [162]. BB may be used for controlling ventricular rate in patients with HCM who develop AF either in acute if hemodynamically stable, or chronic settings but has no value in the prevention of recurrences of AF [163].

## Long QT Syndromes (LQTS)

There are 13 genetic forms of LQTS, implying mutations in genes responsible for coding proteins of sodium-channels, potassium-channels, calcium-channels or membrane factors. The prevalence among Caucasians is estimated at 1:2000 [164]. The triggers for arrhythmic events differ among the types of LQTS: in LQTS1 they appear during the effort, in LQTS2 during emotional stress or rest, and in LQTS 3 during sleep. These patterns may explain why BB therapy was more efficient in the prevention of VT in patients with LQTS1 compared to LQTS2 and LQTS3 [165]. The current consensus recommends BB therapy for all patients with LQTS with an emphasis on long-acting agents [164]. Also, a recent publication based on 606 patients with different LQTS of which 82% were treated with BB demonstrated a very low incidence of arrhythmic deaths (0.3% in the entire population) which emphasizes the beneficial role of this treatment [166]. However, there is data suggesting there is a difference in efficacy among BB agents in relation to the type of LQTS. A study of 1530 patients with LQTS1 and 2 compared the efficacy of atenolol, metoprolol, propranolol and nadolol regarding the rate of arrhythmic events [167]. All agents were similar for the risk reduction of the first event in LQTS1, but only nadolol was efficient in LQTS2. Also, propranolol was the least efficient drug in those patients experiencing an arrhythmic event while under treatment with BB. A similar study based on 382 patients with LQTS1/2 showed a lesser efficacy of metoprolol compared to propranolol or nadolol in symptomatic patients [168]. However, it should be mentioned that only 27% of patients were symptomatic and only 35 patients received metoprolol.

## Catecholaminergic Polymorphic Ventricular Tachycardia (CPVT)

CPVT is an inherited arrhythmogenic disease characterized by polymorphic ventricular tachycardia related to stress. CPTV1, the most frequent, it is determined by mutations type gain-of-function in the ryanodine receptor 2 genes, while CPTV2 is a result of mutation in calsequestrin-2 (*CASQ2*) genes [169]. CPVT has a low prevalence of 1:10.000 but associates a high risk of SCD in young individuals. The relationship between CPVT and sympathetic activation points toward the beneficial role of BB in the management of these patients. A meta-analysis of 11 studies with a total of 403 patients with CPVT from which 88% were treated with BB showed an estimated arrhythmic events rate of 18.6% at 4 years of follow-up and of 37.2% at 8 years of follow-up [170]. The absence of BB therapy is an independent predictor for cardiac events [171]. Among class drugs, it seems nadolol has superior efficacy in the prevention of VT in patients with CPVT [171, 172]. The explanation of this observed effect is unclear. The hypothesis includes the stronger chronotropic inhibition, a small sodium-blocking effect, the long half-life time of 20–24 h which reduces the risk of events in the case of nonadherence [172].

## Adverse Reactions and Contraindications

### *Adverse Reactions*

Side effects of BB could manifest at cardiovascular, pulmonary, peripheral and CNS levels. Also, there are some adverse effects on exercise capacity and sexual life.

#### Cardiovascular

BB could lead to severe bradyarrhythmias. This could be more frequent in patients with preexisting conduction defects or sick sinus syndrome, or if associated with other bradyarrhythmic drugs. If necessary, BB could be administered in such cases when a pacemaker is implanted.

The administration of BB in heart failure needs caution. In stable heart failure, the treatment with BB increases both the quality of life and life expectancy when dosing is gradual. The abrupt dosage could exaggerate heart failure in such patients or in patients with a severe cardiac substrate like significant aortic stenosis, acute myocardial infarction or cardiomegaly.

In patients chronically treated with BB, the abrupt discontinuation could lead to exacerbation of angina or heart failure [173–175]. Also, this negative effect was demonstrated in perioperative patients [176, 177]. However, the analysis performed by Teichert et al. on a large cohort found an increase of myocardial infarction only after cessation of beta-selective betablockers but not in other subgroups [178]. The withdrawal effect could be determined by the increased sensitivity to norepinephrine because of upregulation of beta-receptors.

## Pulmonary

The blockade of β2 receptors in the bronchial smooth muscle could lead to severe bronchospasm and to aggravation of bronchospastic pulmonary diseases. This effect could be less frequent with the use of beta-selective BB. A systematic review of β1-selective BB in patients with chronic obstructive pulmonary disease showed no changes in symptoms or spirometric parameters [179].

## Central Nervous System

The CNS side effects of BB are rare and may manifest as depression, nightmares, and visual hallucinations. BB drugs with high lipophilic profile, like propranolol, are more prone to determine CNS adverse reactions [180]. However, this lipophilic hypothesis is not the only explanation. For example, pindolol (non-selective and moderate ISA) has a higher incidence of CNS side effects compared to metoprolol (selective, no ISA), both drugs being moderately lipophilic [181].

## Peripheral

BB may provoke an exacerbation of the Raynaud phenomenon. Also, some patients complain of cold extremities when treated with BB which could be alleviated by administering a beta-selective drug or a BB with ISA [182]. Regarding the peripheral artery disease, a systematic review stated there is no evidence that BB adversely affects clinical parameters in patients with intermittent claudication [183]. It should be mentioned though the data is scarce and data from large randomized trials is necessary.

## Metabolism

BB may determine weight gain and hyperlipemia [184]. Also, BB promote hyperglycemia [185], but those which promotes nitric oxide formation, like nebivolol and carvedilol, may have a better glycemic profile [186, 187]. Another concern is related to the patients prone to hypoglycemia as BB therapy may blunt its clinical manifestations.

#### Sexual Life

In male patients, chronic treatment with BB could lead to erectile dysfunction in an age-dependent manner [188, 189]. The erectile dysfunction seems to be more frequent in patients with coronary artery disease [190] and in those treated with BB which undergone by-pass cardiac surgery [191] reflecting atherosclerotic involvement of the narrow penile artery and less a selective action. Among BB, nebivolol has some evidence of a better profile regarding this aspect [192, 193].

### *Contraindications*

BB therapy is contraindicated in case of severe bradycardia, high-grade atrioventricular blocks, cardiogenic shock, acute or aggravated heart failure, severe bronchospasm, severe depression, or symptomatic peripheral arterial disease (rest pain, tissue loss) [73, 112]. However, all contraindications are relative if the benefit of the therapy outweighs the potential risk of adverse effects or if the latter may be counteracted (e.g. implantation of a pacemaker in case of advanced bradyarrhythmias) [112].

## Conclusions

With a history which started more 50 years ago, the BB class remains one of the most useful medication for a wide range of cardiovascular diseases, including arrhythmias. An overview of the clinical use of BB as antiarrhythmic drugs, shown in Fig. 4.5, emphasizes the role of this class as a mainstream therapy in a plethora of clinical situations. The multiple BB agents currently in use share a common mechanism of action, namely β1-receptor blocking, but the differences in

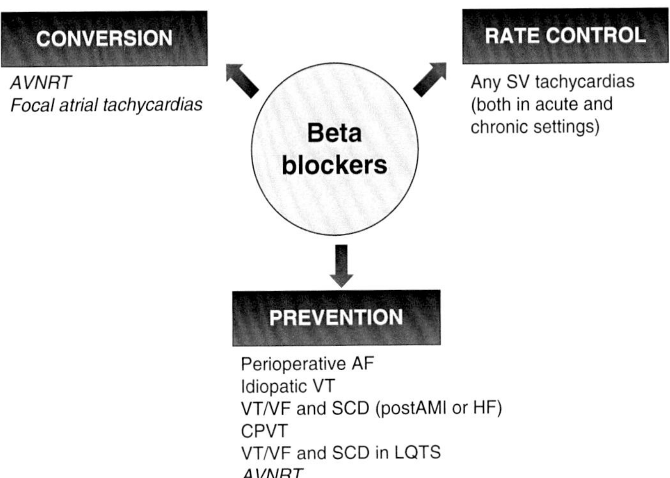


FIGURE 4.5 Overview of clinical benefits of BB therapy in arrhythmias. *AVNRT* atrioventricular nodal reentrant tachycardia, *SV* supraventricular, *AF* atrial fibrillation, *VT* ventricular tachycardia, *VF* ventricular fibrillation, *SCD* sudden cardiac death, *AMI* acute myocardial infarction, *HF* heart failure, *CPVT* catecholaminergic polymorphic ventricular tachycardia LQTS long QT syndromes

pharmacokinetics, adrenergic receptor selectivity, or presence of additional mechanisms like nitric oxide production or intrinsic sympathomimetic activity make this class a heterogeneous one. This diversity permitted a more detailed knowledge of sympathetic molecular pathophysiology and helps the clinician to choose the right beta-blocker for the right patient.

## References

1. Kawashima T. The autonomic nervous system of the human heart with special reference to its origin, course, and peripheral distribution. Anat Embryol. 2005;209:425–38. https://doi.org/10.1007/s00429-005-0462-1.

2. Coote JH, Chauhan RA. The sympathetic innervation of the heart: important new insights. Auton Neurosci. 2016;199:17–23. https://doi.org/10.1016/j.autneu.2016.08.014.
3. Franciosi S, Perry FKG, Roston TM, et al. The role of the autonomic nervous system in arrhythmias and sudden cardiac death. Auton Neurosci. 2017;205:1–11. https://doi.org/10.1016/j.autneu.2017.03.005.
4. Kimura K, Ieda M, Fukuda K. Development, maturation, and transdifferentiation of cardiac sympathetic nerves. Circ Res. 2012;110:325–36. https://doi.org/10.1161/CIRCRESAHA.111.257253.
5. Chiou CW, Eble JN, Zipes DP. Efferent vagal innervation of the canine atria and sinus and atrioventricular nodes. The third fat pad. Circulation. 1997;95:2573–84.
6. Vaseghi M, Shivkumar K. The role of the autonomic nervous system in sudden cardiac death. Prog Cardiovasc Dis. 2008;50:404–19. https://doi.org/10.1016/j.pcad.2008.01.003.
7. Armour JA. Functional anatomy of intrathoracic neurons innervating the atria and ventricles. Hear Rhythm. 2010;7:994–6. https://doi.org/10.1016/j.hrthm.2010.02.014.
8. Hou Y, Scherlag BJ, Lin J, et al. Ganglionated plexi modulate extrinsic cardiac autonomic nerve input: effects on sinus rate, atrioventricular conduction, refractoriness, and inducibility of atrial fibrillation. J Am Coll Cardiol. 2007;50:61–8. https://doi.org/10.1016/j.jacc.2007.02.066.
9. Wake E, Brack K. Characterization of the intrinsic cardiac nervous system. Auton Neurosci. 2016;199:3–16. https://doi.org/10.1016/j.autneu.2016.08.006.
10. Bristow MR. Changes in myocardial and vascular receptors in heart failure. J Am Coll Cardiol. 1993;22:61A–71A.
11. Ihl-Vahl R, Eschenhagen T, Kübler W, et al. Differential regulation of mRNA specific for beta 1- and beta 2-adrenergic receptors in human failing hearts. Evaluation of the absolute cardiac mRNA levels by two independent methods. J Mol Cell Cardiol. 1996;28:1–10.
12. Brodde OE. Beta 1- and beta 2-adrenoceptors in the human heart: properties, function, and alterations in chronic heart failure. Pharmacol Rev. 1991;43:203–42.
13. Schäfers RF, Poller U, Pönicke K, et al. Influence of adrenoceptor and muscarinic receptor blockade on the cardiovascular effects of exogenous noradrenaline and of endogenous noradrenaline

released by infused tyramine. Naunyn Schmiedeberg's Arch Pharmacol. 1997;355:239–49.

14. Rubart M, Zipes DP. Science in medicine mechanisms of sudden cardiac death. J Clin Invest. 2005;115 https://doi.org/10.1172/JCI26381.
15. Rodefeld M, Beau S, Schuessler R, et al. Beta-adrenergic and muscarinic cholinergic receptor densities in the human sinoatrial node: identification of a high beta 2-adrenergic receptor density. J Cardiovasc Electrophysiol. 1996;7:1039–49. https://doi.org/10.1111/j.1540-8167.1996.tb00479.x.
16. Gordan R, Gwathmey JK, Xie L-H. Autonomic and endocrine control of cardiovascular function. World J Cardiol. 2015;7:204. https://doi.org/10.4330/wjc.v7.i4.204.
17. Brodde OE, Bruck H, Leineweber K, Seyfarth T. Presence, distribution and physiological function of adrenergic and muscarinic receptor subtypes in the human heart. Basic Res Cardiol. 2001;96:528–38.
18. Gardner RT, Ripplinger CM, Myles RC, Habecker BA. Molecular mechanisms of sympathetic remodeling and arrhythmias. Circ Arrhythm Electrophysiol. 2016;9:1–9. https://doi.org/10.1161/CIRCEP.115.001359.
19. Cao JM, Fishbein MC, Han JB, et al. Relationship between regional cardiac hyperinnervation and ventricular arrhythmia. Circulation. 2000b;101:1960–9.
20. Kim DT, Luthringer DJ, Lai AC, et al. Sympathetic nerve sprouting after orthotopic heart transplantation. J Heart Lung Transplant. 2004;23:1349–58. https://doi.org/10.1016/j.healun.2003.10.005.
21. Li W, Knowlton D, van Winkle DM, Habecker BA. Infarction alters both the distribution and noradrenergic properties of cardiac sympathetic neurons. Am J Physiol Heart Circ Physiol. 2004;286:H2229–36. https://doi.org/10.1152/ajpheart.00768.2003.
22. Zhou S, Chen LS, Miyauchi Y, et al. Mechanisms of cardiac nerve sprouting after myocardial infarction in dogs. Circ Res. 2004;95:76–83. https://doi.org/10.1161/01.RES.0000133678.22968.e3.
23. Abe T, Morgan DA, Gutterman DD. Protective role of nerve growth factor against postischemic dysfunction of sympathetic coronary innervation. Circulation. 1997;95:213–20.

24. Hasan W, Jama A, Donohue T, et al. Sympathetic hyperinnervation and inflammatory cell NGF synthesis following myocardial infarction in rats. Brain Res. 2006;1124:142–54. https://doi.org/10.1016/j.brainres.2006.09.054.
25. Meloni M, Caporali A, Graiani G, et al. Nerve growth factor promotes cardiac repair following myocardial infarction. Circ Res. 2010;106:1275–84. https://doi.org/10.1161/CIRCRESAHA.109.210088.
26. Ieda M, Kanazawa H, Kimura K, et al. Sema3a maintains normal heart rhythm through sympathetic innervation patterning. Nat Med. 2007;13:604–12. https://doi.org/10.1038/nm1570.
27. Chen R-H, Li Y-G, Jiao K-L, et al. Overexpression of sema3a in myocardial infarction border zone decreases vulnerability of ventricular tachycardia post-myocardial infarction in rats. J Cell Mol Med. 2013;17:608–16. https://doi.org/10.1111/jcmm.12035.
28. Jacobson AF, Senior R, Cerqueira MD, et al. Myocardial iodine-123 meta-iodobenzylguanidine imaging and cardiac events in heart failure. J Am Coll Cardiol. 2010;55:2212–21. https://doi.org/10.1016/j.jacc.2010.01.014.
29. Stanton MS, Tuli MM, Radtke NL, et al. Regional sympathetic denervation after myocardial infarction in humans detected noninvasively using I-123-metaiodobenzylguanidine. J Am Coll Cardiol. 1989;14:1519–26.
30. Kohn J, Aloyz RS, Toma JG, et al. Functionally antagonistic interactions between the TrkA and p75 neurotrophin receptors regulate sympathetic neuron growth and target innervation. J Neurosci. 1999;19:5393–408.
31. Gardner RT, Habecker BA. Infarct-derived chondroitin sulfate proteoglycans prevent sympathetic reinnervation after cardiac ischemia-reperfusion injury. J Neurosci. 2013;33:7175–83. https://doi.org/10.1523/JNEUROSCI.5866-12.2013.
32. Boogers MJ, Borleffs CJW, Henneman MM, et al. Cardiac sympathetic denervation assessed with 123-iodine metaiodobenzylguanidine imaging predicts ventricular arrhythmias in implantable cardioverter-defibrillator patients. J Am Coll Cardiol. 2010;55:2769–77. https://doi.org/10.1016/j.jacc.2009.12.066.
33. Fallavollita JA, Heavey BM, Luisi AJ, et al. Regional myocardial sympathetic denervation predicts the risk of sudden cardiac arrest in ischemic cardiomyopathy. J Am Coll Cardiol. 2014;63:141–9. https://doi.org/10.1016/j.jacc.2013.07.096.

34. Cuculi F, Herring N, de Caterina AR, et al. Relationship of plasma neuropeptide Y with angiographic, electrocardiographic and coronary physiology indices of reperfusion during ST elevation myocardial infarction. Heart. 2013;99:1198–203. https://doi.org/10.1136/heartjnl-2012-303443.
35. Kammerling JJ, Green FJ, Watanabe AM, et al. Denervation supersensitivity of refractoriness in noninfarcted areas apical to transmural myocardial infarction. Circulation. 1987;76:383–93.
36. Warner MR, Wisler PL, Hodges TD, et al. Mechanisms of denervation supersensitivity in regionally denervated canine hearts. Am J Physiol Circ Physiol. 1993;264:H815–20. https://doi.org/10.1152/ajpheart.1993.264.3.H815.
37. Inoue H, Zipes DP. Results of sympathetic denervation in the canine heart: supersensitivity that may be arrhythmogenic. Circulation. 1987;75:877–87.
38. Coumel P, Attuel P, Lavallée J, et al. The atrial arrhythmia syndrome of vagal origin. Arch Mal Coeur Vaiss. 1978;71:645–56.
39. Chen P-S, Tan AY. Autonomic nerve activity and atrial fibrillation. Heart Rhythm. 2007;4:S61–4. https://doi.org/10.1016/j.hrthm.2006.12.006.
40. Coumel P. Autonomic influences in atrial tachyarrhythmias. J Cardiovasc Electrophysiol. 1996;7:999–1007.
41. de Vos CB, Nieuwlaat R, Crijns HJGM, et al. Autonomic trigger patterns and anti-arrhythmic treatment of paroxysmal atrial fibrillation: data from the Euro Heart Survey. Eur Heart J. 2008;29:632–9. https://doi.org/10.1093/eurheartj/ehn025.
42. Dimmer C, Tavernier R, Gjorgov N, et al. Variations of autonomic tone preceding onset of atrial fibrillation after coronary artery bypass grafting. Am J Cardiol. 1998;82:22–5.
43. Huang JL, Wen ZC, Lee WL, et al. Changes of autonomic tone before the onset of paroxysmal atrial fibrillation. Int J Cardiol. 1998;66:275–83.
44. Kapa S, Venkatachalam KL, Asirvatham SJ. The autonomic nervous system in cardiac electrophysiology. Cardiol Rev. 2010;18:275–84. https://doi.org/10.1097/CRD.0b013e3181ebb152.
45. Verrier RL, Josephson ME. Impact of sleep on arrhythmogenesis. Circ Arrhythm Electrophysiol. 2009;2:450–9. https://doi.org/10.1161/CIRCEP.109.867028.
46. Sharifov OF, Fedorov VV, Beloshapko GG, et al. Roles of adrenergic and cholinergic stimulation in spontaneous atrial

fibrillation in dogs. J Am Coll Cardiol. 2004;43:483–90. https://doi.org/10.1016/j.jacc.2003.09.030.
47. Ogawa M, Zhou S, Tan AY, et al. Left stellate ganglion and vagal nerve activity and cardiac arrhythmias in ambulatory dogs with pacing-induced congestive heart failure. J Am Coll Cardiol. 2007;50:335–43. https://doi.org/10.1016/j.jacc.2007.03.045.
48. Tan AY, Zhou S, Ogawa M, et al. Neural mechanisms of paroxysmal atrial fibrillation and paroxysmal atrial tachycardia in ambulatory canines. Circulation. 2008;118:916–25. https://doi.org/10.1161/CIRCULATIONAHA.108.776203.
49. Shen MJ, Zipes DP. Role of the autonomic nervous system in modulating cardiac arrhythmias. Circ Res. 2014;114:1004–21. https://doi.org/10.1161/CIRCRESAHA.113.302549.
50. Cao JM, Chen LS, KenKnight BH, et al. Nerve sprouting and sudden cardiac death. Circ Res. 2000a;86:816–21.
51. Chen PS, Chen LS, Cao JM, et al. Sympathetic nerve sprouting, electrical remodeling and the mechanisms of sudden cardiac death. Cardiovasc Res. 2001;50:409–16.
52. Schwartz PJ. The autonomic nervous system and sudden death. Eur Heart J. 1998;19(Suppl F):F72–80.
53. Zipes DP, Rubart M. Neural modulation of cardiac arrhythmias and sudden cardiac death. Heart Rhythm. 2006;3:108–13. https://doi.org/10.1016/j.hrthm.2005.09.021.
54. Janse MJ, Schwartz PJ, Wilms-Schopman F, et al. Effects of unilateral stellate ganglion stimulation and ablation on electrophysiologic changes induced by acute myocardial ischemia in dogs. Circulation. 1985;72:585–95.
55. Jiang H, Hu X, Lu Z, et al. Effects of sympathetic nerve stimulation on ischemia-induced ventricular arrhythmias by modulating Connexin43 in rats. Arch Med Res. 2008;39:647–54. https://doi.org/10.1016/j.arcmed.2008.07.005.
56. Opthof T, Misier AR, Coronel R, et al. Dispersion of refractoriness in canine ventricular myocardium. Effects of sympathetic stimulation. Circ Res. 1991;68:1204–15.
57. Albert CM, Mittleman MA, Chae CU, et al. Triggering of sudden death from cardiac causes by vigorous exertion. N Engl J Med. 2000;343:1355–61. https://doi.org/10.1056/NEJM200011093431902.
58. Billman GE. Heart rate response to onset of exercise: evidence for enhanced cardiac sympathetic activity in animals susceptible to ventricular fibrillation. Am J Physiol Circ Physiol. 2006;291:H429–35. https://doi.org/10.1152/ajpheart.00020.2006.

59. Corrado D, Basso C, Rizzoli G, et al. Does sports activity enhance the risk of sudden death in adolescents and young adults? J Am Coll Cardiol. 2003;42:1959–63.
60. Verrier RL, Lown B. Behavioral stress and cardiac arrhythmias. Annu Rev Physiol. 1984;46:155–76. https://doi.org/10.1146/annurev.ph.46.030184.001103.
61. Ziegelstein RC. Acute emotional stress and cardiac arrhythmias. JAMA. 2007;298:324. https://doi.org/10.1001/jama.298.3.324.
62. Ng GA, Mantravadi R, Walker WH, et al. Sympathetic nerve stimulation produces spatial heterogeneities of action potential restitution. Heart Rhythm. 2009;6:696–706. https://doi.org/10.1016/j.hrthm.2009.01.035.
63. Swissa M, Zhou S, Gonzalez-Gomez I, et al. Long-term subthreshold electrical stimulation of the left stellate ganglion and a canine model of sudden cardiac death. J Am Coll Cardiol. 2004;43:858–64. https://doi.org/10.1016/j.jacc.2003.07.053.
64. Shusterman V, Aysin B, Gottipaty V, et al. Autonomic nervous system activity and the spontaneous initiation of ventricular tachycardia. ESVEM investigators. Electrophysiologic study versus electrocardiographic monitoring trial. J Am Coll Cardiol. 1998;32:1891–9.
65. Zhou S, Jung B-C, Tan AY, et al. Spontaneous stellate ganglion nerve activity and ventricular arrhythmia in a canine model of sudden death. Heart Rhythm. 2008;5:131–9. https://doi.org/10.1016/j.hrthm.2007.09.007.
66. Frishman WH. Beta-adrenergic blockers: a 50-year historical perspective. Am J Ther. 2008;15:565–76. https://doi.org/10.1097/MJT.0b013e318188bdca.
67. Westfall T, Macarthur H, Westfall D. Adrenergic agonists and antagonists. In: Brunton L, Hilal-Dandan R, Knollmann B, editors. Goodman & Gilman's: the pharmacological basis of therapeutics. 13th ed. New York: McGraw-Hill; 2017. p. 1423.
68. Egan BM, Basile J, Chilton RJ, Cohen JD. Cardioprotection: the role of beta-blocker therapy. J Clin Hypertens (Greenwich). 2005;7:409–16.
69. Pedersen ME, Cockcroft JR. The vasodilatory beta-blockers. Curr Hypertens Rep. 2007;9:269–77.
70. Kozlovski VI, Lomnicka M, Chlopicki S. Nebivovol and carvedilol induce NO-dependent coronary vasodilatation that is unlikely to be mediated by extracellular ATP in the isolated Guinea pig heart. Pharmacol Rep. 2006;58(Suppl):103–10.

71. Dandona P, Ghanim H, Brooks DP. Antioxidant activity of carvedilol in cardiovascular disease. J Hypertens. 2007;25:731–41. https://doi.org/10.1097/HJH.0b013e3280127948.
72. Toda N. Vasodilating beta-adrenoceptor blockers as cardiovascular therapeutics. Pharmacol Ther. 2003;100:215–34.
73. Opie L. Drugs for the heart. Amsterdam: Elsevier; 2013.
74. Zicha S, Tsuji Y, Shiroshita-Takeshita A, Nattel S. Beta-blockers as antiarrhythmic agents. Handb Exp Pharmacol. 2006:235–66.
75. Han W, Wang Z, Nattel S. Slow delayed rectifier current and repolarization in canine cardiac Purkinje cells. Am J Physiol Circ Physiol. 2001;280:H1075–80. https://doi.org/10.1152/ajpheart.2001.280.3.H1075.
76. Li G-R, Lau C-P, Ducharme A, et al. Transmural action potential and ionic current remodeling in ventricles of failing canine hearts. Am J Physiol Circ Physiol. 2002;283:H1031–41. https://doi.org/10.1152/ajpheart.00105.2002.
77. Tsuji Y, Opthof T, Kamiya K, et al. Pacing-induced heart failure causes a reduction of delayed rectifier potassium currents along with decreases in calcium and transient outward currents in rabbit ventricle. Cardiovasc Res. 2000;48:300–9.
78. Dan G-A, Martinez-Rubio A, Agewall S, et al. Antiarrhythmic drugs–clinical use and clinical decision making: a consensus document from the European Heart Rhythm Association (EHRA) and European Society of Cardiology (ESC) Working Group on Cardiovascular Pharmacology, endorsed by the Heart Rhythm Society (HRS), Asia-Pacific Heart Rhythm Society (APHRS) and International Society of Cardiovascular Pharmacotherapy (ISCP). Europace. 2018;20:731–732an. https://doi.org/10.1093/europace/eux373.
79. Li GR, Feng J, Wang Z, et al. Adrenergic modulation of ultrarapid delayed rectifier K+ current in human atrial myocytes. Circ Res. 1996;78:903–15.
80. Knobloch K, Brendel J, Rosenstein B, et al. Atrial-selective antiarrhythmic actions of novel Ikur vs. Ikr, Iks, and IKAch class Ic drugs and beta blockers in pigs. Med Sci Monit. 2004;10:BR221–8.
81. Koumi S, Backer CL, Arentzen CE, Sato R. Beta-adrenergic modulation of the inwardly rectifying potassium channel in isolated human ventricular myocytes. Alteration in channel response to beta-adrenergic stimulation in failing human hearts. J Clin Invest. 1995;96:2870–81. https://doi.org/10.1172/JCI118358.

82. Tomaselli GF, Marbán E. Electrophysiological remodeling in hypertrophy and heart failure. Cardiovasc Res. 1999;42:270–83.
83. Tristani-Firouzi M, Jensen JL, Donaldson MR, et al. Functional and clinical characterization of KCNJ2 mutations associated with LQT7 (Andersen syndrome). J Clin Invest. 2002;110:381–8. https://doi.org/10.1172/JCI15183.
84. Dobrev D, Wettwer E, Kortner A, et al. Human inward rectifier potassium channels in chronic and postoperative atrial fibrillation. Cardiovasc Res. 2002;54:397–404.
85. Workman AJ, Kane KA, Rankin AC. The contribution of ionic currents to changes in refractoriness of human atrial myocytes associated with chronic atrial fibrillation. Cardiovasc Res. 2001;52:226–35.
86. Kharche SR, Stary T, Colman MA, et al. Effects of human atrial ionic remodelling by β-blocker therapy on mechanisms of atrial fibrillation: a computer simulation. Europace. 2014;16:1524–33. https://doi.org/10.1093/europace/euu084.
87. Baruscotti M, Bucchi A, DiFrancesco D. Physiology and pharmacology of the cardiac pacemaker ("funny") current. Pharmacol Ther. 2005;107:59–79. https://doi.org/10.1016/j.pharmthera.2005.01.005.
88. Pogwizd SM, Bers DM. Cellular basis of triggered arrhythmias in heart failure. Trends Cardiovasc Med. 2004;14:61–6. https://doi.org/10.1016/j.tcm.2003.12.002.
89. del Monte F, Lebeche D, Guerrero JL, et al. Abrogation of ventricular arrhythmias in a model of ischemia and reperfusion by targeting myocardial calcium cycling. Proc Natl Acad Sci. 2004;101:5622–7. https://doi.org/10.1073/pnas.0305778101.
90. Hume JR, Duan D, Collier ML, et al. Anion transport in heart. Physiol Rev. 2000;80:31–81. https://doi.org/10.1152/physrev.2000.80.1.31.
91. Nagel G, Hwang T-C, Nastiuk KL, et al. The protein kinase A-regulated cardiac Cl– channel resembles the cystic fibrosis transmembrane conductance regulator. Nature. 1992;360:81–4. https://doi.org/10.1038/360081a0.
92. Mulvaney AW, Spencer CI, Culliford S, et al. Cardiac chloride channels: physiology, pharmacology and approaches for identifying novel modulators of activity. Drug Discov Today. 2000;5:492–505. https://doi.org/10.1016/S1359-6446(00)01561-0.
93. Tamargo J, Delpón E. Pharmacologic bases of antiarrhythmic therapy. In: Zipes D, Jalife J, editors. Cardiac electrophysiology:

from cell to bedside. 6th ed. Amsterdam: Saunders Elsevier; 2014. p. 533.

94. Brodde O-E, Bruck H, Leineweber K. Cardiac adrenoceptors: physiological and pathophysiological relevance. J Pharmacol Sci. 2006;100:323–37.
95. Penela P, Murga C, Ribas C, et al. Mechanisms of regulation of G protein-coupled receptor kinases (GRKs) and cardiovascular disease. Cardiovasc Res. 2006;69:46–56. https://doi.org/10.1016/j.cardiores.2005.09.011.
96. Reiken S, Wehrens XHT, Vest JA, et al. Beta-blockers restore calcium release channel function and improve cardiac muscle performance in human heart failure. Circulation. 2003;107:2459–66. https://doi.org/10.1161/01.CIR.0000068316.53218.49.
97. Page RL, Joglar JA, Caldwell MA, et al. 2015 ACC/AHA/HRS guideline for the management of adult patients with supraventricular tachycardia. Circulation. 2016;133 https://doi.org/10.1161/CIR.0000000000000311.
98. Priori SG, Blomström-Lundqvist C, Mazzanti A, et al. 2015 ESC guidelines for the management of patients with ventricular arrhythmias and the prevention of sudden cardiac death. Eur Heart J. 2015;36:2793–867. https://doi.org/10.1093/eurheartj/ehv316.
99. Blomström-Lundqvist C, Scheinman MM, Aliot EM, et al. ACC/AHA/ESC guidelines for the management of patients with supraventricular arrhythmias--executive summary. A report of the American college of cardiology/American heart association task force on practice guidelines and the European society of cardiology. J Am Coll Cardiol. 2003;42:1493–531.
100. Olshansky B, Sullivan RM. Inappropriate sinus tachycardia. J Am Coll Cardiol. 2013;61:793–801. https://doi.org/10.1016/j.jacc.2012.07.074.
101. Shirey-Rice JK, Klar R, Fentress HM, et al. Norepinephrine transporter variant A457P knock-in mice display key features of human postural orthostatic tachycardia syndrome. Dis Model Mech. 2013;6:1001–11. https://doi.org/10.1242/dmm.012203.
102. Fedorowski A, Li H, Yu X, et al. Antiadrenergic autoimmunity in postural tachycardia syndrome. EP Eur. 2017;19:1211–9. https://doi.org/10.1093/europace/euw154.
103. Li H, Yu X, Liles C, et al. Autoimmune basis for postural tachycardia syndrome. J Am Heart Assoc. 2014;3:e000755. https://doi.org/10.1161/JAHA.113.000755.

104. Arnold AC, Okamoto LE, Diedrich A, et al. Low-dose propranolol and exercise capacity in postural tachycardia syndrome: a randomized study. Neurology. 2013;80:1927–33. https://doi.org/10.1212/WNL.0b013e318293e310.
105. Sidhu B, Obiechina N, Rattu N, Mitra S. Postural orthostatic tachycardia syndrome (POTS). Case Rep. 2013;2013:bcr2013201244. https://doi.org/10.1136/bcr-2013-201244.
106. Grubb BP. Postural tachycardia syndrome. Circulation. 2008;117:2814–7. https://doi.org/10.1161/CIRCULATIONAHA.107.761643.
107. Saoudi N, Cosío F, Waldo A, et al. A classification of atrial flutter and regular atrial tachycardia according to electrophysiological mechanisms and anatomical bases; a statement from a Joint Expert Group from The Working Group of Arrhythmias of the European Society of Cardiology and the North American Society of Pacing and Electrophysiology. Eur Heart J. 2001;22:1162–82. https://doi.org/10.1053/euhj.2001.2658.
108. Porter MJ, Morton JB, Denman R, et al. Influence of age and gender on the mechanism of supraventricular tachycardia. Heart Rhythm. 2004;1:393–6. https://doi.org/10.1016/j.hrthm.2004.05.007.
109. Poutiainen AM, Koistinen MJ, Airaksinen KE, et al. Prevalence and natural course of ectopic atrial tachycardia. Eur Heart J. 1999;20:694–700.
110. Ko JK, Deal BJ, Strasburger JF, Benson DW. Supraventricular tachycardia mechanisms and their age distribution in pediatric patients. Am J Cardiol. 1992;69:1028–32.
111. Wren C. Incessant tachycardias. Eur Heart J. 1998;19(Suppl E):E32-6–54-9.
112. López-Sendón J, Swedberg K, McMurray J, et al. Expert consensus document on beta-adrenergic receptor blockers. Eur Heart J. 2004;25:1341–62. https://doi.org/10.1016/j.ehj.2004.06.002.
113. Arsura EL, Solar M, Lefkin AS, et al. Metoprolol in the treatment of multifocal atrial tachycardia. Crit Care Med. 1987;15:591–4.
114. Hazard PB, Burnett CR. Treatment of multifocal atrial tachycardia with metoprolol. Crit Care Med. 1987;15:20–5.
115. Schwartz M, Rodman D, Lowenstein SR. Recognition and treatment of multifocal atrial tachycardia: a critical review. J Emerg Med. 1994;12:353–60.

116. Hill GA, Owens SD. Esmolol in the treatment of multifocal atrial tachycardia. Chest. 1992;101:1726–8. https://doi.org/10.1378/chest.101.6.1726.
117. Brubaker S, Long B, Koyfman A. Alternative treatment options for atrioventricular-nodal-reentry tachycardia: an emergency medicine review. J Emerg Med. 2018;54:198–206. https://doi.org/10.1016/j.jemermed.2017.10.003.
118. Sung RJ, Blanski L, Kirshenbaum J, et al. Clinical experience with esmolol, a short-acting beta-adrenergic blocker in cardiac arrhythmias and myocardial ischemia. J Clin Pharmacol. 1986;26:A15–26. https://doi.org/10.1002/j.1552-4604.1986.tb02983.x.
119. Gupta A, Naik A, Vora A, Lokhandwala Y. Comparison of efficacy of intravenous diltiazem and esmolol in terminating supraventricular tachycardia. J Assoc Physicians India. 1999;47:969–72.
120. Issa ZF, John MM, Douglas ZP. Clinical arrhythmology and electrophysiology: a companion to braunwalds heart disease. 2nd ed. Amsterdam: Elsevier Saunders; 2012.
121. Granada J, Uribe W, Chyou P-H, et al. Incidence and predictors of atrial flutter in the general population. J Am Coll Cardiol. 2000;36:2242–6. https://doi.org/10.1016/S0735-1097(00)00982-7.
122. Platia EV, Michelson EL, Porterfield JK, Das G. Esmolol versus verapamil in the acute treatment of atrial fibrillation or atrial flutter. Am J Cardiol. 1989;63:925–9.
123. Schwartz M, Michelson EL, Sawin HS, MacVaugh H. Esmolol: safety and efficacy in postoperative cardiothoracic patients with supraventricular tachyarrhythmias. Chest. 1988;93:705–11.
124. January CT, Wann LS, Alpert JS, et al. 2014 AHA/ACC/HRS guideline for the management of patients with atrial fibrillation: executive summary: a report of the American College of Cardiology/American Heart Association Task Force on practice guidelines and the Heart Rhythm Society. Circulation. 2014;130:2071–104. https://doi.org/10.1161/CIR.0000000000000040.
125. Kirchhof P, Benussi S, Kotecha D, et al. 2016 ESC guidelines for the management of atrial fibrillation developed in collaboration with EACTS. Eur Heart J. 2016;37:2893–962. https://doi.org/10.1093/eurheartj/ehw210.
126. Anderson S, Blanski L, Byrd RC, et al. Comparison of the efficacy and safety of esmolol, a short-acting beta blocker, with

placebo in the treatment of supraventricular tachyarrhythmias. The Esmolol vs Placebo Multicenter Study Group. Am Heart J. 1986;111:42–8.

127. Plewan A, Lehmann G, Ndrepepa G, et al. Maintenance of sinus rhythm after electrical cardioversion of persistent atrial fibrillation; sotalol vs bisoprolol. Eur Heart J. 2001;22:1504–10. https://doi.org/10.1053/euhj.2000.2546.
128. Katritsis DG, Panagiotakos DB, Karvouni E, et al. Comparison of effectiveness of carvedilol versus bisoprolol for maintenance of sinus rhythm after cardioversion of persistent atrial fibrillation. Am J Cardiol. 2003;92:1116–9.
129. Lafuente-Lafuente C, Valembois L, Bergmann J-F, Belmin J. Antiarrhythmics for maintaining sinus rhythm after cardioversion of atrial fibrillation. Cochrane Database Syst Rev. 2015;3:CD005049. https://doi.org/10.1002/14651858.CD005049.pub4.
130. Dagres N, Lewalter T, Lip GYH, et al. Current practice of antiarrhythmic drug therapy for prevention of atrial fibrillation in Europe: the European Heart Rhythm Association survey. Europace. 2013;15:478–81. https://doi.org/10.1093/europace/eut063.
131. Brieger D, Amerena J, Attia J, et al. National Heart Foundation of Australia and the Cardiac Society of Australia and New Zealand: Australian clinical guidelines for the diagnosis and management of atrial fibrillation 2018. Heart Lung Circ. 2018;27:1209–66. https://doi.org/10.1016/j.hlc.2018.06.1043.
132. Devereaux P, Yang H, Yusuf S, et al. Effects of extended-release metoprolol succinate in patients undergoing non-cardiac surgery (POISE trial): a randomised controlled trial. Lancet. 2008;371:1839–47. https://doi.org/10.1016/S0140-6736(08)60601-7.
133. Fleisher LA, Fleischmann KE, Auerbach AD, et al. 2014 ACC/AHA guideline on perioperative cardiovascular evaluation and management of patients undergoing noncardiac surgery. Circulation. 2014;130:2215–45. https://doi.org/10.1161/CIR.0000000000000106.
134. Danelich IM, Lose JM, Wright SS, et al. Practical management of postoperative atrial fibrillation after noncardiac surgery. J Am Coll Surg. 2014;219:831–41. https://doi.org/10.1016/j.jamcollsurg.2014.02.038.
135. Bessissow A, Khan J, Devereaux PJ, et al. Postoperative atrial fibrillation in non-cardiac and cardiac surgery: an overview.

J Thromb Haemost. 2015;13:S304–12. https://doi.org/10.1111/jth.12974.
136. Arsenault KA, Yusuf AM, Crystal E, et al. Interventions for preventing post-operative atrial fibrillation in patients undergoing heart surgery. Cochrane Database Syst Rev. 2013; https://doi.org/10.1002/14651858.CD003611.pub3.
137. Burgess DC, Kilborn MJ, Keech AC. Interventions for prevention of post-operative atrial fibrillation and its complications after cardiac surgery: a meta-analysis. Eur Heart J. 2006;27:2846–57. https://doi.org/10.1093/eurheartj/ehl272.
138. Mathew JP, Fontes ML, Tudor IC, et al. A multicenter risk index for atrial fibrillation after cardiac surgery. JAMA. 2004;291:1720–9. https://doi.org/10.1001/jama.291.14.1720.
139. Blessberger H, Kammler J, Domanovits H, et al. Perioperative beta-blockers for preventing surgery-related mortality and morbidity. Cochrane Database Syst Rev. 2018; https://doi.org/10.1002/14651858.CD004476.pub3.
140. Rienstra M, Damman K, Mulder BA, et al. Beta-blockers and outcome in heart failure and atrial fibrillation. A meta-analysis. JACC Heart Fail. 2013;1:21–8. https://doi.org/10.1016/j.jchf.2012.09.002.
141. Kotecha D, Flather MD, Altman DG, et al. Heart rate and rhythm and the benefit of beta-blockers in patients with heart failure. J Am Coll Cardiol. 2017;69:2885–96. https://doi.org/10.1016/j.jacc.2017.04.001.
142. Cadrin-Tourigny J, Shohoudi A, Roy D, et al. Decreased mortality with beta-blockers in patients with heart failure and coexisting atrial fibrillation. JACC Heart Fail. 2017;5:99–106. https://doi.org/10.1016/j.jchf.2016.10.015.
143. Al-Khatib SM, Stevenson WG, Ackerman MJ, et al. 2017 AHA/ACC/HRS guideline for management of patients with ventricular arrhythmias and the prevention of sudden cardiac death. Circulation. 2018;138:e272–391. https://doi.org/10.1161/CIR.0000000000000549.
144. Ling Z, Liu Z, Su L, et al. Radiofrequency ablation versus antiarrhythmic medication for treatment of ventricular premature beats from the right ventricular outflow tract: prospective randomized study. Circ Arrhythm Electrophysiol. 2014;7:237–43. https://doi.org/10.1161/CIRCEP.113.000805.
145. Piccini JP, Hranitzky PM, Kilaru R, et al. Relation of mortality to failure to prescribe beta blockers acutely in patients with sustained ventricular tachycardia and ventricular fibrillation

following acute myocardial infarction (from the VALsartan in acute myocardial iNfarcTion trial [VALIANT] Registry). Am J Cardiol. 2008;102:1427–32. https://doi.org/10.1016/j.amjcard.2008.07.033.

146. Teo KK, Yusuf S, Furberg CD. Effects of prophylactic antiarrhythmic drug therapy in acute myocardial infarction. An overview of results from randomized controlled trials. JAMA. 1993;270:1589–95.
147. Nademanee K, Taylor R, Bailey WE, et al. Treating electrical storm: sympathetic blockade versus advanced cardiac life support-guided therapy. Circulation. 2000;102:742–7.
148. Kettering K, Mewis C, Dornberger V, et al. Efficacy of metoprolol and sotalol in the prevention of recurrences of sustained ventricular tachyarrhythmias in patients with an implantable cardioverter defibrillator. Pacing Clin Electrophysiol. 2002;25:1571–6. https://doi.org/10.1046/j.1460-9592.2002.01571.x.
149. Brodine WN, Tung RT, Lee JK, et al. Effects of beta-blockers on implantable cardioverter defibrillator therapy and survival in the patients with ischemic cardiomyopathy (from the Multicenter Automatic Defibrillator Implantation Trial-II). Am J Cardiol. 2005;96:691–5. https://doi.org/10.1016/j.amjcard.2005.04.046.
150. Freemantle N, Cleland J, Young P, et al. Beta blockade after myocardial infarction: systematic review and meta regression analysis. BMJ. 1999;318:1730–7. https://doi.org/10.1136/bmj.318.7200.1730.
151. Boutitie F, Boissel JP, Connolly SJ, et al. Amiodarone interaction with beta-blockers: analysis of the merged EMIAT (European Myocardial Infarct Amiodarone Trial) and CAMIAT (Canadian Amiodarone Myocardial Infarction Trial) databases. The EMIAT and CAMIAT investigators. Circulation. 1999;99:2268–75.
152. Cleland JGF, Bunting KV, Flather MD, et al. Beta-blockers for heart failure with reduced, mid-range, and preserved ejection fraction: an individual patient-level analysis of double-blind randomized trials. Eur Heart J. 2018;39:26–35. https://doi.org/10.1093/eurheartj/ehx564.
153. Packer M, Bristow MR, Cohn JN, et al. The effect of carvedilol on morbidity and mortality in patients with chronic heart failure. N Engl J Med. 1996;334:1349–55. https://doi.org/10.1056/NEJM199605233342101.

154. MERIT-HF Study Group. Effect of metoprolol CR/XL in chronic heart failure: Metoprolol CR/XL randomised intervention trial in congestive heart failure (MERIT-HF). Lancet. 1999;353:2001–7.
155. CIBIS-II Investigators and Committees. The Cardiac Insufficiency Bisoprolol Study II (CIBIS-II): a randomised trial. Lancet. 1999;353:9–13.
156. Cleophas TJ, Zwinderman AH. Beta-blockers and heart failure: meta-analysis of mortality trials. Int J Clin Pharmacol Ther. 2001;39:383–8.
157. Al-Gobari M, Khatib C El, Pillon F, Gueyffier F (2013) Beta-blockers for the prevention of sudden cardiac death in heart failure patients: a meta-analysis of randomized controlled trials. BMC Cardiovasc Disord 13:52. doi: https://doi.org/10.1186/1471-2261-13-52
158. Fauchier L, Pierre B, de Labriolle A, Babuty D (2007) Comparison of the beneficial effect of beta-blockers on mortality in patients with ischaemic or non-ischaemic systolic heart failure: a meta-analysis of randomised controlled trials. Eur J Heart Fail 9:1136–1139. doi: https://doi.org/10.1016/j.ejheart.2007.09.003.
159. Remme WJ, Cleland JG, Erhardt L, et al. Effect of carvedilol and metoprolol on the mode of death in patients with heart failure. Eur J Heart Fail. 2007;9:1128–35. https://doi.org/10.1016/j.ejheart.2007.07.014.
160. Corrado D, Wichter T, Link MS, et al. Treatment of arrhythmogenic right ventricular cardiomyopathy/dysplasia. Circulation. 2015;132:441–53. https://doi.org/10.1161/CIRCULATIONAHA.115.017944.
161. Marcus GM, Glidden DV, Polonsky B, et al. Efficacy of antiarrhythmic drugs in arrhythmogenic right ventricular cardiomyopathy. J Am Coll Cardiol. 2009;54:609–15. https://doi.org/10.1016/j.jacc.2009.04.052.
162. Ammirati E, Contri R, Coppini R, et al. Pharmacological treatment of hypertrophic cardiomyopathy: current practice and novel perspectives. Eur J Heart Fail. 2016;18:1106–18. https://doi.org/10.1002/ejhf.541.
163. Elliott PM, Anastasakis A, Borger MA, et al. 2014 ESC guidelines on diagnosis and management of hypertrophic cardiomyopathy: the task force for the diagnosis and management of hypertrophic cardiomyopathy of the European Society of

Cardiology (ESC). Eur Heart J. 2014;35:2733–79. https://doi.org/10.1093/eurheartj/ehu284.
164. Priori SG, Wilde AA, Horie M, et al. HRS/EHRA/APHRS expert consensus statement on the diagnosis and management of patients with inherited primary arrhythmia syndromes. Heart Rhythm. 2013;10:1932–63. https://doi.org/10.1016/j.hrthm.2013.05.014.
165. Schwartz PJ, Priori SG, Spazzolini C, et al. Genotype-phenotype correlation in the long-QT syndrome: gene-specific triggers for life-threatening arrhythmias. Circulation. 2001;103:89–95.
166. Rohatgi RK, Sugrue A, Bos JM, et al. Contemporary outcomes in patients with long QT syndrome. J Am Coll Cardiol. 2017;70:453–62. https://doi.org/10.1016/j.jacc.2017.05.046.
167. Abu-Zeitone A, Peterson DR, Polonsky B, et al. Efficacy of different beta-blockers in the treatment of long QT syndrome. J Am Coll Cardiol. 2014;64:1352–8. https://doi.org/10.1016/j.jacc.2014.05.068.
168. Chockalingam P, Crotti L, Girardengo G, et al. Not all beta-blockers are equal in the management of long QT syndrome types 1 and 2. J Am Coll Cardiol. 2012;60:2092–9. https://doi.org/10.1016/j.jacc.2012.07.046.
169. Roston TM, Yuchi Z, Kannankeril PJ, et al. The clinical and genetic spectrum of catecholaminergic polymorphic ventricular tachycardia: findings from an international multicentre registry. Europace. 2018;20:541–7. https://doi.org/10.1093/europace/euw389.
170. van der Werf C, Zwinderman AH, Wilde AAM. Therapeutic approach for patients with catecholaminergic polymorphic ventricular tachycardia: state of the art and future developments. Europace. 2012;14:175–83. https://doi.org/10.1093/europace/eur277.
171. Hayashi M, Denjoy I, Extramiana F, et al. Incidence and risk factors of arrhythmic events in catecholaminergic polymorphic ventricular tachycardia. Circulation. 2009;119:2426–34. https://doi.org/10.1161/CIRCULATIONAHA.108.829267.
172. Leren IS, Saberniak J, Majid E, et al. Nadolol decreases the incidence and severity of ventricular arrhythmias during exercise stress testing compared with β1-selective β-blockers in patients with catecholaminergic polymorphic ventricular tachycardia. Heart Rhythm. 2016;13:433–40. https://doi.org/10.1016/j.hrthm.2015.09.029.

173. Fonarow GC, Abraham WT, Albert NM, et al. Influence of beta-blocker continuation or withdrawal on outcomes in patients hospitalized with heart failure. J Am Coll Cardiol. 2008;52:190–9. https://doi.org/10.1016/j.jacc.2008.03.048.
174. Frishman WH. Beta-adrenergic blocker withdrawal. Am J Cardiol. 1987;59:26F–32F.
175. Psaty BM, Koepsell TD, Wagner EH, et al. The relative risk of incident coronary heart disease associated with recently stopping the use of beta-blockers. JAMA. 1990;263:1653–7.
176. Shammash JB, Trost JC, Gold JM, et al. Perioperative β-blocker withdrawal and mortality in vascular surgical patients. Am Heart J. 2001;141:148–53. https://doi.org/10.1067/mhj.2001.111547.
177. Wallace AW, Au S, Cason BA. Association of the pattern of use of perioperative β-blockade and postoperative mortality. Anesthesiology. 2010;113:794–805. https://doi.org/10.1097/ALN.0b013e3181f1c061.
178. Teichert M, de Smet PAGM, Hofman A, et al. Discontinuation of beta-blockers and the risk of myocardial infarction in the elderly. Drug Saf. 2007;30:541–9. https://doi.org/10.2165/00002018-200730060-00008.
179. Salpeter SR, Ormiston TM, Salpeter EE. Cardioselective beta-blockers for chronic obstructive pulmonary disease. Cochrane Database Syst Rev. 2005;4:CD003566. https://doi.org/10.1002/14651858.CD003566.pub2.
180. Conant J, Engler R, Janowsky D, et al. Central nervous system side effects of beta-adrenergic blocking agents with high and low lipid solubility. J Cardiovasc Pharmacol. 1989;13:656–61.
181. McAinsh J, Cruickshank JM. Beta-blockers and central nervous system side effects. Pharmacol Ther. 1990;46:163–97.
182. Heintzen MP, Strauer BE. Peripheral vascular effects of beta-blockers. Eur Heart J. 1994;15(Suppl C):2–7.
183. Paravastu SCV, Mendonca DA, da Silva A. Beta blockers for peripheral arterial disease. Cochrane Database Syst Rev. 2013;9:CD005508. https://doi.org/10.1002/14651858.CD005508.pub3.
184. Frishman WH, Clark AJB. Effects of cardiovascular drugs on plasma lipids and lipoproteins. In: Frishman WHSE, editor. Cardiovascular pharmacotherapeutics. New York: McGraw Hill; 1997. p. 1515–59.

185. Elliott WJ, Meyer PM. Incident diabetes in clinical trials of antihypertensive drugs: a network meta-analysis. Lancet. 2007;369:201–7. https://doi.org/10.1016/S0140-6736(07)60108-1.
186. Celik T, Iyisoy A, Kursaklioglu H, et al. Comparative effects of nebivolol and metoprolol on oxidative stress, insulin resistance, plasma adiponectin and soluble P-selectin levels in hypertensive patients. J Hypertens. 2006;24:591–6. https://doi.org/10.1097/01.hjh.0000209993.26057.de.
187. Lithell H, Andersson PE. Metabolic effects of carvedilol in hypertensive patients. Eur J Clin Pharmacol. 1997;52:13–7.
188. Fogari R, Zoppi A, Poletti L, et al. Sexual activity in hypertensive men treated with valsartan or carvedilol: a crossover study. Am J Hypertens. 2001;14:27–31.
189. Wassertheil-Smoller S, Oberman A, Blaufox MD, et al. The trial of antihypertensive interventions and management (TAIM) study. Final results with regard to blood pressure, cardiovascular risk, and quality of life. Am J Hypertens. 1992;5:37–44.
190. Solomon H, Man JW, Wierzbicki AS, Jackson G. Relation of erectile dysfunction to angiographic coronary artery disease. Am J Cardiol. 2003;91:230–1.
191. Gür Ö, Gurkan S, Yumun G, Turker P. The comparison of the effects of nebivolol and metoprolol on erectile dysfunction in the cases with coronary artery bypass surgery. Ann Thorac Cardiovasc Surg. 2017;23:91–5. https://doi.org/10.5761/atcs.oa.16-00242.
192. Brixius K, Middeke M, Lichtenthal A, et al. Nitric oxide, erectile dysfunction and beta-blocker treatment (MR NOED study): benefit of nebivolol versus metoprolol in hypertensive men. Clin Exp Pharmacol Physiol. 2007;34:327–31. https://doi.org/10.1111/j.1440-1681.2007.04551.x.
193. van Nueten L, Taylor FR, Robertson JI. Nebivolol vs atenolol and placebo in essential hypertension: a double-blind randomised trial. J Hum Hypertens. 1998;12:135–40.

# Chapter 5
# Modulation of Calcium Handling: Calcium-Channel Modulators

**Erol Tülümen and Martin Borggrefe**

## L-Type $Ca^{2+}$ Channels: Verapamil and Diltiazem

### *Electrophysiological Properties. Differences*

Several calcium channels (L, N, T, P, Q and R) were identified in humans. Of these channels, voltage-sensitive L-type and T-type calcium channels are mainly operative in cardiovascular system. There are five classes of calcium channel blocking drugs: phenylalkylamines, dihydropyridines, benzothiazepines, diphenylpiperazines, and a diarylaminopropylamine. Clinically available calcium channel blockers are dihydropyridines, benzothiazepines and phenylalkylamines. These calcium channel

E. Tülümen (✉) · M. Borggrefe
Department of Medicine, University Medical Center Mannheim, Mannheim, Germany

German Center for Cardiovascular Research (DZHK), Partner Site Heidelberg/Mannheim, Mannheim, Germany
e-mail: erol.tueluemen@umm.de



A. Martínez-Rubio et al. (eds.), *Antiarrhythmic Drugs*, Current Cardiovascular Therapy,
https://doi.org/10.1007/978-3-030-34893-9_5

blockers (CCB) are selective and inhibit voltage–sensitive L-type slow calcium channels mediated calcium influx in cardiac myocytes and in smooth muscle by slowing the activation of the L-type calcium channel and also delay its recovery from inactivation. To show its effect, the drugs travel through the slow channel and bind to channel from the inner side of the membrane. They bind more effectively when the channels are in open and in inactivated state and reduce opening frequency of the channels. Verapamil and diltiazem block calcium channels in use (frequency)-dependent (effect is more apparent at faster rates) and in voltage-dependent fashion (more effective blockage in depolarized fibers).

Whereas phenylalkilamines are relatively selective for myocardial cells, dihydropyridines are relatively selective for smooth muscle cells, especially in arterial beds. Benzothiazepine CCB (diltiazem) has an intermediate effect between phenylalkylamine and dihydropyridines in their selectivity for vascular and myocardial cells (Table 5.1).

As sinus node/AV node cells and working myocardial cells have different electrophysiological properties, verapamil and diltiazem (non-dihydropyridine CCB, ND-CCB) exert different effects on nodal cells, fibers and working myocardial cells. By blocking calcium current through L-Type channel ($I_{CaL}$) in nodal cells, ND-CCBs reduce maximum diastolic potential, the slope of spontaneous diastolic depolarization in phase 4, and maximal action potential amplitude of phase 0. Thus, ND-CCBs prolong conduction time and refractory periods of the AV node (prolonged AH interval and lengthened AV nodal anterograde/retrograde refractory periods). Nevertheless, ND-CCBs show no effect on atrial and ventricular activation time, i.e. P wave duration, HV interval and QRS duration (ND-CCBs do not have a significant effect on action potential amplitude, V max of phase 0, resting membrane voltage or refractoriness of atrial, myocardial working cells as well as purkinje fibers as these cells have fast-response characteristics related to $I_{Na}$) [1].

However, ND-CCBs by blocking $I_{Ca}$ in Phase 2 and 3 reduces the plateau height of the action potential in phase 2,

TABLE 5.1 Selectivity of calcium channel blockers

| | **Arterial vasodilation** | **Negative inotropy** | **Sinus node depression** | **AV node depression** |
|---|---|---|---|---|
| Dihydropiridine CCB (e.g. Nifedipine) | ↑↑↑↑↑ | ↑ | 0 or reflex tachycardia | Neutral |
| Diltiazem | ↑↑↑ | ↑↑ | ↑↑↑↑↑ | ↑↑↑↑↑ |
| Verapamil | ↑↑↑↑ | ↑↑↑↑ | ↑↑↑↑↑ | ↑↑↑↑↑ |

Dihydropyridine CCB (nifedipine) is the most selective for arterial vasodilatation, while diltiazem and verapamil have more effects on the heart (negative inotropy, sinus node and AV node depression) may shorten the action potential slightly in all cardiac fibers, and prolong the it slightly in Purkinje fibers. Verapamil suppresses triggered activity by reducing diastolic calcium load and hence early and late afterdepolarizations [1].

Verapamil is a racemic mixture of d- and l-isomer of verapamil. D-isomer of verapamil shows to some extent $I_{Na}$ blocking effect, therefore some anaesthetic activity. Clinical effect of verapamil is through the l-isomer of verapamil. Verapamil may also block the alfa receptors and increase the vagal effect on AV node. As verapamil does not block beta receptors, reflex sympathetic stimulation that occurs as a response to peripheral vasodilation and transient hypotension (by $I_{CaL}$ blockage of smooth muscle cells) may diminish its direct effect on sinus node (slowing the sinus rate).

Similar to working myocardium, ND-CCBs have no direct effect on refractoriness of accessory pathways. Moreover, via reflex sympathetic stimulation they may enhance the conduction over the accessory pathway in patients with Wolff-Parkinson-White syndrome (along with direct AV-Nodal blocking effect, verapamil may increase ventricular response over the accessory pathway during atrial fibrillation).

## *Pharmacokinetics*

ND-CCBs can be administered per os or by the intravenous route. Both of the drugs show high first-pass effect, high plasma protein binding, and extensive hepatic metabolism. Although enteral absorption of these drugs is almost complete, bioavailability of ND-CCBs is substantially reduced (~20–35% for verapamil and ~40% for diltiazem) by high first pass effect and extensive hepatic metabolism. The begin of the effect of these drugs by oral administration depends on formulation. Diltiazem and verapamil are available in a variety of preparations from different manufacturers, and those preparations may have different pharmacokinetics. Therefore, dosing may vary depending on type of preparation and manufacturer. The first effect of conventional tablets is usually seen in 30–60 min, however the beginning of effect and peak effect are delayed in slow releasing, long acting forms. The peak effect of intravenous administration is within first 15 min. ND-CCBs are extensively bound to plasma proteins (70–85% for diltiazem and 90% for verapamil). They are metabolized rapidly and almost completely in liver into several active and inactive metabolites via CYP enzyme system (mainly via CYP3A4). Principal metabolite of diltiazem is desacetyldiltiazem (20% of the effect of diltiazem), and major metabolite of verapamil is norverapamil (20% of the effect of verapamil). Half-life of ND-CCBs is between 2 and 11 h and is prolonged in elderly, in patients with hepatic disease, or when they are administered repeatedly due to saturation of hepatic enzymes. Excretion is for mainly in urine as metabolites (>70%); and approximately 2–4% of a dose is excreted unchanged (Table 5.2).

## *Adverse Effects, Drug Interactions and Contraindications*

Most of the adverse effects of ND-CCBs are due to the extension of their pharmacological effects.

*Cardiac side effects:* Excessive inhibition of calcium influx in SA node, AV node and myocardial cells can cause serious bradycardia, atrioventricular block, cardiac depression, heart failure and cardiac arrest. Concomitant use of other cardiodepressant drugs like β-blocking drugs increase the susceptibility to side effects and also the severity of side effects.

*Extracardiac side effects:* Extracardiac side effects are usually rare. The most commonly reported side effects are constipation, dizziness, and headache.

TABLE 5.2 Pharmacokinetics of verapamil and diltiazem

| | **Verapamil** | **Diltiazem** |
|---|---|---|
| Absorption (oral, %) | >90 | >90 |
| Bioavailability (%) | 20–35 | 40 |
| Onset of action[a], oral (min) | 90–120 | <30 |
| Peak effect[a], h | 1–6 | 2–4 |
| Protein binding (%) | 90 | 70–85 |
| Plasma half-life, h[b] | 4–8 | 3–4 |
| Distribution volume (Lt/kg) | 5.0 ± 2.1 | 3.3 ± 1.2 |
| Metabolism | 80% first pass effect, active metabolites | 60% first pass effect |
| Active metabolite | Nor-verapamil | Desacetyldiltiazem, N-Desmethyldiltiazem |
| Excretion (%) | | |
| Renal | 70 (3–4% unchanged) | 35(2–4% unchanged) |
| Fecal | 16 | 65 |

[a]Onset of action and peak effect depend on the formulation of drug. Diltiazem is available in a range of formulations, including standard (onset of action 15 min, peak plasma concentrations after 2–4 h, and plasma t1/2 of 3–4 h) and longer-acting (peak plasma concentrations approximately 8–11 h after dosing, and average plasma t1/2 of 6–8 h). With verapamil, the time to maximal concentration is ~80–90 min with the immediate-release; and ~7–8 h with modified-release preparations

[b]Plasma half-life of verapamil increases during long term administration

*Verapamil*

- Very common (10% or more): Headache
- Common (1–10%): Dizziness, lethargy, constipation (particularly in the elderly up to 10%), dyspepsia, nausea, diarrhoea, flatulence
- Uncommon (0.1–1%): Abdominal discomfort/pain, oedema.
- Rare: gynecomastia, reversible hepatic impairment, paresthesia, gingival hyperplasia, erythromelalgia, hyperprolactinemia.

*Diltiazem:* generally mild side effects.

- Common (1–10%): Headache, fatigue, tiredness/malaise, accidental injury, pain, scalp irritation, rash
- Rare: gingival hyperplasia, exfoliative dermatitis, angioneurotic edema, erythema multiforme, vasculitis, transient increased liver transaminases

## Drug Interactions

ND-CCBs are frequently administered concomitantly with other medications (antihypertensive drugs, vasodilators etc.). ND-CCBs may affect absorption, distribution, metabolism, and excretion of concomitant drug, and may interact with drug transport proteins (Table 5.3).

Concomitant use of CYP3A4 inducers (e.g. carbamazepine, phenytoin, rifampicin) may reduce plasma levels and CYP3A4 inhibitors (e.g. ketoconazole, itraconazole, ritonavir, erythromycin, fluoxetine, valproic acid, cimetidine, other CCBs, HIV protease inhibitors, grapefruit juice) may increase verapamil's plasma levels. Therefore, caution is advised when administered concomitantly with such drugs.

Similarly, due to competitive inhibition of CYP3A4 with ND-CCBs may lead to an increase of plasma levels of other CYP3A4 metabolized drugs (e.g. cyclosporin, tacrolimus, ketoconazole, carbamazepine, sildenafil).

TABLE 5.3 Drug interactions with verapamil

| Mechanism of interaction | Tissue distribution | Substrates |
|---|---|---|
| Drugs absorption and elimination via MDR1 (ABCB1, P-gp1): *Verapamil inhibits P-gp and affects oral absorption and renal excretion of the listed drugs*[a] | Liver<br>Kidney<br>Intestine<br>BBB<br>BTB<br>BPB | Amitriptyline, Amiodarone, Amprenavir, Anticancer agents, Apixaban, Atorvastatin, Cefoperazone, Chorambucil, Chlorpromazine, Cimetidine, Ciprofloxacin, Cisplatin, Clarithromycin, Colchicine, Cyclosporine, Dabigatran, Dexamethasone, Digoxin, Diltiazem, Domperidone, Doxorubicin, Erythromycin, Edoxaban, Estradiol, Etoposide, Fentanyl, Fexofenadine, Grepafloxacin, Hydrocortisone, Imatinab mesylate, Indinavir, Itraconazole, Ketoconazole, Lansoprazole, Levofloxacin, Lidocaine, Loperamide, Losartan, Lovastatin, Methadone, Methotrexate, Methylprednisolone, Morphine, Nadolol, Nelfinavir, Norfloxacin, Nortriptyline, Ondansetron, Omeprazole, Pantoprazole, Phenytoin, Pravastatin, Propranolol, Progesterone, Quinidine, Ranitidine, Ritonavir, Rivaroxaban, Rhodamine 123, Saquinavir, Tacrolimus, Testosterone, Timolol, Trimethoprim, Verapamil, Vincristine |

Table 5.3 (continued)

| Mechanism of interaction | Tissue distribution | Substrates |
|---|---|---|
| Metabolism of drugs via CYP3A4: *Verapamil is a moderate inhibitor of CYP3A4, it decreases the metabolism of the listed drugs and thus increases the plasma level and clinical effect*[a] | Liver | Alprazolam, Amiodarone, Atorvastatin, Buspirone, Carbamazepine, Cisapride, Clarithromycin, Cyclosporine, Dapsone, Dihydropyridine calcium, channel blockers, Diltiazem, Efavirenz, Erythromycin, Ergot alkaloids, Estrogens, Fentanyl, Lovastatin, Midazolam, Nefazodone, Phosphodiesterase, inhibitors, Pioglitazone, Prednisolone, Progesterone, Protease Inhibitors, Quinidine, (R)-, Warfarin, Rifampin, Sertraline, Sirolimus, Simvastatin, Tacrolimus, Testosterone, Trazadone, Triazolam |
| Pharmacodynamical interactions: *Verapamil potentiates the effects of drugs with similar pharmacodynamics* | Heart | Beta blockers, Digoksin, Amiodarone, Clonidine, Alfa Adrenergic Blockers, Disopyramide, Neuromuscular Blocking Agents |

*P-glycoprotein 1* (permeability glycoprotein, P-gp) also known as multidrug resistance protein 1 (*MDR1*) or ATP-binding cassette sub-family B member 1 (*ABCB1*) or cluster of differentiation 243 (*CD243*). It is an important protein of the cell membrane that pumps (ATP-dependent efflux pump with broad substrate specificity) many foreign substances out of cells. *BBB* blood-brain barrier, *BPB* blood-placental barrier, *BTB* blood-testis-barrier

[a]The list does not represent all of the drugs metabolized via CYP3A4

Combination of ND-CCBs with drugs that exert similar effects may potentiate effect of these drugs. This combination (e.g. combination of ND-CCBs with beta blockers, antiarrhythmic drugs or cardiac glycosides) may pose an increased risk of deep bradycardia, heart block, hypotension and/or decreased cardiac contractility, congestive heart failure. ND-CCBs increase the depression of cardiac contractility, conduction and automaticity and the vasodilatation produced by general anesthetics, or effect of neuromuscular blocking agent.

ND-CCBs increase the plasma levels of quinidine, lovastatin, atorvastatin, simvastatin, increase the risk of lithium toxicity. Verapamil is also an inhibitor of P-glycoprotein that decreases the clearance of digoxin and increases its plasma levels (50–75%); thus, the maintenance dose of digoxin should be reduced to avoid the risk of bradycardia or AV block. Unlike verapamil, diltiazem does not interact with digoxin. New oral anticoagulants (dabigatran, rivaroxaban, apixaban, edoxaban) are substrates of P- glycoprotein, thus concomitant verapamil treatment can affect the bioavailability of these drugs (i.e. increase of plasma concentrations). Interaction between verapamil and new oral anticoagulants can be minimized if NOACs are administered 2 h prior to verapamil; or alternatively dose reduction of NOAC (dabigatran and edoxaban) should be considered.

Elevated serum calcium levels due to high doses of vitamin D and/or high intake of calcium salts may reduce the response to diltiazem.

Verapamil may increase blood alcohol concentrations and prolong its effects.

## Pregnancy

There are no well controlled studies with ND-CCBs in pregnant or in breastfeeding women. In animal studies, CCBs were shown to have some teratogenic effects. Therefore,

ND-CCBs are classified as *pregnancy category C* by FDA. Thus, during the pregnancy or breastfeeding period ND-CCBs should only be used if the potential benefits to the pregnant woman outweigh any possible risks to the foetus.

## *Clinical Uses*

### Treatment and Prophylaxis of Paroxysmal SVT and Control of Ventricular Rate in Atrial Flutter/ Atrial Fibrillation

Intravenous verapamil or diltiazem may be used in hemodynamically stable supraventricular tachycardias (SVT) either for rate control or to terminate the tachycardia (class IIa indication, level of evidence B) [2]. ND-CCBs have been shown to successfully terminate SVTS in 64–98% of patients [2]. These agents are especially helpful in patients who cannot tolerate beta blockers or have recurrence after conversion with adenosine. Diltiazem and verapamil should not be used in patients with suspected systolic heart failure.

In patients with broad complex tachycardias, it is critical to distinguish SVT with aberrant conduction (or SVT with pre-existing bundle brunch block) from ventricular tachycardia or pre-excitation. The administration of intravenous verapamil or diltiazem in patients with either VT or a pre-excited AF may lead to hemodynamic compromise or may accelerate the ventricular rate and lead to ventricular fibrillation.

#### Parenteral (in Acute Treatment)

*Diltiazem:* 0.25 mg/kg over 2 min (under monitoring of blood pressure and ECG); may be repeated after 15 min (0.25–0.35 mg/kg over 2 min) or maintenance dose: 5–15 mg/h IV.

*Verapamil:* 5–10 mg (0.075–0.15 mg/kg) over 2 min; may be repeated after 30 min as 10 mg (0.15 mg/kg) over 2 min.

Oral

Verapamil (Immediate release tablets): 240–480 mg/day in 3 or 4 divided doses.

## Treatment of Hypertension

In the contemporary guidelines for the management of high blood pressure, calcium channel blockers are referred as first line therapy along with ACE inhibitors/Angiotensin receptor blockers, diuretics (and beta blockers) [3]. However, guidelines essentially refer to long acting dyhidropyridine–CCBs (vasoselective CCBs) rather than verapamil or diltiazem. Verapamil or diltiazem is mostly used as an alternative to beta blockers in patients who have contraindications to beta blockers or cannot tolerate beta blockers.

Diltiazem

*Extended Release Capsules*

- Initial dose: 120–240 mg orally once a day
- Maintenance dose: 120–540 mg orally once a day
- Maximum dose: 540 mg/day

*Extended Release Coated Capsules*

- Initial dose: 180–240 mg orally once a day, increasing the dose as needed
- Maintenance dose: 240–360 mg orally once a day
- Maximum dose: 480 mg/day

*Extended Release Tablets*

- Initial dose: 180–240 mg orally once a day, increasing the dose as needed
- Maximum dose: 540 mg/day

Verapamil

*Immediate Release Tablets*

- Initial dose: 40–80 mg orally three times a day
- Maintenance dose: If adequate response is not obtained with the initial dose, dose may be titrated upward to max. dose of 480 mg/day

*Extended Release Capsules*

- Initial dose: 100–200 mg orally once a day (preferentially at bedtime)
- Maintenance dose: If adequate response is not obtained with the initial dose, dose may be titrated upward to max. dose of 400 mg/day.

*Extended Release Tablets*

- Initial dose: 180 mg orally once a day (preferentially at bedtime)
- Maintenance dose: If adequate response is not obtained with the initial dose, dose may be titrated upward to max. dose of 480 mg/day

*Sustained Release Capsules*

- Initial dose: 120–240 mg orally once a day (preferentially in the morning)
- Maintenance dose: If adequate response is not obtained with the initial dose, dose may be titrated upward to max. dose of 480 mg/day

*Sustained Release Tablets*

- Initial dose: 120–180 mg orally once a day (preferentially in the morning with food)
- Maintenance dose: If adequate response is not obtained with the initial dose, dose may be titrated upward to max. dose of 480 mg/day

Verapamil SR is also available as a fixed combination with trandolapril for treatment of arterial hypertension.

## Treatment of Chronic Stable and Vasospastic Angina Pectoris

ND-CCBs are effective in patients with angina acting by relieving coronary vasoconstriction, lowering heart rate, negative inotropic effect and peripheral vasodilatation [1]. Verapamil has been approved for all kind of anginas (effort, vasospastic, unstable). Compared to beta blockers, verapamil has similar anti-anginal effect in patients with chronic stable angina, however with less new diabetes, fewer angina attacks and less psychological depression. Diltiazem has similar effect like verapamil with more favorable side-effect profile. There is no study comparing the antianginal effect of verapamil with diltiazem.

Combination of ND-CCBs with beta blockers should be avoided due to increased risk of heart block, sinus bradycardia, and heart failure. ND-CCBs should not be used in patients with stable angina and left ventricular dysfunction. Beta blocker may be combined with dyhidropyridine CCBs like amlodipine, long acting nifedipine, felodipine, lacidipine or lercanidipine.

### Dosis

*Diltiazem*

*Immediate Release Tablets*

- Initial dose: 30 mg orally four times a day (before meals and bedtime), increasing gradually every 1–2 days until the optimal response is attained
- Maintenance dose: 180–360 mg orally per day in divided doses (3–4 times a day)

*Extended Release Capsules*

- Initial dose: 120–180 mg orally once a day, increase the dose every 7–14 days as needed
- Maximum dose: 540 mg/day

*Extended Release Coated Capsules*

- Initial dose: 120–180 mg orally once a day, increase the dose every 7–14 days as needed
- Maximum dose: 480 mg/day

*Extended Release Tablets*

- Initial dose: 180 mg orally once a day, increase the dose every 7–14 days as needed
- Maximum dose: 360 mg/day

*Verapamil*

*Immediate Release Tablets*

- Initial dose: 40–120 mg orally three times a day
- Maintenance dose: If adequate clinical response is not obtained with the initial dose, dose may be titrated upward to max. dose of 480 mg/day

*Extended Release Tablets*

- Initial dose: 180 mg orally once a day (preferentially at bedtime)
- Maintenance dose: If adequate response is not obtained with the initial dose, dose may be titrated upward to max. dose of 480 mg/day

Contraindications

- Cardiogenic shock, severe hypotension, HF, AMI with pulmonary congestion.
- LV Dysfunction (LVEF <40%), severe aortic stenosis
- 2nd and 3d-degree AV block, sick sinus syndrome, SA block, or severe sinus bradycardia (in patients without pacemaker)
- Atrial fibrillation or atrial flutter associated with an accessory pathway
- Hypersensitivity to drug
- Pregnancy and lactation (relative contraindication)

## Modulation of Abnormal $Ca^{2+}$ Homeostasis/Cycling

### *Abnormal $Ca^{2+}$ Homeostasis/Cycling and Arrhythmia Risk*

Calcium ions are plays important role not only in generation of action potential but also in excitation-contraction coupling and in various other cellular processes through calcium regulated enzymes or calcium sensitive ion channels. Disorders of calcium handling (either due to dysfunction of calcium channels or due to dysfunction in regulatory proteins) result in disorders in depolarization, in repolarization and also calcium overload in myocardial cells.

Calcium ions play a pivotal role in excitation-contraction coupling. Cardiac excitation-contraction coupling is initiated by opening of voltage dependent $Na^+$ channels, which mediates an influx of $Na^+$ ions and depolarizes the myocytes membrane. The action potential spreads along the membranes of transvers tubules (T-Tubules) to the interior of muscle fiber. Depolarization of cell membrane activates voltage-gated (slow) L-type $Ca^{2+}$ channels during phase 1 and especially phase 2 of action potential and allow inward $Ca^{2+}$ current which creates plateau in the action potential. These "trigger $Ca^{2+}$" ions bind to ryanodine receptor in the sarcoplasmic reticulum (storage organelle of calcium ions) membrane and induce "$Ca^{2+}$-induced $Ca^{2+}$ release" of the sarcoplasmic reticulum [4]. The T-tubules of cardiac muscle, are much more developed and have five times greater diameter than that of the skeletal muscle T-tubules, however sarcoplasmic reticulum is less well developed. Therefore, the strength of contraction depends to a great extent on the concentration of calcium ions in the T-tubules (i.e. extracellular fluid). Sudden 500-fold increase of cytosolic $Ca^{2+}$ concentration induces the contraction of myofilaments by binding of calcium to the troponin C. In heart muscle, calcium pulse lasts longer than skeletal muscle and is about 300 ms. At the end of phase 2, L-type $Ca^{2+}$ channels are inactivated and influx of calcium ions ends abruptly. Subsequently, calcium ions rapidly pumped out of the sarcoplasm back into the sarcoplasmic reticulum (re-uptake via sarco–/–endoplasmic reticulum calcium-ATPase, SERCA) and T-tubule (via sodium-calcium exchanger and Na/K-ATPase). The removal of calcium ions from sarcoplasm is an energy dependent (active) process.

Abnormal calcium homeostasis appears in various cardiac diseases like chronic heart failure, myocardial ischemia, left ventricular hypertrophy, or channelopathies and plays crucial role in development or arrhythmias. Up- or down regulation of channels, dysfunctions (functional or structural) in any of those channels or in regulatory proteins lead to "calcium-leak" or "calcium sparks" which triggers early (EAD) and delayed afterdepolarizations (DAD). EADs and DADs represent a substantial function in triggering of arrhythmias [5, 6].

## *SERCA2a, NCX, RyR2 Channels*

### Sarcoplasmic/Endoplasmic Reticulum Calcium ATPase (SERCA2a)

In cardiac muscle, the removal of intracellular calcium from sarcoplasm is essential part of the regulation of cardiac contractility. After contraction of myofilaments, calcium ions are pumped out from sarcoplasm, and maintaining low cytosolic calcium concentration relies upon SERCA (into SR) and plasma membrane calcium ATPase and $Na^{+}/Ca^{2+}$ Exchanger-NCX (into extracellular fluid) pumps.

There are three human SERCA genes encoding up to ten isoforms of calcium channels. The SERCA1 isoform is specific for the SR in fast-twitch skeletal muscle. SERCA2 has been found in the SR of slow-twitch skeletal muscle and in other tissues. The SERCA2a isoform is expressed in the SR of cardiac muscle. SERCA2b is the major isoform expressed in smooth muscle and non-muscle tissues and also has a housekeeping function (essential for most mammalian cells). SERCA2a may play a role in the pathogenesis of cardiac hypertrophy and failure. SERCA2a activity is regulated by phospholamban.

The function of SERCA is controlled by the regulatory protein phospholamban (PLB/PLN). PLB operates as a subunit and inhibits SERCA. Increased β-adrenergic stimulation via cAMP induced protein kinase A pathway phosphorylates the PL and due to increased phosphorylation reduces the association between SERCA and PLB. Phosphorylation of PL leads to dissociation of PLB, interrupts the inhibition and hence increases the SERCA mediated calcium transport. Another regulatory protein is calcium binding protein calsequestrin. Calsequestrin is located in SR and helps the SR to store an extraordinarily high amount of calcium ions by binding 18–50 $Ca^{2+}$ ions to each molecule of calsequestrin. As Calsequestrin binds calcium ions with very low affinity, they can also easily be released back to sarcoplasm. Reduction of free calcium concentration within the SR enhances the pump function of SERCA by decreasing the high concentration gradient between sarcoplasm and SR. Phosphorylation of calsequestrin increases the calcium binding capacity of calsequestrin nearly twofold. Under pathological circumstances SERCA2 can also be regulated by microRNAs (miR-25 suppresses SERCA2 in heart failure).

Experimental inhibitor of SERCA is thapsigargin and experimental stimulator is istaroxime.

SERCA3 is expressed in many tissues. SERCA3 is associated with the relaxation of vascular smooth muscle and may also play a role in insulin secretion in beta cell through the regulation of calcium signalling.

## Natrium/Calcium Exchanger (NCX)

NCX is a dimeric transporter of ten transmembrane helices. It is an antiporter membrane protein that removes calcium from sarcoplasm. It uses the energy that is stored in the large concentration gradient of sodium (higher concentrations in extracellular fluid) by allowing sodium to flow down across the plasma membrane into sarcoplasm and in exchange counter transport calcium ions into extracellular fluid. The NCX removes a single calcium ion in exchange for the import of three sodium ions.

NCX may reverse direction of flow along with the changes in sodium gradient. Most of the time NCX is in the $Ca^{2+}$ efflux position. Nevertheless, during the upstroke of the cardiac action potential there is a large influx of Na ions and results in a large increase in intracellular sodium for a very short of time. This causes the reversal of the flow via NCX (pump sodium ions out of the cell and $Ca^{2+}$ ions into the cell). Subsequent activation of L-type calcium channel and influx of $Ca^{2+}$ results in rise of sarcoplasmic calcium concentration and NCX returns to its calcium efflux position.

Na/K-ATPase indirectly contributes to calcium homeostasis. It rectifies the sodium influx by pumping actively sodium ions out of sarcoplasm and prevents the increase of sodium concentration.

Several pathological conditions may abnormally switch the NCX to reverse the flow in $Ca^{2+}$ influx position. (1) Higher internal sodium than usual (when cardiac glycoside blocks Na/K -ATPase pump, which results in an increase of sarcoplasmic $Na^{+}$ concentration) (2) the sarcoplasmic reticulum release of calcium is inhibited (results in a decrease in sarcoplasmic calcium concentration) (3) other calcium influx channels are inhibited (results in a decrease in sarcoplasmic $Ca^{2+}$ concentration) (4) when the action potential duration is prolonged.

## RyR2 Channels

Ryanodine receptors (RyRs) are huge intracellular calcium channels [7]. RyR2 is the cardiac ryanodine receptor and consists of high molecular weight homotetramer. Each monomer has at least six transmembrane segments to form the pore region of the channel and also a large cytoplasmic regulatory domain that serves as a docking platform for multiple regulatory proteins and enzymes (including calmodulin, the FK506-binding protein FKBP12.6/calstabin2, protein kinase A, CaM-dependent kinase II, protein phosphatases 1 and 2A, phosphodiesterase, junctin, triadin, and calsequestrin).

RyRs take part in different signalling pathways in different tissues. In cardiac muscle, cardiac isoform (RyR2) plays a crucial role in excitation contraction coupling by mediating major calcium release from the intracellular calcium store, the sarcoplasmic reticulum (other minor source of calcium ions is the extracellular fluid largely via $I_{CaL}$). The depolarization of cell membrane activates voltage-gated L-type $Ca^{2+}$ channels and leads inward calcium current ($I_{CaL}$). As calcium ions are primary physiological ligand of RyRs, calcium binding to ryanodine receptor triggers the opening of RyRs and thus induces enormous "calcium-induced calcium release".

RyR2 activity is also modulated by multiple other subunit proteins and enzymes. Caffeine, low concentration of ryanodine (<10 μM) or cyclic ADP-ribose activate the channel. On the contrary, magnesium, ruthenium red, or higher concentrations of ryanodine (≥100 μM) inhibit the channel. In muscle cells, calcium-free calmodulin (apoCalmodulin) activates the RyR channel, and calcium bound calmodulin inhibits the channel. Phosphorylation of the RyR by cAMP-dependent protein kinase and by Calcium/calmodulin-dependent protein kinase II dissociates FKBP12 or FKBP12.6 from the RyR complex. When by FKBP12 or FKBP12.6 is dissociated from the FKBP-RyR complex, the RyR2 channel is activated.

Furthermore, calcium release from RyR has been shown to regulate ATP production in heart and pancreas cells.

The mutations of RyR2 and its regulatory proteins are shown to be associated with catecolaminergic polymorphic ventricular arrhythmias and sudden cardiac death.

## *Arrhythmogenic Substrate Is Disease-Specific: AF, HF, Channelopathies*

### Atrial Fibrillation (AF)

AF is a complex, multifactorial arrhythmia. Major arrhythmogenic mechanisms are ectopic activity (as a trigger and driver of AF) and re-entry (different types of functional and/or structural re-entries, play role in maintenance of AF). Abnormal calcium handling plays critical role not only in promoting the ectopic activity, but also facilitating the maintenance of atrial fibrillation by enhancing the re-entry [8]. Rapid atrial rate during AF causes several progressive structural (increased fibrosis, cellular disarray etc.) and functional changes (further alterations in calcium handling, abbreviated AP duration and wavelength, changes in cellular physiology etc.) as well. Abnormal calcium handling is pivotal in AF pathophysiology by enhancing AF, and as a mediator which leads to functional and structural changes of AF (AF begets AF).

Focal ectopic activities in atria are mostly due to DADs (i.e. triggered activity). DADs are oscillations of the membrane potential occurring after phase 3 of action potential. DADs are results mainly from spontaneous diastolic SR calcium releases through RyR2, which increases cytoplasmic calcium levels and hence activates NCX and generates depolarizing transient-inward current. When transient-inward current sufficiently depolarizes the membrane potential, voltage-gated sodium channels are activated and a triggered action potential is generated. Initially, DADs occur as result of increased SR calcium load and higher RyR2-protein expression. Thereafter, additionally functional and structural changes occur (like increase in CaMKII-dependent RyR2 phosphorylation, reduced activity of protein phosphatase 1, reduced levels of regulatory proteins like sarcolipin and FKBP12.6, and increased calcium sensitivity and expression of NCX) which further increase the susceptibility to cellular DADs.

Re-entry is facilitated by shortening of effective refractory period and slowing in atrial conduction. At initial phase of AF, high atrial rate related cellular calcium overload reduces inward calcium current through L-type calcium channels (LTCC) to protect cell from cytotoxic calcium overload which results in action potential shortening and wavelength abbreviation. Reduction of inward calcium current may result from calcium-dependent reduction in gene expression, from posttranslational modifications like LTCC hypophosphorylation and from calpain-mediated breakdown of channel subunits. Through several calcium dependant pathways, density of the inward rectifier kalium current $IK_1$ and the acetylcholine-dependent inward-rectifier kalium current ($IK_{ACh}$) are also increased which in turn further shorten action potential duration and cause a more negative resting membrane potential, thereby increasing atrial excitability and facilitate the formation of rotors.

Moreover, re-entry is also enhanced by fibroblast-to-myofibroblast transition and myofibroblast proliferation which is triggered through several calcium dependant pathways as well.

## Heart Failure

Calcium is the pivotal intracellular mediator between sarcolemmal action potential and myofilament activation, contraction and relaxation. Apart from excitation contraction coupling, calcium is crucial for physiological stress adaptation. A higher diastolo-systolic calcium gradient increases force generation and cardiac output. In heart failure, independent from the cause of myocardial injury, several compensatory mechanisms like myocardial hypertrophy, increasing the filling pressure and activation of neuro-hormonal pathways are activated to overcome the depressed cardiac function. However, a chronic hyperactivation of neuro-hormonal pathways contributes to progressive maladaptive remodelling of the heart, progressive deterioration of pump function, and arrhythmias. These maladaptive responses are associated with abnormal intracellular calcium metabolism, and show important similarities beyond the reason of heart failure (decreased calcium transients, enhanced diastolic SR calcium leak and diminished SR calcium sequestration, that lead to defective excitation contraction coupling i.e. impaired contractility and relaxation) [9]. Despite preserved calcium influx current density through L-type calcium channel, the ability of any given calcium current to activate SR calcium sparks (i.e. impaired calcium induced calcium release) was significantly diminished which leads to reduction in yield of excitation contraction coupling (ECC). Along with reduced SR calcium release via RyR2 and subsequent reduced calcium re-uptake and sequestration via SERCA2a, there is an increase in open probability of RyR2 and SR diastolic calcium leak. Elevated diastolic calcium level further contribute to reduced contractile force generation, impaired relaxation, and abnormal force–frequency relationship.

In addition, due to chronic hyperadrenergic state, desensitization of beta-adrenoreceptors and thus reduced global intracellular cAMP synthesis occur. Alterations of second messenger system leads to alterations in expression and functions of regulatory proteins (like calmodulin-dependent protein kinase II, Protein kinase A, protein kinase C, Calcineurin, and S100A1) [10]. The ratio of phospholamban to SERCA2 is increased and contributes to increased diastolic calcium levels and cardiac dysfunction. Furthermore, due to the changes in the expression and function of NCX and SERCA2, there is a shift toward increased outward calcium current via NCX to the extracellular space and a net decrease in SR calcium re-uptake.

Beside electrical remodelling, there is a structural remodelling (structural changes of the T-tubules, SR storage organelles, and/or the architecture of the dyads) as well which contributes to defective EC coupling by altering the geometry of the calcium release unit.

## *Channelopathies*

### Catecholaminergic Polymorphic Ventricular Tachycardia (CPVT)

CPVT is an inherited arrhythmia syndrome characterized by physical or emotional stress triggered polymorphic ventricular tachycardia in patients with structurally normal hearts. CPVT is caused by mutations in RyR2 or CASQ2 which result in defective intracellular/sarcoplasmic calcium handling [11, 12]. Two forms of CPVT have been described resulting from mutations in either the RyR2 or CASQ2. Mutations in RyR2 (CPVT type 1) are identified in about half of the patients with CPVT and are inherited in an autosomal dominant form. Mutations in CASQ2 (CPVT type 2) are inherited in autosomal recessive pattern and found only 1–2% of patients with CPVT. Some other rare mutations in other genes (such as Ank2, TRDN and CALM1) related to intracellular calcium handling have also been identified in patients with clinical features similar to CPVT.

Mutations in CPVT-1 cause a gain of function in the RyR, and mutations in CASQ2 result in a decreased calcium binding affinity leading to higher levels of free SR calcium which triggers store-overload induced calcium release. As a result, mutations in these two genes precipitate diastolic calcium leak into sarcoplasma under adrenergic stimulation. Increased amount of diastolic calcium leads to an activation of the NCX resulting in a depolarizing positive inward current that induces delayed afterdepolarizations (DAD), triggered activity, premature ventricular beats and bidirectional/polymorphic VT. Corresponding to the intensity of exercise, the complexity of arrhythmias will increase from single ventricular extrasystoles (mostly polymorphic) to bidirectional VT or to polymorphic VT.

## Brugada Syndrome/Short QT Syndrome

Brugada syndrome is a rare genetic disease, characterized by coved type ST-segment elevations in the right precordial leads, increased risk of fatal ventricular arrhythmias and sudden cardiac death. Short QT syndrome is also rare genetic disease characterized by very short QT intervals on ECG, increased risk of fatal ventricular arrhythmias and sudden cardiac death. In 2007, two missense mutations in the CACNA1C (A39V and G490R) and one in the CACNB2

(S481L) which are encoding the alpha1- and beta2b-subunits of the L-type calcium channel were reported in patients with Brugada pattern ECG and short QT interval (QTc < 360 s) [13]. Both mutations result in a loss of function of Cav1.2 that leads to diminished depolarizing inward calcium in plateau phase, shortening of the action potential (short QT phenotype) and loss of the action potential dome (Brugada syndrome phenotype).

In 2011, a loss-of-function mutation in the CACNA2D1 (nucleotide c.2264G > C; amino acid p. Ser755Thr), the gene encoding Cav$\alpha$2$\delta$-1 subunit of calcium channel was found in a patient with short QT interval and documented VF.

## Long QT Syndrome (LQTS 8, Timothy Syndrome)

Long QT syndrome is rare genetic disease which causes abnormal, prolonged repolarization and thus increased risk of fatal arrhythmias. The Timothy Syndrome (TS) is a rare, autosomal dominant inherited form of the LQTS and is classified as LQTS type 8. In TS, gain of function mutations of the gene CACNA1c (chromosome 12p13.33) which encodes the calcium channel Cav1.2 (voltage-dependent L-type calcium channel subunit alpha-1C) is responsible for prolongation of action potential [14]. The mutations result in reduced Cav1.2 channel inactivation, which leads to sustained depolarizing inward calcium currents during the plateau phase and thus prolonged plateau phase and action potential (prolonged QT interval). This prolongation in turn leads to increased risk of spontaneous, abnormal secondary depolarizations (after-depolarizations), lethal arrhythmias, and sudden death. Since the calcium channel Cav1.2 is highly expressed in many tissues like brain, patients with TS have many cardiac (QT prolongation, congenital heart diseases like patent ductus arteriosus, patent foramen ovale, hypertrophic or dilated cardiomyopathy, bradycardia, atrioventricular block) and also extracardiac manifestations (syndactyly, craniofacial findings like low-set ears, depressed nasal bridge, premaxillary underdevelopment, baldness at birth, as well as intermittent hypoglycemia, immune deficiency, autism spectrum disorders and language, motor, and generalized developmental delays).

## *Modulation of Abnormal $Ca^{2+}$ Homeostasis*

- $Ca^{2+}$ channel blockers (diltiazem, verapamil): mechanism of action, clinical uses

Mechanism of action and clinical uses of NDCCB are discussed in details in previous chapter.

- RyR2 blockers/stabilizers, dantrolene, rycals, CaMKII inhibitors, SERCA2a, Flecainide

### RyR2 Blockers/Stabilizers

Dysfunctions or dysregulations of ryanodine receptors in heart (RyR2) cause fatal arrhythmias and is involved in heart failure, whereas dysfunctions in ryanodine receptors in skeletal muscle (RyR1) result in malignant hyperthermia and myopathies like central core or minicore myopathy.

Mutations, defective regulation and distorted subunit composition of ryanodine channels cause diastolic calcium leakage from the sarcoplasmic reticulum, which in turn triggers arrhythmias and weaken cardiac contractility. Hence, modulation of RyR2 mediated abnormal calcium homestasis have emerged as a potential therapeutic target for arrhythmias. Pharmacological agents known to modulate RyR2 are listed in Table 5.4 [15].

Ryanodine is a plant alkaloid, which binds with high affinity and specificity to its receptor in the SR (ryanodine receptor has been named after this alkaloid). RyR2 has both a high- and low-affinity binding site for ryanodine, which are responsible for the concentration dependent effects of ryanodine on the activity of RyR. At nanomolar concentrations ryanodine increases the open probability without affecting

TABLE 5.4 RyR2 modulating agents

| **Agonists** | **Antagonists** |
|---|---|
| Purine derivatives (caffeine)[a] | Ruthenium red[b] |
| Digitalis glycosides (digoxin)[a] | Dantrolene[a] |
| Suramin[a] | Ryanoids (ryanodine)[a,b] |
| Volatile anesthetics (halothane)[a] | Local anesthetics (tetracaine)[b] |
| 4-Chloro-m-cresol (4-CMC)[a] | 1,4-Benzothiazepines (JTV519/ K201)[c] |
| Peptide toxins (IpTx)[a] | |
| Macrocyclic compounds (FK506)[c] | |

[a]Modulators of channel gating
[b]Modulators of ion translocation
[c]Allosteric modulator subunit interactions

rates of ion movement, at submicromolar concentrations locks the RyR, and increases open probability to almost 100%, leads to a long-lasting subconductance (~50% of the normal conductance), however at micromolar concentration fully closes them and inhibits SR calcium release.

Ruthenium red, is a water-soluble dye that inhibit SR calcium release from both the cytosolic and luminal sides of the channel. As ruthenium red is neurotoxic, it is not an ideal candidate for drug development.

Charged local anaesthetics (tertiary amines like procaine, tetracaine, and lidocaine or quaternary amines like QX572, QX314) also inhibit RyR2 channels. Procaine appears to be more selective for RyR2 compared to RyR1. They show their effects by stabilizing RyR2 in a closed transformational state and decrease the open probability of the channels (tetracaine and procaine), or by voltage dependent blockade of channels and reduce the conductance without an effect on open probality of channel (lidocaine and quaternary amines).

## Dantrolene

Dantrolene is a hydantoin derivative used for the treatment of malignant hyperthermia and is the only currently approved drug for clinical use [16]. In skeletal muscle, 10–100 micromolar dantrolene inhibits abnormal calcium release from the SR. The sensitivity to dantrolene to RyR2 is lower than RyR1. Dantrolene prevents aberrant calcium release by stabilizing interdomain interactions within the RyR2.

## Stabilizers of Calsitabin-RyR2 Complex (1,4-Benzothiazepines Derivatives/Rycals)

Rycals are JTV519, S44121/Arm036 and S107. They stabilize the interaction between inhibitory subunit calstabin2 (FK506 binding protein 12.6, FKBP12.6) and hyperphosphorylated RyR2 (closed conformational state), reduce the channel-opening probability, and hence prevent arrhythmgenetic diastolic calcium leak, contractile dysfunction and calcium overload [17]. JTV519 prevents triggered ectopic activity triggered by a SR calcium leak through FKBP12.6-depleted RyR2 in ventricular and in pulmonary vein cardiomyocytes. Nonetheless, JTV519 also blocks voltage-gated sodium, voltage gated L-type calcium, and kalium channels (Ikr, Ik1, IAch) and its effectiveness in treatment of clinical arrhythmias is yet uncertain.

## CaMKII Inhibitors

KN-93 is a potent and specific inhibitor of calcium/calmodulin-dependent protein kinase II (CaMKII). Dysregulation of CaMKII pathway is considered to be associated not only with arrhythmias but also with Alzheimer's disease and Angelman syndrome. In hearts, CaMKIIδ enhances calcium current via L-type channels by augmentation of peak calcium influx and slowed inactivation of the calcium current, thus it may act pro-arrhythmic by triggering early afterdepolarizations (EADs).

### SERCA2a Activator (N106)

In heart failure, activity and expression of the cardiac sarcoplasmic reticulum calcium ATPase (SERCA2a) is characteristically decreased. The small ubiquitin-like modifier type 1 (SUMO-1) is a regulator of SERCA2a and SUMOylation of SERCA2a improves its function. N106 is a small molecule that directly activates the SUMO-activating enzyme and consequently increases SUMOylation of SERCA2a.

### Flecainide/Propafenone

Flecainide and propafenone are class Ic antiarrhythmics and blocks sodium channels. However, both of these drugs also block the open state of RyR2, prevent diastolic calcium leak, and hence supress DADs and triggered arrhythmias [18]. Furthermore, their sodium channel blocking properties also contribute to RyR2 blocking effect by preventing DADs reaching to threshold potential and trigger premature beats.

## Medical Treatment of Inherited Cardiac Arrhythmias Syndromes Associated to Mutations in Calcium Handling

### *Idiopathic VT*

Ventricular tachycardias in structurally normal hearts are mostly focal in origin and underlying mechanisms are triggered activity, abnormal automaticity, or rarely re-entry within the Purkinje fibers. Idiopathic VTs most commonly originate from the RV outflow tract. Other locations of focal idiopathic VTs include the LV outflow tract, aortic cusps, mitral and tricuspid annuli, papillary muscles. Treatment options for idiopathic VTs are catheter ablation and medical therapy. Medical therapy may be indicated in patients with mild to moderate symptoms. As the underlying mechanism mostly is cAMP-mediated EADs or DADs, medical treatment include beta-blockers, verapamil, diltiazem (rate of efficacy of 20 to 50%) that supress cAMP mediated pathways and triggered activity. Alternative therapy includes class IA, IC and III agents.

## *CPVT*

CPVT is resulted from mutations in RyR2 or CASQ2 which result in stress induced diastolic calcium leak into sarcoplasma and DADs mediated triggered activity. Medical treatment includes β-blockers, verapamil, or a combination of both to reduce diastolic calcium and to prevent DADs. In addition, ryanodine channel blocker flecainide and sympathetic denervation may be added to therapy in some patients who are refractory to β-blocker/verapamil therapy.

## *Brugada/Short QT Overlap Syndrome*

Quinidine is the only drug used in long term medical treatment of Brugada/Short QT Syndrome. Although quinidine is class I antiarrhythmic agent (blockers of the fast inward sodium current), it also displays inhibitory effect on the slowly inactivating, tetrodotoxin-sensitive Na current, slow inward calcium current (ICa), rapid (IKr) and slow ($I_{Ks}$) components of the delayed potassium rectifier current, inward potassium rectifier current ($I_{KI}$), the ATP-sensitive potassium channel ($I_{KATP}$) and Ito.

## *Long QT Syndrome Type 8*

In long QT syndrome 8, there is a progressive prolongation of action potential duration and QT interval, induction of DADs, and both DAD and EADs-mediated triggered activities due to gain of function mutations of the calcium channel

Cav1.2. Antiarrhythmic treatment includes β-blocker, verapamil, mexilatine, and ranolazine to maintain repolarization stability and to prevent DADs and EADs.

## References


1. Thomas Michel BH. Calcium channel antagonists. In: Knollman LBBCB, editor. Goodman & Gilman's the pharmacological basisi of therapeutics. 12th ed. New York: McGraw Hill; 2011. p. 755–60.
2. Page RL, Joglar JA, Caldwell MA, Calkins H, Conti JB, Deal BJ, et al. 2015 ACC/AHA/HRS guideline for the management of adult patients with supraventricular tachycardia: executive summary: a report of the American College of Cardiology/American Heart Association Task Force on Clinical Practice Guidelines and the Heart Rhythm Society. Circulation. 2016;133(14):e471–505.
3. James PA, Oparil S, Carter BL, Cushman WC, Dennison-Himmelfarb C, Handler J, et al. 2014 evidence-based guideline for the management of high blood pressure in adults: report from the panel members appointed to the eighth Joint National Committee (JNC 8). JAMA. 2014;311(5):507–20.
4. Fabiato A. Calcium-induced release of calcium from the cardiac sarcoplasmic reticulum. Am J Phys. 1983;245(1):C1–14.
5. Milberg P, Fink M, Pott C, Frommeyer G, Biertz J, Osada N, et al. Blockade of I(Ca) suppresses early afterdepolarizations and reduces transmural dispersion of repolarization in a whole heart model of chronic heart failure. Br J Pharmacol. 2012;166(2):557–68.
6. Cheng H, Lederer WJ. Calcium sparks. Physiol Rev. 2008;88(4):1491–545.
7. Fleischer S, Ogunbunmi EM, Dixon MC, Fleer EA. Localization of Ca2+ release channels with ryanodine in junctional terminal cisternae of sarcoplasmic reticulum of fast skeletal muscle. Proc Natl Acad Sci U S A. 1985;82(21):7256–9.
8. Heijman J, Voigt N, Nattel S, Dobrev D. Cellular and molecular electrophysiology of atrial fibrillation initiation, maintenance, and progression. Circ Res. 2014;114(9):1483–99.
9. Lehnart SE, Maier LS, Hasenfuss G. Abnormalities of calcium metabolism and myocardial contractility depression in the failing heart. Heart Fail Rev. 2009;14(4):213–24.

10. Gorski PA, Ceholski DK, Hajjar RJ. Altered myocardial calcium cycling and energetics in heart failure--a rational approach for disease treatment. Cell Metab. 2015;21(2):183–94.
11. Priori SG, Napolitano C, Tiso N, Memmi M, Vignati G, Bloise R, et al. Mutations in the cardiac ryanodine receptor gene (hRyR2) underlie catecholaminergic polymorphic ventricular tachycardia. Circulation. 2001;103(2):196–200.
12. Lahat H, Pras E, Olender T, Avidan N, Ben-Asher E, Man O, et al. A missense mutation in a highly conserved region of CASQ2 is associated with autosomal recessive catecholamine-induced polymorphic ventricular tachycardia in Bedouin families from Israel. Am J Hum Genet. 2001;69(6):1378–84.
13. Antzelevitch C, Pollevick GD, Cordeiro JM, Casis O, Sanguinetti MC, Aizawa Y, et al. Loss-of-function mutations in the cardiac calcium channel underlie a new clinical entity characterized by ST-segment elevation, short QT intervals, and sudden cardiac death. Circulation. 2007;115(4):442–9.
14. Splawski I, Timothy KW, Sharpe LM, Decher N, Kumar P, Bloise R, et al. Ca(V)1.2 calcium channel dysfunction causes a multisystem disorder including arrhythmia and autism. Cell. 2004;119(1):19–31.
15. Santonastasi M, Wehrens XH. Ryanodine receptors as pharmacological targets for heart disease. Acta Pharmacol Sin. 2007;28(7):937–44.
16. Mickelson JR, Louis CF. Malignant hyperthermia: excitation-contraction coupling, Ca2+ release channel, and cell Ca2+ regulation defects. Physiol Rev. 1996;76(2):537–92.
17. Kaneko N, Matsuda R, Hata Y, Shimamoto K. Pharmacological characteristics and clinical applications of K201. Curr Clin Pharmacol. 2009;4(2):126–31.
18. Hilliard FA, Steele DS, Laver D, Yang Z, Le Marchand SJ, Chopra N, et al. Flecainide inhibits arrhythmogenic Ca2+ waves by open state block of ryanodine receptor Ca2+ release channels and reduction of Ca2+ spark mass. J Mol Cell Cardiol. 2010;48(2):293–301.

# Chapter 6
# Other Antiarrhythmic Drugs

**Juan Tamargo**

In previous chapters of this book several authors analyze in detail the antiarrhythmic drugs (AADs) classified in groups I-IV according to the Vaughan-Williams classification. However, some old (adenosine, digoxin) and new AADs (ivabradine, ranolazine, vernakalant) were not listed in any of the original four classes. Therefore, in this chapter, I shall review the electrophysiological effects of these drugs (Table 6.1). Their electrophysiological and pharmacokinetic properties, adverse effects, doses drug interactions, cautions, contraindications and clinical indications are summarized in Tables 6.2, 6.3, 6.4, 6.5, 6.6, and 6.7.

J. Tamargo (✉)
Department of Pharmacology, School of Medicine, Universidad Complutense, CIBERCV, Madrid, Spain
e-mail: jtamargo@med.ucm.es



A. Martínez-Rubio et al. (eds.), *Antiarrhythmic Drugs*, Current Cardiovascular Therapy,
https://doi.org/10.1007/978-3-030-34893-9_6

TABLE 6.1 Other antiarrhythmic drugs

1. Adenosine

- Adenosine A1 receptor agonists: Capadenoson (AF, angina), Selodenoson (AF, discontinued), Tecadenoson (PSVT, AF)
- Other: Neladenoson bialanate (HF with reduced ejection fraction), Regadenoson (pharmacologic stress testing)

2. Cardiac glycosides: Digoxin, Digitoxin

3. Atrial-selective blocking drugs: Ranolazine, Vernakalant

4. Selective $I_f$ blockers: Ivabradine

5. Other drugs:

- GAP junction modifiers: Rotigaptide (GAP486, ZP123: discontinued), Danegaptide (GAP134, ZP1609: AF, myocardial reperfusion injury)
- $Na^+$-$Ca^{2+}$-exchanger inhibitors: KB-R7943, SEA0400, SN-6, YM-244769

*AF* atrial fibrillation, *HF* heart failure, *PSVT* paroxysmal supraventricular tachycardia

## Adenosine

Adenosine is a ubiquitous endogenous purine nucleoside. Activation of $G_{i/o}$ protein–bound cardiac adenosine A1 receptors present in atrial muscle, sino-atrial (SAN) and atrio-ventricular nodal (AVN) cells [1–3]: (a) activates the acetylcholine-gated inward rectifying $K^+$ current ($I_{KACh}$/$I_{KAdo}$) that hyperpolarizes the membrane potential, slows SAN pacemaker rate and shortens atrial action potential duration (APD) and refractoriness. (b) Inhibits the mixed $Na^+$-$K^+$ inward pacemaker current ($I_f$) generated via non-selective hyperpolarization-activated cyclic nucleotide-gated cation (HCN) channels, which regulates the rate of the spontaneous depolarization of the SAN cells. (c) Reduces adenyl cyclase activity and intracellular cAMP levels, which indirectly inhibits the L-type calcium current

Table 6.2 Effect of antiarrhythmic drugs on ECG parameters and cardiac effective refractory periods

| Drug | RR | PR | QRS | QTc | JT | ARP | VRP | AVNRP |
|---|---|---|---|---|---|---|---|---|
| Adenosine[a] | –/then + | + | 0 | 0 | 0 | – | 0 | + |
| Digoxin | 0/+ | + | 0/+ | 0/– | 0 | – | 0/– | + |
| Ivabradine | + | 0 | 0 | 0 | 0 | 0 | 0 | 0 |
| Ranolazine | 0 | 0 | 0 | 0/+ | 0 | + | + | 0 |
| Vernakalant[a] | 0/+ | 0 | 0/+ | 0 | 0 | + | 0 | 0 |

RR, PR and QRS intervals of the ECG. ARP, VRP and AVNRP: atrial, ventricular and atrio-ventricular refractory periods. PRVAcc: refractory period of the accessory pathway

0: unchanged, –: decrease, +: increase

[a]Changes are transient and values return to normal within 30 s (adenosine) or 2 h (vernakalant)

Table 6.3 Pharmacokinetic properties

| Drug | F (%) | $T_{max}$ (h) | PPB (%) | Vd (L/kg) | $t_{1/2}$ (h) | Excretion H/R (%) | Dose |
|---|---|---|---|---|---|---|---|
| Adenosine (IV) | 100 | – | – | – | <10 s | Red blood cells | Rapid IV bolus of 6 mg (1–2 s) followed by saline flush (≤3 mg in patients taking verapamil, diltiazem, β-blockers or dipyridamole, or in the elderly). Another bolus of 12 mg after 1–2 min; this 12 mg bolus can be repeated in 1–2 min if SVT persist. Pediatric dosing: 0.1–0.3 mg/kg |
| Digoxin (oral/IV) | 60–75 | PO: 3–6<br>IV: 1–3 | 25 | 4 | 35 (30–48; up to 3–5 days in CKD) | 25/75 | • IV: 0.5–1 mg over 12–24 h in divided doses depending on age, lean body weight and renal function. Half of the total dose given as the first dose; further doses should be given by IV infusion over a period of 10–20 minutes at intervals of 4–8 h. Maximum loading dose: 8–12 mcg/kg given at 6–8-h intervals<br>• Oral: (1) loading: 0.5–1 mg, with additional 0.125–0.25 mg tid for 1 day; (2) maintenance: 0.125–0.375 mg od (0.0625 mg in renal impairment) |

| | | | | | | | |
|---|---|---|---|---|---|---|---|
| Digitoxin (oral) | 95 | 1 | >90 | 0.61 | 6–9 days | 75/25 | IV bolus: 0.4–0.6 mg. Oral: 0.05–0.3 mg/day |
| Ivabradine[a] (oral) | 40 | 1–1.5 | 70 | 1.3 | 11 | 95/5[b] CYP3A4 | 2.5–7.5 mg bid |
| Ranolazine (oral) | 35–55 | 4–6 | 65 | 2.5 | 7 | 25/75 (5[b]) CYP3A4 (70–85%) CYP2D6 (10–15%) | Initial dose 375 mg bid. The dose should be titrated to a maximum dose of 750 mg bid (EMA) or 1000 mg bid (FDA) |
| Vernakalant (IV) | – | 1–5 min | 45–60 | 2.3 | 3–5.5 | 7/93 CYP2D6 | 3 mg/kg IV over 10 min. Then, 2 mg/kg over 10 min after waiting for 15 min. If conversion does not occur within 15 min, a second 10-min infusion of 2 mg/kg can be administered |

*CKD* chronic kidney disease, *F* oral bioavailability, *h* hours, *H* hepatic/biliar, *IV* intravenous, *min* minutes, *PPB* protein plasma binding, *R* renal, *s* seconds, *SVT* supraventricular tachycardia, *t1/2* drug half-life, *Tmax* time to peak plasma levels, *Vd* volume of distribution

[a]Off-label use

[b]Renal excretion without biotransformation

TABLE 6.4 Most common adverse effects

| | |
|---|---|
| Adenosine | • >10%: Flushing, shortness of breath/dyspnea<br>• 1–10%: Headache, chest pressure, light-headedness, nausea, sweating, palpitations, hypotension, bronchospasm. Seizures in susceptible patients. In patients with asthma or COPD adenosine-induced bronchospam may last more than 30 min<br>• Sinus pauses, AV block and atrial/ventricular extrasystoles immediately after conversion that can reinitiate PSVT or degenerate to AF, sustained or non-sustained VT |
| Digoxin<br>Digitoxin | • Gastrointestinal (anorexia, nausea, vomiting, abdominal pain), neurological (headache, fatigue, dizziness, drowsiness), ocular (blurred and colored vision), psychiatric (disorientation, mental confusion, depression), rash<br>• Supraventricular or ventricular tachyarrhythmias and bradyarrhythmias (bradycardia, heart block), coronary steal<br>• At plasma levels >2 ng/mL digoxin is toxic, produces proarrhythmia and can aggravate HF, particularly with co-existent hypokalemia. However, symptoms can appear at lower levels |
| Ivabradine | • Phosphenes, diplopia; bradycardia, sinus arrest and heart block, palpitations, AF; hypotension. Dizziness, fatigue |
| Ranolazine | • Dyspepsia, anorexia; tinnitus; bradycardia, palpitations, hypotension; hyperhydrosis. Small increases in serum creatinine without changing the glomerular filtration rate. QTc prolongation (6–15 ms) but cases of torsades de pointes are very rare |
| Vernakalant | • Dysgeusia, sneezing, paresthesias, nausea, cough, pruritus, hypotension, bradycardia, complete AV block, AF/AFl, PVCs, non-sustained VT |

*AF* atrial fibrillation, *AFl* atrial flutter, *AV* atrio-ventricular, *COPD* chronic obstructive pulmonary disease, *HF* heart failure, *PSVT* paroxysmal supraventricular tachycardia, *PVCs* premature ventricular beats, *VT* ventricular tachycardia

Table 6.5 Drug interactions, cautions and contraindications

| Drug | Drug interactions | Cautions | Contraindications |
|---|---|---|---|
| Adenosine | Digoxin, BBs, diltiazem or verapamil potentiate the bradycardiac and/or hypotensive effects. Dipyridamole inhibits the reuptake of adenosine and potentiates its effects (lower doses needed). Methylxanthines (theophylline, caffeine) antagonize its effects (higher doses needed). Higher degrees of heart block with carbamazepine. Any influence of recent intake of caffeinated beverages is disputed | It should only be used with full resuscitative equipment available. Immediate drug discontinuation in the presence of angina, severe bradycardia, hypotension, respiratory failure or cardiac arrest. Adenosine may trigger convulsions in susceptible patients. Patients who develop high-level AV block at a particular dose should not be given further dosage increments. Atrial flutter because of the risk of 1:1 conduction and serious VT | Symptomatic bradycardia, sick sinus syndrome, second- or third-degree AV block (in absence of pacemaker), known pre-excitation, long QT syndrome, severe hypotension, decompensated HF, severe bronchospasm or asthma, ACS or <2–4 days after an acute MI. Tachycardia with a wide QRS complex (unless the diagnosis of SVT with aberrancy is certain). Concomitant use of dipyridamole. Discontinue adenosine in patients who develop severe respiratory difficulties |

(continued)

Table 6.5 (continued)

| Drug | Drug interactions | Cautions | Contraindications |
|---|---|---|---|
| Digoxin | See Table 6.6<br>Monitor SDC with clarithromycin, cyclosporine, erythromycin, flecainide, itraconazole, posaconazole, propafenone, verapamil or voriconazole. Reduce the dose of digoxin when coadministered with amiodarone (30%–50%) or dronedarone (50%) | Advanced age, renal failure, hypokalemia, hypercalcemia, hypoxemia, hypothyroidism, severe myocarditis, amyloidosis and acute MI increase digitalis-related arrhythmias. Lower doses in hypothyroidism; higher doses in hyperthyroidism. Withheld digoxin for 24 h before cardioversion | Digitalis toxicity. Intermittent complete heart block or second-degree AV block, especially if there is a history of Stokes-Adams attacks, bradycardia or sick sinus syndrome (in absence of pacemaker). Hypertrophic obstructive cardiomyopathy, unless there is concomitant atrial fibrillation and HF. Supraventricular arrhythmias associated with a known or suspected accessory AV pathway (WPW); VPCs, VT and/or VT; arrhythmias caused by cardiac glycoside intoxication. Severe hypokalemia. IV digoxin in the early-phase of MI. High SDC associated with increased risk of death |

| | | | |
|---|---|---|---|
| Ivabradine | The risk of bradycardia increases when coadministered with amiodarone, BBs, verapamil or diltiazem. Potent CYP3A4 inhibitors and inducers markedly increased or decreased ivabradine plasma levels, respectively | Avoid use with verapamil or diltiazem. Patients with hypotension, retinitis pigmentosa and moderate hepatic or severe renal impairment. Ivabradine-induced bradycardia is a risk factor for QT prolongation. With moderate CYP3A4 inhibitors: initial dose of 2.5 mg if resting heart rate is above 70 bpm, with monitoring of heart rate. | Heart rate <60 bpm, sick sinus syndrome, sino-atrial block, third-degree AV block, AF, acute MI, unstable angina, cardiogenic shock, unstable or acute HF, severe hypotension (<90/50 mmHg), severe hepatic impairment. Avoid potent CYP3A4 inhibitors/inducers and QT prolonging drugs. Pregnancy, lactation and women of child-bearing potential not using appropriate contraceptive measures |
| Ranolazine | Potent CYP3A4 inhibitors/inducers increase/decrease ranolazine exposure, respectively. Potent CYP2D6 inhibitors may increase ranolazine plasma levels. | The dose should be limited to 500 mg bid in patients treated with moderate CYP3A inhibitors. Careful dosing in patients with mild-moderate renal impairment (crCl <60 mL/min), mild hepatic impairment and HF (NYHA class III–IV). | Coadministration of potent CYP3A4 inhibitors/inducers or with class I or class III anti-arrhythmics other than amiodarone Pre-existing QT prolongation, co-administration of QT-prolonging drugs, severe renal impairment (crCL <30 mL/min), moderate-severe hepatic impairment, treatment with QTc-prolonging drugs |

(continued)

Table 6.5 (continued)

| Drug | Drug interactions | Cautions | Contraindications |
|---|---|---|---|
| Vernakalant | No formal interaction studies have been conducted | Hypotension, hypertrophic obstructive, restrictive cardiomyopathies, or constrictive pericarditis, advanced hepatic impairment and HF (NYHA class I or II) due to the higher risk of hypotension and ventricular arrhythmias. Hypotension responds to drug discontinuation and intravenous fluid administration | Severe aortic stenosis, SBP <100 mmHg, NYHA class III–IV HF, recent (<30 days) ACS (including MI), basal QT >440 ms, severe bradycardia, sinus node dysfunction or second- and third-degree heart block in the absence of a pacemaker. Use of IV class I and III AADs 4 h prior/after vernakalant |

*AADs* antiarrrhythmics, *ACS* acute coronary syndromes, *AF* atrial fibrillation, *AFl* atrial flutter, *AVN* atrio-ventricular node, *AVRT* atrioventricular reentrant tachycardia, *BB* beta-blockers, *CKD* chronic kidney disease, *COPD* chronic obstructive lung disease, *crCl* creatinine clearance, *HF* heart failure, *MI* myocardial infarction, *NYHA* New York Heart Association, *PSVT* paroxysmal supraventricular tachycardia, *SAN* sino-atrial node, *SBP* systolic blood pressure, *SDC* serum digoxin concentration, *SVT* supraventricular tachycardia, *TdP* torsades de pointes, *VPC* ventricular extrasystoles, *VT* ventricular tachycardia, *WPW* Wolf-Parkinson-White syndrome.

Potent CYP3A4 inhibitors: azole antifungals (ketoconazole, itraconazole, posaconazole, voriconazole), boceprevir, macrolide antibiotics (clarithromycin, josamycin, telithromycin), HIV protease inhibitors (indinavir, lopinavir, nelfinavir, ritonavir, saquinavir), nefazodone, telaprevir. Mild CYP3A4 inhibitors: diltiazem, erythromycin, fluconazole, verapamil, grapefruit juice.

CYP3A4 inducers: carbamazepin, phenobarbital, phenytoin, rifampicin, St John's worth

TABLE 6.6 Effects of drugs and medical conditions on serum digoxin concentrations (SDC)

| | |
|---|---|
| *Decrease SDC (it may be necessary to increase the daily dose of digoxin)* | |
| Decrease drug absorption | • Acarbose, adrenaline, antiacids, bupropion, cholestyramine, high-bran diet, kaolin-pectin, some bulk laxatives metoclopramide, neomycin, salbutamol, sulfasalazine, supplemental enteral nutrition<br>• Chemotherapy drugs: cyclophosphamide, cytarabine, methotrexate, vincristine<br>• Other drugs: phenytoin, rifampicin, St John's wort |
| Increase renal excretion | • Bupropion, hydralazine, nitroprusside, sympathomimetic drugs (dopamine, dobutamine) |
| Increase *digitalis resistance* | • Reduced oral bioavailability, inadequate intestinal absorption, increased metabolic degradation in the gut<br>• Neonates and infants<br>• Hyperthyroidism |
| *Increase SDC (reduce the daily dose of digoxin)* | |
| Increase oral absorption | • Antibiotics that inhibit intestinal microflora: macrolides (e.g. clarithromycin[a], erythromycin, telithromycin[a]), tetracyclines, gentamicin, trimethoprim<br>• Anticholinergic drugs (propantheline, diphenoxylate), omeprazole |
| Decreased renal and non-renal excretion | • Alprazolam, atorvastatin, epoprostenol, lapatinib, potassium-sparing diuretics, propafenone, spironolactone<br>• Decrease renal blood flow: β-blockers, heart failure<br>• ARBs, ACEIs, NSAIDs, and COX-2 inhibitors may modify renal function in some patients leading to an indirect increase in SDC<br>• Decreased glomerular filtration rate: elderly, renal impairment |

(continued)

TABLE 6.6 (continued)

| | |
|---|---|
| P-glycoprotein inhibitors[a] | • Amiodarone, cyclosporine, dronedarone, itraconazole, ketoconazole, lapatinib, nefazodone, quinidine, quinine, ranolazine, telmisartan, ticagrelor, verapamil<br>• Antiretroviral HIV-1 protease inhibitors: atazanavir, darunavir, indinavir, lopinavir, nelfi-navir, ritonavir, saquinavir, telaprevir, tipranavir |
| Increase cardiac sensitivity to digoxin-induced proarrhythmia | • Advanced age, hypothyroidism, electrolyte disturbances (hypokalemia, hypomagnesemia, hypercalcemia), IV calcium<br>• Sympathomimetic agents: induce cardiac arrhythmias and may also lead to hypokalaemia<br>• Acute myocardial infarction, acute rheumatic or viral carditis, severe myocarditis, amyloidosis<br>• Chronic kidney disease<br>• Hypoxemia due to chronic lung disease<br>• Drugs producing hypokalemia: thiazides and loop diuretics, amphotericin B, β-adrenergic agonists, carbenoxolone, corticosteroids, laxatives, lithium salts, NSAIDs (diclofenac, indometacin), pancuronium, suxamethonium<br>• Amiodarone, beta-blockers, diltiazem, verapamil: increase the risk of bradycardia and AV block<br>• Class IA and IC AADs: increase the risk of bradycardia, intracardiac conduction block and proarrhythmia |

*AADs* antiarrhythmic drugs, *ACEIs* angiotensin converting enzyme inhibitors, *ARBs* angiotensin receptor blockers, *NSAIDs* nonsteroidal anti-inflammatory drugs

[a]P-glycoprotein inhibitors can enhance digoxin absorption and/or reduce its renal clearance

TABLE 6.7 Clinical recommendations of adenosine, digoxin and vernakalant in clinical guidelines

| *Adenosine* [10, 11] | Class | Level |
|---|---|---|
| Adenosine is recommended for the acute treatment of narrow QRS tachycardia in the absence of an established diagnosis | I | B |
| Adenosine is recommended for acute treatment in patients with regular SVT, with AVNRT due to manifest or concealed accessory pathways or with orthodromic AVRT | I | B |
| Adenosine is recommended for acute treatment in ACHD patients and SVT | I | B |
| Adenosine can terminate some forms of focal AT due to a triggered mechanism in ACHD | I | B |
| Adenosine is recommended for acute treatment in pregnant patients with SVT | I | C |
| Adenosine is recommended to either restore SR or diagnose the tachycardia mechanism in patients with suspected focal AT | IIa | B |
| Adenosine is recommended for the acute treatment of wide QRS tachycardia if there is no pre-excitation on a resting ECG | IIa | C |
| Adenosine in patients with WPW syndrome who have pre-excited AF is potentially harmful because it accelerates the ventricular rate | III | B |
| *Digoxin* | | |
| In the absence of pre-excitation, IV digoxin is recommended to acutely control heart rate in patients with HF [13, 27] | I | B |
| Digoxin is recommended to control heart rate in AF patients with LVEF ≥40% [13] | I | B |
| Digoxin is recommended to control heart rate in AF patients with LVEF <40% [13] | I | B |

TABLE 6.7 (continued)

| | | |
|---|---|---|
| Digoxin is effective to control resting heart rate in patients with HFrEF, with dosage appropriate to avoid bradycardia [27] | I | C |
| A combination of digoxin and a β-blocker (or a nondihydropyridine calcium channel antagonist for patients with HFpEF), is reasonable to control resting and exercise heart rate in patients with AF [27] | IIa | B |
| Intravenous digoxin in the latest pocket Gls version should be considered for rate control of AT if beta-blockers fail [13] | IIa | C |
| Digoxin can be effective for ongoing management in pregnant patients with highly symptomatic SVT [11] | IIa | C |
| Digoxin should be considered for rate control of AT if beta-blockers fail in patients without WPW syndrome [11] | IIa | C |
| Oral digoxin may be reasonable for treatment of AVNRT in patients who are not candidates for, or prefer not to undergo, catheter ablation [10] | IIb | B |
| Digoxin may be considered to slow a rapid ventricular response in patients with ACS and AF associated with severe LV dysfunction and HF or hemodynamic instability [27] | IIb | C |
| Oral digoxin may be reasonable for ongoing management in patients with symptomatic SVT of unknown mechanism without pre-excitation who are not candidates for, or prefer not to undergo, catheter ablation [10] | IIb | C |
| Oral digoxin may be reasonable for ongoing management of orthodromic AVRT in patients without pre-excitation on their resting ECG who are not candidates for, or prefer not to undergo, catheter ablation [10] | IIb | C |
| Digoxin is potentially harmful for ongoing management in patients with AVRT or AF and pre-excitation on their resting ECG [10, 11, 13] | III | C |

TABLE 6.7 (continued)

| | | |
|---|---|---|
| *Ivabradine* | | |
| Ivabradine is reasonable for ongoing management in patients with symptomatic IST [10, 11] | IIa | B |
| The combination of beta blockers and ivabradine may be considered for ongoing management in patients with IST [10, 11] | IIb | C |
| Ivabradine may be considered in patients with postural orthostatic tachycardia syndrome [11] | IIb | C |
| Ivabradine with a beta-blocker may be considered for the chronic treatment of recurrent focal AT when other measures fail [11] | IIb | C |
| *Ranolazine* | | |
| Ranolazine may be considered as add-on therapy to shorten the QT interval in LQTS3 patients with a QTc >500 ms [51] | IIb | C |
| *Vernakalant* | | |
| In patients with no history of ischemic or structural heart disease, vernakalant is recommended for PCV of recent-onset AF [13] | I | A |
| Intravenous vernakalant is an alternative to amiodarone for PCV of AF in patients without hypotension, severe HF or severe structural heart disease (especially aortic stenosis) [13] | IIb | B |
| Intravenous vernakalant may be considered for cardioversion of postoperative AF in patients without severe HF, hypotension, or severe structural heart disease (especially aortic stenosis) [13] | IIb | B |

ACHD adult c.ongenital heart disease, ACS acute coronary syndromes, AF atrial fibrillation, AT atrial tachycardia, AVNRT atrioventricular nodal reentrant tachycardia, AVRT atrioventricular reentrant tachycardia, GI gastrointestinal, HFrEF heart failure with reduced ejection fraction, HF heart failure, IST inappropriate sinus tachycardia, LVEF left ventricular ejection fraction, PCV pharmacological cardioversion, SR sinus rhythm, SVT supraventricular tachycardia, WPW Wolff-Parkinson-White

($I_{Ca}$) during sympathetic stimulation. As a consequence, adenosine decreases SAN pacemaker activity and in the AVN slows conduction velocity and increases refractoriness. (d) Activates presynaptic purinergic receptors located on sympathetic nerve terminals decreasing the release of nor-epinephrine. These two later effects explain why adenosine terminates some atrial and ventricular arrhythmias and abolishes both early (EADs) and delayed (DADs) afterde-polarizations induced by catecholamines.

Activation of the Gs protein–bound A2 receptors increases adenyl cyclase activity and cAMP levels, inhibits $Ca^{2+}$ entry and myosin light chain kinase and stimulates ATP-sensitive potassium ($K_{ATP}$) channels which hyperpolarizes vascular smooth muscle cells [1–3]. As a result, adenosine decreases coronary and peripheral vascular resistances, vasodilates coronary microvessels (<150 mm in diameter), adequates coronary blood flow to cardiac metabolic demands playing a key role in ischemic pre-conditioning and attenuates isch-emia-reperfusion injury. Because of its coronary vasodilator properties, adenosine is indicated for stress radionuclide myocardial perfusion imaging in patients unable to undergo adequate exercise stress. Adenosine has also been used to produce controlled hypotension.

**Pharmacodynamics** An intravenous (IV) bolus of adenosine, preferable through a large venous or central line, rapidly (within 10–30 s) and transiently slows AV conduction velocity [due to effects on the atrial-His (AH) interval, but not on the H-V interval] and increases AV refractoriness (prolongs the PR and A-H intervals) leading to a transient AV block that is then responsible for tachycardia termination [4, 5]. Thus, adenosine the drug of choice to terminate supraventricular tachycardias (SVT) using the AVN as a portion of the reentrant circuit, such as AV nodal re-entry tachycardias (AVNRT) and AV reentrant tachycardias (AVRT). Success rates range from 78% to 96% (similar to verapamil) in acute episodes of SVT [3–11]. Adenosine also slows sinus rate, may cause sinus exit block and can terminate

SAN reentry. The effects of adenosine on the SAN and AVN are of greater and longer in patients with recent heart transplantation (<1 year). Adenosine is effective in terminating some focal atrial tachycardias (AT) due to a triggered mechanism in adult congenital heart disease patients, but does not interrupt macro-re-entrant ATs unless the reentrant circuit involves the AVN [7, 12]. Adenosine is unlikely to terminate atrial fibrillation (AF) or atrial flutter (AFl) [13], but it can produce a transient AV block, which unmask atrial activity and helps to diagnosis. Adenosine does not affect conduction velocity through the His-Purkinje or normal accessory pathways, but conduction can be blocked in accessory pathways with long conduction times or decremental conduction. Ventricular tachycardias (VT) do not respond to adenosine, but it can terminate idiopathic right outflow tract VT caused by a cAMP-mediated triggered activity caused by delayed afterdepolarizations; idiopathic left septal VT rarely responds.

Adenosine terminates AVNRT, SVT using an accessory pathway, and some forms of focal AT which account for <25% of SVT in adults with repaired congenital disease. However, evwn when it is unlikely to terminate atrial reentry tachycardia or atrial flutter, which represents >70% of SVT episodes in this population, adenosine may help to the diagnosis by producing transient AV block, which would make the atrial activity visible [1, 4, 7, 10–12].

Adenosine can help to the diagnosis of narrow-complex tachyarrhythmias [1, 4, 5, 8–12]. The appearance of transient AVN block with persistent AT can help to differentiate focal AT from AVNRT and AVRT [7]. In wide-QRS tachycardias of uncertain origin, adenosine can help to differentiate SVT (with aberrant conduction) from VT; adenosine is likely to terminate SVT with aberrancy or reveals the underlying atrial mechanism, while the VT continues. When an accessory by-pass tract is present, adenosine may increase conduction down the anomalous pathway revealing latent pre-excitation in patients with suspected Wolff-Parkinson-White (WPW) syndrome. A normal response occurs if transient high-grade AV block is observed; the presence of an anterograde conduction accessory pathway is inferred if adenosine produces a PR shortening-QRS widening without interruption of AV conduction. Adenosine can also differentiate conduction over the AVN from that over an accessory pathway during ablative procedures of the accessory pathway, and can provide a diagnosis in VT with retrograde conduction by blocking the P wave.

Adenosine may also promote arrhythmogenesis [2, 14]. It often produces bradycardia, sinus arrest and several degrees of AVN block, and even when prolonged bradycardia is unusual, caution is recommended in patients with known sinus node disease [2, 5, 15]. The risk of bradycardia increases in recipients of denervated orthotropic heart transplants, in whom SVT is common [5, 16]. Adenosine may induce AF with fast ventricular conduction and even VT by several mechanisms as it heterogeneously shortens atrial APD and refractoriness, produces transient sympathetic stimulation (tachycardia) through baroreflex activation in response to hypotension and it can hyperpolarize dormant pulmonary vein myocytes increasing their excitability and automaticity [17, 18]; the risk of AF appears more commonly associated with AVRT than AVNRT [8]. Patients with orthodromic AVRT often present atrial or ventricular premature complexes immediately after conversion that ocassionally may induce further episodes of AVRT. In this situation, an antiarrhythmic drug may be required to prevent acute reinitiation of tachycardia [1, 9–11]. Adenosine may also occasionally cause or accelerate pre-excited atrial arrhythmias [5, 19]. Because of the risk of proarrhythmia, adenosine should be used only in-hospital and with full resuscitative equipment available.

**Pharmacokinetics** After IV administration adenosine is rapidly cleared from circulation via cellular uptake by erythrocytes and vascular endothelial cells, where it is metabolized by the adenosine deaminase to inosine and adenosine monophosphate which are excreted by the kidneys. Its half-life ($t_{1/2}$) is <20 s, which explains why adverse effects even when frequent, they rapidly disappear and the repeated administration is safe within 1 min of the last dose.

The starting dose required for efficient rhythm correction is ~6 mg, given as a rapid bolus (1–2 sec) followed by a rapid saline flush. Large, centrally located (e.g. antecubital) veins are likely to deliver more effective drug concentrations to the heart than smaller distal veins [10, 11]. Another bolus of 12 mg can be administered after 1–2 min; this 12 mg bolus can be repeated in 1–2 min if SVT persist (Table 6.3).

**Adverse Effects** (Table 6.4) The most common include flushing, dyspnea (most likely secondary to stimulation of vagal C fibers in the lungs), chest discomfort, headache, dizziness, numbness or nausea, AV block and arrhythmias, but serious adverse adverse effects are rare because of the drug's very short half-life [2, 20]. Chest discomfort begins at approximately the same time as the delay in AV conduction and is immediately preceded by a marked increase in coronary-sinus flow, suggesting that the pain has a myocardial origin [5, 11]. Adenosine may precipitate or aggravate bronchospasm; thus, it may be reasonable to replace adenosine by verapamil in asthmatic patients.

**Indications** Adenosine is the drug of choice to rapidly terminate regular narrow-QRS-complex PSVT using the AVN as part of the reentry circuit when vagal manoeuvres fail, except for patients with severe asthma or angina pectoris [10, 11]. Because of its rapid onset and short duration of action, adenosine is preferable to verapamil or diltiazem, particularly in patients treated with IV β-adrenergic blockers or with history of heart failure (HF) or severe hypotension, and in neonates. Adenosine is the drug of choice for termination of SVT in pregnant patients when vagal manoeuvres fail; adverse effects to the fetus would not be expected and maternal side effects are transient given its short half-life [10, 11, 21]. Adenosine can also terminate AT, sinus node reentry and idiopathic right outflow tract VT commonly triggered by sympathetic stimulation.

**Selective A1R Agonists** (Table 6.1) They slow conduction velocity and prolong refractoriness in the AVN without affecting intraventricular conduction or reducing blood pressure or causing bronchospasm, two common side effects of adenosine [22]. They are effective for the conversion of PSVT to sinus rhythm (SR) and for ventricular rate control in AF without the negative inotropic and vasodilator effects of β-blockers, verapamil or diltiazem. Tecadenoson dose-dependently prolongs the AH interval (peak effect within 1 min, but returned to baseline after 10 min) without an effect on the HV interval, presents a longer $t_{1/2}$ than adenosine (20–30 min) and converts PSVT to SR in 90% of patients even after the first bolus, coincident with anterograde AV conduction block. Patients with a history of asthma or chronic obstructive pulmonary disease tolerated tecadenoson without bronchospasm. Other A1 adenosine receptor-selective full agonists and partial agonists are under development for multiple clinical indications.

## Cardiac Glycosides

Cardiac glycosides (digoxin and digitoxin) increase cardiac contractility and slow AVN conduction and have been used for decades to treat patients with symptomatic heart failure (HF) or impaired left ventricular (LV) function and for ventricular rate control in patients with supraventricular arrhythmias, mainly permanent and persistent AF, respectively. However, their use have declined over the past years because of its narrow therapeutic window and multiple interactions (Table 6.7), the increasing number of evidence-based therapies for HF and the results of the DIG trial [23], where digoxin therapy was shown to reduce all-cause and HF-specific hospitalizations but had no effect on survival.

**Mechanism of Action** Digoxin inhibits the $Na^+/K^+$-ATPase (3 $Na^+$ out – 2 $K^+$ in) [24, 25]. This inhibition increases the intracellular $Na^+$ concentration ($[Na^+]_i$), which in turn, activates the reverse mode of the $Ca^{2+}$-$Na^+$ exchanger (NCX, $Na^+$ efflux/$Ca^{2+}$ influx) leading to an increase in intracellular $Ca^{2+}$ concentration ($[Ca^{2+}]_i$). This increase in $[Ca^{2+}]_i$ at the level of contractile proteins might account for the positive inotropic effect and the proarrhythmic effects during digitalis intoxication. Furthermore, digitalis form calcium-conductance pathways and cation-selective $Ca^{2+}$ channels which may play a role in $Ca^{2+}$-dependent cardiotoxicity [26].

*At therapeutic concentrations* the electrophysiologic effects of digoxin are mediated indirectly by enhancing both central and peripheral vagal and inhibiting sympathetic tone, and to a lesser extent through a direct cardiac effect [24, 25]. The increase in vagal tone: (a) inhibits $I_f$ and accelerates the inactivation of the $I_{Ca}$ due to the higher $[Ca^{2+}]_i$, producing a mild resting bradycardia that may increase LV performance; (b) activates the $I_{KACh}$ leading to a nonuniform shortening of atrial APD and refractoriness; and (c) slows conduction and prolongs refractoriness in the AVN (prolongs the PR interval). This latter effect is the basis to use digoxin to control ventricular rate in patients with AF, particularly in unstabilized HF patients in whom β-blockers and calcium antagonists are contraindicated and to terminate reentrant tachyarrhythmias involving the AVN. However, digoxin exerts minimal effects on the His-Purkinje and ventricular muscle and the QRS and QT intervals are unaffected. Inhibition of $Na^+/K^+$-ATPase in the vagal afferent fibers restores cardiac baroreceptor sensitivity, leading to a decrease in peripheral sympathetic nerve activity; digoxin also reduces renin and angiotensin II plasma levels. This neurohumoral inactivation may play a key role at these therapeutic concentrations.

*At toxic concentrations*, digoxin directly causes sinus bradycardia and different degrees of AVN block, shortens atrial and ventricular APD and refractoriness, but increases $[Ca^{2+}]_i$ and sympathetic cardiac activity; these later effects increase the automaticity of cardiac pacemakers (AVN, His-Purkinje system) [24, 25]. Additionally, the inhibition of the $Na^+/K^+$-ATPase depolarizes the resting membrane potential, partially inactivates $Na^+$ channels and decreases intracardiac conduction velocity. Additionally, digoxin increases $[Ca^{2+}]_i$ and induces the spontaneous release of $Ca^{2+}$ from the sarcoplasmic reticulum during the diastole, which, in turn, activates the forward mode of the NCX ($Na^+$ influx/$Ca^{2+}$ efflux) leading to a net inward transient depolarizing current ($I_{Ti}$) that can generate EADs and DADs. All these effects predispose to both bradyarrhythmias and supraventricular and ventricular tachyarrhythmias that may degenerate in VT and ventricular fibrillation (VF). The increase in $[Ca^{2+}]_i$ in vascular smooth muscle cells can cause a direct vasoconstriction that may cause mesenteric artery occlusion or ischemia.

**Electrophysiological Effects** Digoxin effectively slows ventricular rate at rest when vagal tone predominates and in sedentary elderly patients with persistent/permanent AF [24, 25]. However, when sympathetic activity increases (i.e., during exercise, serious illness, fever, HF, hyperthyroidism, chronic lung disease, postoperative) its beneficial effects on AV conduction are reduced. Thus, digoxin is rarely used as a single agent for ventricular rate control in AF, but a satisfactory rate control can be achieved both at rest and during exercise when combined with β-blockers, verapamil or diltiazem. The ongoing RATE-AF trial is the first randomised clinical trial comparing digoxin and beta-blockers in AF.

Digoxin produces a nonuniform shortening of atrial APD and refractoriness that may explain why digoxin may increase the duration of AF, predisposes to early relapses of AF after restoration of SR and can convert the AFl to AF [24, 25]. Digoxin is no more effective than placebo to terminate AF or facilitate direct current cardioversion and may even induce episodes of AF in patients with so-called vagal AF [27]. Digoxin is contraindicated in patients with pre-excited AF because it slows AVN conduction but can accelerate anterograde conduction via the bypass tract increasing the ventricular rate during AF and the risk of provoking a life-threatening ventricular arrhythmia [13, 27–29].

In the ACC/AHA/HRS Guideline for the management of adult patients with supraventricular tachycardia oral digoxin is recommended for ongoing management in patients with symptomatic SVT without pre-excitation or with AVNRT who are not candidates for, or prefer not to undergo, catheter ablation [10]. However, digoxin should be reserved for patients who are unresponsive to, or are not candidates for β-blockers, diltiazem, or verapamil or a class IC agents (flecainide or propafenone) and it be used with caution in the presence of renal dysfunction. Interestingly, in the 2019 ESC Guidelines for the management of patients with SVT digoxin is not mentioned [11].

Because of its positive inotropic agent, digoxin is recommended for heart rate control in patients with AF and LVEF <40%, particularly in unstabilized patients in whom both β-blockers, diltiazem or verapamil are contraindicated. The combination of digoxin and carvedilol leads to better ventricular rate control than either agent, reduces symptoms, improves exercise tolerance and LV function [30]. In patients with AF (25% of the patients in NYHA class III) the IV administration of digoxin and esmolol produces a rapid rate control and conversion to SR occurs in 25% of patients [31]. In the AF-CHF trial [32], including patients with AF and LVEF ≤35%, adequate rate control was achieved in 82–88% of patients using adjusted doses of β-blockers with digoxin and in the CHF-STAT trial [33], amiodarone improved ventricular rate control when added to background therapy with digoxin in patients with AF and HF.

Several observational studies and meta-analysis associated digoxin therapy with excess mortality in patients with AF, but this finding was not confirmed in other studies [34–36]. The association is hampered by selection and prescription biases, because digoxin is commonly prescribed in sicker patients, with more comorbidities (HF, diabetes) and a higher baseline risk of mortality. A recent meta-analysis of 52 studies including over 600,000 patients with AF and concomitant HF, concluded that digoxin had a neutral effect on mortality but reduced hospital admission [36]. Thus, until proper randomized controlled trials are available, digoxin remains a suitable treatment option for rate control in patients with AF and HF.

**Digoxin Plasma Levels** Digoxin presents a narrow therapeutic window. Routine monitoring of serum digoxin concentrations (SDC) is not warranted in AF patients with controlled ventricular rate and without symptoms of toxicity, but is justified in patients with suspected digoxin intoxication, impaired renal excretion, variable cardiac responses, altered volume of distribution (Vd), hyperthyroidism, or suspected drug interactions, and to monitor compliance with therapy (Table 6.7). A retrospective analysis of the DIG trial found that low SDC (0.6–0.9 ng/mL) provided hemodynamic benefit and a small decrease in all-cause mortality, while at higher SDC (≥1.2 ng/mL) digoxin increased mortality (12%) [37]. Thus, SDC should be maintained between 0.6 and 1 ng/mL.

Doses should be based on age, gender, lean body mass, serum creatinine, serum electrolytes and presence of other drugs as digoxin presents multiple pharmacodynamic/pharmacokinetic interactions (Table 6.6). In elderly patients digoxin presents a lower Vd due to a loss of lean muscle mass and decline in renal function. Renal impairment decreases digoxin clearance and prolongs its $t_{1/2}$. Thus, doses, clinical response and SDC should be carefully titrated in elderly and in patients with chronic kidney disease. No dosage adjustments are recommended for patients with hepatic impairment. Digoxin is a substrate of P-glycoprotein (P-gp) and P-gp inhibitors can enhance digoxin absorption and/or reduce its renal clearance.

**Adverse Effects** Digoxin presents a narrow therapeutic index and SDC should be maintained between 0.5 and 0.9 ng/mL (Table 6.7). Cardiac glycosides can produce any type of arrhythmia, including bradyarrhythmias related to an increase in vagal tone (sinus bradycardia or arrest, AV block) and supraventricular (paroxysmal AT with variable AV block,

AVN tachycardias) and ventricular tachyarrhythmias (ventricular bideminy, VT, VF), particularly when electrolyte disorders are present.

If there is suspicion of toxicity, digoxin should be discontinued and ECG and SDC monitored. Electrolyte disorders, thyroid dysfunction and drugs/factor increasing SDC should be corrected (Table 6.7). Potassium salts should be avoided in the presence of bradycardia or conduction disturbances. Bradyarrhythmias or AV block respond to atropine but a temporary cardiac pacing may be required if symptomatic; ventricular arrhythmias may respond to lidocaine. Life-threatening arrhythmias can be treated with antidigoxin Fab fragments. Direct-current cardioversion should only be used if necessary using the lowest effective energy because life-threatening VT/VF can result. For elective electrical cardioversion of AF of a patient who is taking digoxin, the drug should be withheld for 1–2 days before cardioversion is performed.

**Indications** Digoxin is no longer a first-line drug for acute or long-term rate control during permanent/persistent AF or AFl, but because of its low cost and accumulated knowledge in prescription during decades, digoxin would remain for rate control AF, especially for elderly-sedentary or patients with HF or LV dysfunction [13, 27].

For *acute heart rate control* in patients without evidence of reduced LVEF, digoxin can be added to β-blockers, verapamil or diltiazem where required [13, 27]. However, β-blockers and diltiazem/verapamil are preferred over digoxin because of their rapid onset of action and effectiveness at rest and/or during exercise. In patients with signs of HF or evidence of reduced LVEF, β-blockers and/or digoxin should be considered as first-line therapy to improve LV function; digoxin is indicated in unstabilized HF patients in whom β-blockers and calcium channel blockers are contraindicated. For *long-term rate control* digoxin, alone or in combination with other AV blocking drugs (beta-blockers, diltiazem, or verapamil) is recommended for long-term rate control in patients with persistent/permanent AF with

LVEF ≥40%, with dosage appropriate to avoid bradycardia, and in AF patients with LVEF <40% [13, 27]. In SVT, digoxin has been replaced by adenosine, β-blockers and verapamil, drugs with faster onset of action and better safety profile. However, in the absence of pre-excitation, digoxin may be reasonable in patients with symptomatic SVT (including pregnant patients), orthodromic AVRT who are not candidates for, or prefer not to undergo, catheter ablation, and in AVNRT in patients with SBP <110 mmHg in whom β-blockers, verapamil or diltiazem may cause symptomatic hypotension or bradycardia [10, 11]. Digoxin has no role in ventricular arrhythmias.

## Atrial-Selective Sodium Channel Blockers

A new strategy for suppression of AF/AFl is the development of the so-called atrial-selective $Na^+$ channel blockers, drugs that predominantly depresses atrial versus ventricular $Na^+$ channel-dependent parameters and suppresses AF at concentrations producing little to no effect in the ventricles, thus reducing the risk of ventricular proarrhythmia. It has been hypothesized [38] that drugs like vernakalant and ranolazine that preferentially bind to the inactivated state of the $Na^+$ channel with fast unbinding kinetics might exhibit atrial selectivity during AF because: (a) atrial cells exhibit a more depolarized (~10 mV) resting membrane potential and a more negative half-inactivation voltage of $Na^+$ channels. Because reactivation depends on membrane potential, fewer $Na^+$ channels recover from the inactivated state during diastole in atrial as compared to ventricular cells and atrial refractoriness persist after the action potential is fully repolarized (postrepolarization refractoriness-PRR). (b) Atrial action potentials present a more gradual phase 3 which at rapid atrial rates results in a progressive disappearance of the diastolic interval in atria but not in ventricles and a less negative take-off potential further increasing the percentage of inactivated $Na^+$ channels. During AF, as the atria fail to fully repolarize, the difference in resting membrane potential between the atria and ventricles increases and less atrial $Na^+$ channels fully recover during diastole and remain in the inactivated state leading to the accumulation of $Na^+$-channel block and PRR.

## *Vernakalant*

Vernakalant is an atrial-selective multichannel blocker that inhibits the peak ($I_{Na}$) and late $Na^+$ ($I_{Na,L}$) currents, resulting in slow intra-atrial conduction and prolongation of atrial refractoriness, and several outward $K^+$ currents that control atrial repolarization: the ultra-rapid delayed rectifier current ($I_{Kur}$), the transient potassium current ($I_{to}$) and the inward rectifier currents $I_{KAch}$ and $I_{KATP}$ [39]. However, vernakalant has no effect on $I_{CaL}$ or the rapid component of the delayed rectifier ($I_{Kr}$). As a consequence, vernakalant blocks $I_{Na}$ in a rate- and voltage-dependent manner, so that $Na^+$ channel blockade increases at depolarized potentials and high heart rates, i.e. during AF, and selectively prolongs atrial APD and refractoriness with minimal effects on ventricular repolarization (QT interval) and refractoriness.

**Pharmacodynamics** The efficacy and safety of IV vernakalant for cardioversion of recent-onset AF was evaluated in six clinical trials [40, 41]. Vernakalant selectively prolongs atrial APD and refractoriness without affecting ventricular repolarization (QT interval) or refractoriness, heart rate or blood pressure. Vernakalant was significantly more effective than placebo for the conversion of AF to SR; the mean time to conversion was 8–14 min and 75–82% of patients converted after the first dose. The highest efficacy of vernakalant was observed for AF lasting for up to 72 h (51–79%), but decreased with the duration of the arrhythmia, being ineffective for the conversion of AF lasting >7 days or AFl. Interestingly, pre-treatment with vernakalant can improve the efficacy of electrical cardioversion. In the AVRO trial [42], vernakalant was more effective than IV amiodarone but the responder rates were lower, probably because of the higher proportion of patients with HF were enrolled in this trial. The probability of conversion to SR is independent of age, sex, LVEF, left atrial size, prior use of AADs, history of coronary artery disease or renal impairment, but there was a trend towards decreased efficacy in elderly patients (aged ≥75 years), those with a history of HF and in patients receiving digoxin or class I AADs. However, vernakalant is ineffective in patients with AFl [13, 40, 41].

Drug exposure is not influenced by age, gender, race, coronary artery disease, HF, renal or hepatic impairment, CP2D6 genotype or coadministration of CYP2D6 inhibitors, AVN blockers or warfarin.

**Indications** Intravenous vernakalant is recommended for the rapid termination of recent-onset AF (≤7 days for non-surgery patients; ≤3 days for post-cardiac surgery patients) to SR in adults without structural heart disease or with hypertension, CAD, abnormal LV hypertrophy or moderate HF (NYHA class I–II) and for cardioversion of postoperative AF, provided they do not present severe HF, hypotension, or severe aortic stenosis [13]. Vernakalant represents a fast and effective alternative to class IC antiarrhythmics and amiodarone, presents few proarrhythmic and extracardiac effects, eliminates the need for conscious sedation or anesthesia and when pharmacological cardioversion has failed it does not modify the efficacy of subsequent electric cardioversion. However, there are no head-to-head comparison with DC cardioversion or class IC AADs.

## *Ranolazine*

Ranolazine is approved for the treatment of chronic stable angina for patients inadequately controlled or intolerant to β-blockers and/or calcium channel blockers.

**Mechanism of Action** In atrial and ventricular muscle and Purkinje fibres, the rapid upstroke of the action potential is due to the activation of the $I_{Na}$. Most cardiac $Na^+$ channels open transiently (1–3 ms) during membrane depolarization, but rapidly inactivate-close and remain closed during the plateau phase of the action potential. However, some $Na^+$ channels do not inactivate or inactivate but reopen during the plateau generating the late $Na^+$ current ($I_{NaL}$) [43, 44]. An enhanced $I_{NaL}$ slows the rate of repolarization, prolongs the APD (QT interval) and increases transmural dispersion of repolarization (TDR) across the ventricular wall. These effects facilitate triggered and re-entrant arrhythmias. The $I_{NaL}$ increases under conditions associated with a high incidence of cardiac arrhythmias, including myocardial ischemia, LV hypertrophy, HF and arrhythmias associated with mutations in the cardiac $Na^+$ channel or their regulatory proteins (e.g. long QT and Brugada syndromes) [43, 44]. Myocardial ischemia increases the $I_{NaL}$ and the $[Na^+]_i$ which, in turn, activates the reverse mode of the NCX, leading to a $Na^+$-mediated $Ca^{2+}$ overload. This increase in $Na^+$ and $Ca^{2+}$ concentrations is a major contributor to the electrical (EADs, DADs, arrhythmias), mechanical (increases diastolic wall tension and $MVO_2$) and metabolic disturbances (increase ATP consumption, decreases ATP formation) in the ischemic myocardium [43, 44].

Ranolazine selectively inhibits the $I_{NaL}$, with almost no inhibition of the peak $I_{Na}$. Thus, it does not widen the QRS complex or slows intracardiac conduction velocity. Ranolazine also inhibits the $I_{Kr}$, but the expected prolongation of the APD and QTc interval secondary to this effect is counteracted by the inhibition of $I_{NaL}$. Indeed, ranolazine suppresses EADs and torsades de pointes induced by selective $I_{Kr}$-blockers and QT-prolonging drugs. Ranolazine prolongs atrial and ventricular refractoriness, induces PRR and reduces TDR. Ranolazine, however, does not modify cardiac contractility, AVN conduction or blood pressure.

**Effects on Atrial Fibrillation** In experimental models, vernakalant dose-dependently prolongs atrial APD and refractoriness, slows intra-atrial conduction, induces PRR, suppresses EADs and DADs elicited in pulmonary vein sleeves and terminates and/or prevents initiation of AF [43]. The combination of ranolazine with dronedarone or amiodarone induces potent synergistic use-dependent atrial-selective depression of $Na^+$ channel-mediated parameters, markedly increases PRR, and prevents the induction of AF.

In small uncontrolled trials, ranolazine (500–1000 mg bid) was effective to maintain SR in patients with recurrent AF despite AF ablation and AAD therapy, facilitates electrical cardioversion in cardioversion-resistant patients, prevents post-operative AF and at high doses (2 g p.o.) produces the conversion of recent-onset AF (<48 h duration) [45, 46]. In patients with unstable angina and non-ST-segment elevation myocardial infarction, ranolazine tended to reduce the episodes of AF as compared with placebo [47].

In a meta-analysis of eight trials in patients with preserved LVEF and recent-onset AF, ranolazine significantly reduces the incidence of AF compared to the control group in various clinical settings (i.e., after cardiac surgery, acute coronary syndromes, post-electrical cardioversion of AF). In the RAFAELLO study, ranolazine (375–750 mg bid) does not prolong the time to AF recurrence as compared to placebo [48], while in the HARMONY trial the combination of ranolazine (750 mg bid) and low doses of dronedarone (225 mg bid), but not each drug in monotherapy, significantly reduces AF burden vs placebo in patients with paroxysmal AF [49].

**Effects on Ventricular Arrhythmias** Ranolazine suppresses experimental ventricular arrhythmias associated with reduced repolarization reserve due to an increased $I_{NaL}$ and/or reduced $I_{Kr}$. In patients with unstable angina and non-ST-segment elevation myocardial infarction, ranolazine significantly reduces the incidence of non-sustained VT, SVT, bradycardias or pauses as compared with placebo, but not sudden cardiac death [47]. In LQT3 patients with the SCN5A-ΔKPQ mutation and an increased $I_{NaL}$, I.V. ranolazine shortens the QTc interval without changes in PR and QRS intervals, AV conduction or blood pressure, and improves diastolic dysfunction [50]. Thus, ranolazine may be considered as add-on therapy to shorten the QT interval in LQTS3 patients with a QTc >500 ms [51].

**Drug Interactions** Ranolazine is a moderate/potent inhibitor of P-gp and a mild inhibitor of CYP3A4 [20]. Avoid the administration of ranolazine with strong CYP3A inhibitors/inducers; limit the dose to 500 mg bid in patients on moderate CYP3A inhibitors (Table 6.5). Dose adjustment of CYP3A4 substrates (atorvastatin, lovastatin, simvastatin; limit the dose of simvastatin to 20 mg od), particularly of drugs with a narrow therapeutic range (e.g. cyclosporin, everolimus, sirolimus, tacrolimus), may be required when coadminstred with ranolazine.Monitortheplasmalevelsoftheimmunosuppressants when coadminstred with ranolazine. Ranolazine increases the exposure to digoxin. Exposure to CYP2D6 substrates (e.g. tricyclic antidepressants, antipsychotics) may be increased by ranolazine, and lower doses of these drugs may be required. Ranolazine also increases plasma levels of digoxin and metformin (metformin dose should not exceed 1700 mg/day when ranolazine is administered at 1000 mg bid). There is a theoretical risk that concomitant treatment of ranolazine with other drugs known to prolong the QTc interval may give rise to a pharmacodynamic interaction and increase the possible risk of ventricular arrhythmias. There is a theoretical risk that concomitant treatment of ranolazine with other drugs known to prolong the QTc interval may give rise to a pharmacodynamic interaction and increase the possible risk of ventricular arrhythmias.

**Clinical Indications** Ranolazine is well tolerated, does not produce significant hemodynamic, organ toxicity or proarrhythmic effects and its effects are more pronounced on atrial than on ventricular myocardium. Thus, it may represent a promising new AAD in patients with paroxysmal and persistent AF and structural heart diseases associated with an increase in $I_{NaL}$, where most AADs are contraindicated, SVT and ventricular arrhythmias. However, long-term RCTs are needed that confirm the efficacy and safety of ranolazine for the cardioversion of AF and the maintenance of SR in these patients.

## Selective $I_f$ Blockers: Ivabradine

Elevated resting heart rate is an independent risk factor of cardiovascular morbidity and mortality in the general population and in patients with cardiovascular diseases. Ivabradine is an antianginal drug that selectively inhibits the cardiac pacemaker current (I) which is responsible for normal automaticity of the sinus node and reduces heart rate in a dose-dependent manner, without influencing intracardiac conduction velocity or refractoriness, myocardial contractility and blood pressure [52].

The off-label use of ivabradine in small trials recruiting patients with inappropriate sinus tachycardia (IST) in response to exercise or orthostatic challenge reduced maximum/minimum heart rate and symptoms during exercise or daily activity and improved exercise tolerance in stress tests and quality of life with an efficacy comparable with placebo or other therapies, but is better tolerated than metoprolol [52–54]. A persistent clinical benefit was observed in some patients even after discontinuing the drug. Thus, ivabradine is recommended for symptomatic patients with IST [10, 11]. However, this is not an FDA/EMA-approved indication of ivabradine. Potential mechanisms of the antiarrhythmic effects of ivabradine includes $I_f$ inhibition, reduction of cardiomyocyte $Ca^{2+}$ overload and APD prolongation induced by heart rate reduction. Ivabradine may also be effective in focal AT, but there are limited data of the efficacy of ivabradine in the treatment of postural orthostatic tachycardia syndrome, sinus tachycardia after ablation of the AVNRT and refractory junction ectopic tachycardia [10, 11, 55]. Thus, larger prospective comparative studies are needed to establish the antiarrhythmic efficacy and safety of ivabradine. However, by breaking the pressure homeostatic loop, the selective blockade of $I_f$ is associated with a reflex increase in the activity of sympathetic efferent fibres [56]. Thus, ideally ivabradine should be preferably co-administered with a β-blocker when possible under close monitoring for the possibility of excess bradycardia; this combination may also be more beneficial than each drug alone for IST [10, 11].

**Drug Interactions** Ivabradine is metabolized via cytochrome CYP3A4 and it should be avoided or used with caution with potent CYP44A inhibitors/inducers (Table 6.5) [20]. Increased plasma concentrations of ivabradine may be associated with excessive bradycardia. Ranolazine is partially metabolised by CYP2D6 and potent CYP2D6 may increase its plasma concentrations. Ranolazine is also a mild inhibitor of CYP2D6 and exposure to CYP2D6 substrates (e.g. cyclophosphamide, efavirenz, flecainide, metoprolol, propafenone or tricyclic antidepressants and antipsychotics) may be increased by ivabradine, so that lower doses of these drugs may be required. Ivabradine should not be taken during pregnancy or breastfeeding [21].

## Gap-Junction Coupling Enhancers

Coordinated cardiac impulse conduction is a function of membrane excitability which depends on $Na^+$ or $Ca^{2+}$ channel activity, intercellular coupling of cardiomyocytes via low resistance connections (gap-junctions), and tissue architecture mainly determined by fibrosis [57]. Gap junction channels are composed of two hemichannels (connexons), formed from six connexin molecules, provided by either of the adjacent cells. The major connexins (Cx40, Cx43, and Cx45) are expressed in a chamber-specific manner. Cx43 is found in ventricles and atria, Cx40 in the atria and specific conduction system and Cx45 in the conduction system, SAN and ANV. Cellular uncoupling due to changes in Cx expression (resulting in irregular activation patterns), location (lateralization) and function occur in many forms of heart disease (i.e., ischemia, cardiac hypertrophy, HF and AF) and contribute to cardiac arrhythmias as they slow intracardiac conduction, increase repolarization heterogeneity and modulate automaticity. Cellular uncoupling together with increased fibrosis and decreased expression of $Na^+$ channels, are implicated in conduction slowing during ischemia, increasing the risk of fatal ventricular arrhythmias [57, 58].

Small-molecules that enhance gap-junction conductance have been developed in an attempt to improve conduction, eliminate functional block and suppress reentry [59]. The hexapepide rotigaptide and its dipeptide analogue danegaptide, increase gap-junction conductance (electrical coupling) acting via Cx43 and Cx45 gap junctions and may represent a novel therapeutic strategy to improve conduction, eliminate functional block and abolish reentry. Both drugs improve conduction during acidosis, acute metabolic stress or myocardial ischemia without affecting sarcolemmal ion channels or cardiac contractility and suppress reentrant ventricular tachyarrhythmias during ischemia-reperfusion. However, rotigaptide partially reverses the loss of Cx43 and does not restore normal conduction or prevent arrhythmias in the healing infarct border zone, i.e. after a prolonged period of gap-junction remodeling, is ineffective against focal ventricular tachyarrhythmias and does not suppress triggered arrhythmias. Gap-junction enhancers can also reduce AF vulnerability in some models (chronic mitral regurgitation, acute ischemia, sterile pericarditis), but not in HF or atrial tachypacing models, and it is unclear whether they are equally effective in chronically remodelled atria. Therefore, gap-junction enhancers may be only effective when alterations in gap-junctions are responsible for conduction slowing, but not when conduction slowing is mainly due to decreased $Na^+$ channel availability or structural remodeling (fibrosis). Furthermore, their electrophysiological effects when connexins are re-distributed but their expression and function remains unaltered is uncertain and there are concerns about their safety because theoretically, pharmacological restoration of intercellular coupling may destabilize re-entry and be proarrhythmic.

## $Na^+/Ca^{2+}$ Exchanger (NCX) Inhibitors

The NCX is a bidirectional electrogenic transporter ($Ca^{2+}$:$3Na^+$) producing a net current in the direction of $Na^+$ transport [60]. During the upstroke of the action potential the large influx of $Na^+$ via the $I_{Na}$ increases the $[Na^+]_i$ and the NCX functions in the *reverse mode* ($Na^+$ out/$Ca^{2+}$ in), generating an outward repolarizing current. During the plateau and early diastole, there is a large influx of $Ca^{2+}$ via the $I_{Ca}$, the $[Ca^{2+}]_i$ raises and the NCX functions in the *forward mode* ($Ca^{2+}$ out/$Na^+$ in) which in conjunction with the sarcoplasmic reticulum $Ca^{2+}$ uptake (via SERCA2a) facilitates cardiac relaxation and maintains intracellular $Ca^{2+}$ balance.

The *reverse mode* is favoured by membrane depolarization and increased $[Na^+]_i$ (rapid pacing, sympathetic stimulation, ischemia/reperfusion, digitalis intoxication) promoting $Ca^{2+}$ influx and cellular $Ca^{2+}$ overload leading to contractile failure (abnormally slow relaxation) and triggered arrhythmias. NCX is overexpressed in patients with HF or cardiac hypertrophy, which enhances $Ca^{2+}$ extrusion, compensates the reduced removal of $Ca^{2+}$ from the cytosol due to reduced SERCA2a activity, prolongs the APD and contributes to the spontaneous release of $Ca^{2+}$ from the sarcoplasmic reticulum and to the appearance of DADs. DADs arise from uncontrolled spontaneous $Ca^{2+}$ release from the sarcoplasmic reticulum under conditions of abnormal $Ca^{2+}$ overload and/or dysfunction of sarcoplasmic reticulum $Ca^{2+}$ release (RYR2) channels (ischemia-reperfusion, HF, LV hypertrophy, catecholamine-induced polymorphic VT) [61]. The increase of $[Ca^{2+}]_i$ activates the forward mode of the NCX and generates a transient inward depolarizing current ($I_{TI}$) that generates DADs and phase 3 EADs.

Inhibition of reverse NCX might be a novel antiarrhythmic strategy to reduce intracellular $Ca^{2+}$ overload and suppress triggered activity under pathological conditions, while blockade of the forward mode at resting membrane potentials reduces $Ca^{2+}$ extrusion and promotes intracellular $Ca^{2+}$ overload [60, 61]. Therefore, a unique desirable property of NCX inhibitors will be the preferential inhibition of the reverse NCX based in the asymmetric nature of the cotransporter (i.e. different sensitivity for $Na^+$ and $Ca^{2+}$ at the opposite sides of the membrane), but the lack of structural information about the mammalian cardiac NCX is a major drawback to achieving this goal. Currently available NCX inhibitors present limited selectivity with additional benefit arising from off-target effects as they inhibit other cardiac channels, which may explain the contradictory results in the treatment of ischemic-reperfusion injury and triggered activity. Additionally, no proof-of-concept clinical studies are not available.

**Acknowledgments** We thank P Vaquero for her invaluable technical assistance. This work was supported by grants from the Ministerio de Ciencia e Innovación (SAF2017-88116-P), Instituto de Salud Carlos III [PI16/00398 and CIBER-Cardiovascular (CB16/11/00303)] and Comunidad de Madrid (B2017/BMD-3738).

## References

1. DiMarco JP. Adenosine and digoxin. In: Zipes DP, Jalife J, editors. Cardiac electrophysiology: from cell to bedside. 3rd ed. Philadelphia: Saunders; 2000. p. 933–8.
2. Layland J, Carrick D, Lee M, Oldroyd K, Berry C. Adenosine. Physiology, pharmacology, and clinical applications. JACC Cardiovasc Interv. 2014;7:581–91.
3. Lerman BB, Markowitz SM, Cheung JW, Liu CF, Thomas G, Ip JE. Supraventricular tachycardia. Mechanistic insights deduced from adenosine. Circ Arrhythm Electrophysiol. 2018;11:e006953.

4. DiMarco JP, Miles W, Akhtar M, Milstein S, Sharma AD, Platia E, et al. Adenosine for paroxysmal supraventricular tachycardia: dose ranging and comparison with verapamil. Assessment in placebo-controlled, multicenter trials. The Adenosine for PSVT Study Group. Ann Intern Med. 1990;113:104–10.
5. Camm AJ, Garratt CJ. Adenosine and supraventricular tachycardia. N Engl J Med. 1991;325:1621–9.
6. Brady WJ, DeBehnke DJ, Wickman LL, Lindbeck G. Treatment of out-of-hospital supraventricular tachycardia: adenosine vs verapamil. Acad Emerg Med. 1996;3:574–85.
7. Markowitz SM, Stein KM, Mittal S, Slotwtner DJ, Lerman BB. Differential effects of adenosine on focal and macroreentrant atrial tachycardia. J Cardiovasc Electrophysiol. 1999;10:489–502.
8. Glatter KA, Cheng J, Dorostkar P, Modin G, Talwar S, Al-Nimri M, et al. Electrophysiologic effects of adenosine in patients with supraventricular tachycardia. Circulation. 1999;99:1034–40.
9. Delaney B, Loy J, Kelly A-M. The relative efficacy of adenosine versus verapamil for the treatment of stable paroxysmal supraventricular tachycardia in adults: a meta-analysis. Eur J Emerg Med. 2011;18:148–52.
10. Page RL, Joglar JA, Caldwell MA, Calkins H, Conti JB, Deal BJ, et al. 2015 ACC/AHA/HRS guideline for the management of adult patients with supraventricular tachycardia: executive summary: a report of the American College of Cardiology/American Heart Association Task Force on Clinical Practice Guidelines and the Heart Rhythm Society. J Am Coll Cardiol. 2016;67:1575–623.
11. Brugada J, Katritsis DG, Arbelo E, Arribas F, Bax JJ, Blomström-Lundqvist C, et al.; ESC Scientific Document Group. 2019 ESC guidelines for the management of patients with supraventricular tachycardia. The Task Force for the management of patients with supraventricular tachycardia of the European Society of Cardiology (ESC). Eur Heart J. 2019. pii: ehz467. https://doi.org/10.1093/eurheartj/ehz467.
12. Kall JG, Kopp D, Olshansky B, Kinder C, O'Connor M, Cadman CS, et al. Adenosine-sensitive atrial tachycardia. Pacing Clin Electrophysiol. 1995;18:300–6.
13. Kirchhof P, Benussi S, Kotecha D, Ahlsson A, Atar D, Casadei B, et al. 2016 ESC guidelines for the management of atrial fibrillation developed in collaboration with EACTS: The Task Force for the management of atrial fibrillation of the European Society

of Cardiology (ESC)Developed with the special contribution of the European Heart Rhythm Association (EHRA) of the ESCEndorsed by the European Stroke Organisation (ESO). Eur Heart J. 2016;37:2893–962.
14. Pelleg A, Pennock RS, Kutalek SP. Proarrhythmic effects of adenosine: one decade of clinical data. Am J Ther. 2002;9:141–7.
15. Fragakis N, Antoniadis AP, Korantzopoulos P, Kyriakou P, Koskinas KC, Geleris P. Sinus nodal response to adenosine relates to the severity of sinus node dysfunction. Europace. 2012;14:859–64.
16. Ellenbogen KA, Thames MD, DiMarco JP, Sheehan H, Lerman BB. Electrophysiological effects of adenosine in the transplanted human heart. Evidence of supersensitivity. Circulation. 1990;81:821–8.
17. Ip JE, Cheung JW, Chung JH, Liu CF, Thomas G, Markowitz SM, et al. Adenosine-induced atrial fibrillation. Insights into mechanism. Circ Arrhythm Electrophysiol. 2013;6:e34–7.
18. Li N, Csepe TA, Hansen BJ, Sul LV, Kalyanasundaram A, Zakharkin SO, et al. Adenosine-induced atrial fibrillation. Localized reentrant drivers in lateral right atria due to heterogeneous expression of adenosine A1 receptors and GIRK4 subunits in the human heart. Circulation. 2016;134:486–98.
19. Garratt CJ, Griffith MJ, O'Nunain S, Ward DE, Camm AJ. Effects of intravenous adenosine on antegrade refractoriness of accessory atrioventricular connections. Circulation. 1991;84:1962–8.
20. Tamargo J, Caballero R, Delpón E. Cardiovascular drugs-from A to Z. In: Kaski JC, Kjeldsen KP, editors. The ESC handbook on cardiovascular pharmacotherapy. Oxford: Oxford University Press; 2019. p. 423–808.
21. Regitz-Zagrosek V, Roos-Hesselink JW, Bauersachs J, Blomström-Lundqvist C, Cıfkova R, De Bonis M, et al. ESC Scientific Document Group. 2018 ESC guidelines for the management of cardiovascular diseases during pregnancy. Eur Heart J. 2018;39:3165–241.
22. Müller C, Jacobson KA. Recent developments in adenosine receptor ligands and their potential as novel drugs. Biochim Biophys Acta. 2011;1808:1290–308.
23. The Digitalis Investigation Group. The effect of digoxin on mortality and morbidity in patients with heart failure. N Engl J Med. 1997;336:525–33.

24. Gheorghiade M, van Veldhuisen DJ, Colucci WS. Contemporary use of digoxin in the management of cardiovascular disorders. Circulation. 2006;113:2556–64.
25. Tamargo J, Delpón E, Caballero R. The safety of digoxin as a pharmacological treatment of atrial fibrillation. Expert Opin Drug Saf. 2006;5:453–67.
26. Arispe N, Diaz JC, Simakova S, Pollard HB. Digitoxin induces calcium uptake into cells by forming transmembrane calcium channels. Proc Natl Acad Sci U S A. 2008;105:2610–5.
27. January CT, Wann LS, Alpert JS, Calkins H, Cigarroa JE, Cleveland JC Jr, et al. ACC/AHA Task Force Members. 2014 AHA/ACC/HRS guideline for the management of patients with atrial fibrillation: executive summary. A report of the American College of Cardiology/American Heart Association Task Force on Practice Guidelines and the Heart Rhythm Society. Circulation. 2014;130:2071–4.
28. Sellers TD Jr, Bashore TM, Gallagher JJ. Digitalis in the pre-excitation syndrome. Analysis during atrial fibrillation. Circulation. 1977;56:260–7.
29. Sheinman BD, Evans T. Acceleration of ventricular rate by fibrillation associated with the Wolff-Parkinson-White syndrome. Br Med J (Clin Res Ed). 1982;285:999–1000.
30. Khand AU, Rankin AC, Martin W, Taylor J, Gemmell I, Cleland JG. Carvedilol alone or in combination with digoxin for the management of atrial fibrillation in patients with heart failure? J Am Coll Cardiol. 2003;42:1944–51.
31. Shettiggar UR, Toole JG, Appunn DO. Combined use of esmolol and digoxin in the acute treatment of atrial fibrillation or flutter. Am Heart J. 1993;126:368–74.
32. Roy D, Talajic M, Nattel S, Atrial Fibrillation and Congestive Heart Failure Investigators, et al. Rhythm control versus rate control for atrial fibrillation and heart failure. N Engl J Med. 2008;358:2667–77.
33. Deedwania PC, Singh BN, Ellenbogen K, Fisher S, Fletcher R, Singh SN. Spontaneous conversion and maintenance of sinus rhythm by amiodarone in patients with heart failure and atrial fibrillation: observations from the veterans affairs congestive heart failure survival trial of antiarrhythmic therapy (CHF-STAT). The Department of Veterans Affairs CHF-STAT Investigators. Circulation. 1998;98:2574–9.
34. Turakhia MP, Santangeli P, Winkelmayer WC, Xu X, Ullal AJ, Than CT, et al. Increased mortality associated with digoxin in

contemporary patients with atrial fibrillation: findings from the TREAT-AF study. J Am Coll Cardiol. 2014;64:660–8.
35. Vamos M, Erath JW, Hohnloser SH. Digoxin-associated mortality: a systematic review and meta-analysis of the literature. Eur Heart J. 2015;36:1831–8.
36. Ziff OJ, Lane DA, Samra M, Griffith M, Kirchhof P, Lip GY, et al. Safety and efficacy of digoxin: systematic review and meta-analysis of observational and controlled trial data. BMJ. 2015;351:h4451.
37. Ahmed A, Rich MW, Love TE, Lloyd-Jones DM, Aban IB, Colucci WS, et al. Digoxin and reduction in mortality and hospitalization in heart failure: a comprehensive post hoc analysis of the DIG trial. Eur Heart J. 2006;27:178–86.
38. Antzelevitch C, Burashnikov A, Sicouri S, Belardinelli L. Electrophysiological basis for the antiarrhythmic actions of ranolazine. Heart Rhythm. 2011;8:1281–90.
39. Fedida D. Vernakalant (RSD1235): a novel, atrial-selective antifibrillatory agent. Expert Opin Investig Drugs. 2007;16:519–32.
40. Guerra F, Matassini MV, Scappini L, Urbinati A, Capucci A. Intravenous vernakalant for the rapid conversion of recent onset atrial fibrillation: systematic review and meta-analysis. Expert Rev Cardiovasc Ther. 2014;12:1067–75.
41. Akel T, Lafferty J. Efficacy and safety of intravenous vernakalant for the rapid conversion of recent-onset atrial fibrillation: a meta-analysis. Ann Noninvasive Electrocardiol. 2018;23:e12508.
42. Camm AJ, Capucci A, Hohnloser SH, Torp-Pedersen C, Van Gelder IC, Mangal B, et al. A randomized active-controlled study comparing the efficacy and safety of vernakalant to amiodarone in recent-onset atrial fibrillation. J Am Coll Cardiol. 2011;57:313–21.
43. Tamargo J, Caballero R, Delpón E. Ranolazine: an antianginal drug with antiarrhythmic properties. Expert Rev Cardiovasc Ther. 2011;9:815–27.
44. Bengel P, Ahmad S, Sossalla S. Inhibition of late sodium current as an innovative antiarrhythmic strategy. Curr Heart Fail Rep. 2017;14:179–86.
45. Gong M, Zhang Z, Fragakis N, Korantzopoulos P, Letsas KP, Li G, et al. Role of ranolazine in the prevention and treatment of atrial fibrillation: a meta-analysis of randomized clinical trials. Heart Rhythm. 2017;14:3–1.

46. White CM, Nguyen E. Novel use of ranolazine as an antiarrhythmic agent in atrial fibrillation. Ann Pharmacother. 2017;51:245–52.
47. Morrow DA, Scirica BM, Karwatowska-Prokopczuk E, Murphy SA, Budaj A, Varshavsky S, et al. Effects of ranolazine on recurrent cardiovascular events in patients with non-ST-elevation acute coronary syndromes: the MERLIN-TIMI 36 randomized trial. JAMA. 2007;297:1775–83.
48. De Ferrari GM, Maier LS, Mont L, Schwartz PJ, Simonis G, Leschke M, et al. RAFFAELLO Investigators. Ranolazine in the treatment of atrial fibrillation: results of the dose-ranging RAFFAELLO (Ranolazine in Atrial Fibrillation Following An ELectricaL CardiOversion) study. Heart Rhythm. 2015;12:872–8.
49. Reiffel JA, Camm AJ, Belardinelli L, Zeng D, Karwatowska-Prokopczuk E, Olmsted A, et al. HARMONY Investigators. The HARMONY Trial: combined ranolazine and dronedarone in the management of paroxysmal atrial fibrillation: mechanistic and therapeutic synergism. Circ Arrhythm Electrophysiol. 2015;8:1048–56.
50. Moss AJ, Zareba W, Schwarz KQ, Rosero S, McNitt S, Robinson JL. Ranolazine shortens repolarization in patients with sustained inward sodium current due to type-3 long-QT syndrome. J Cardiovasc Electrophysiol. 2008;19:1289–93.
51. Priori S, Blomstroöm-Lundqvist C, Mazzanti A, Blom N, Borggrefe M, Camm J, et al. 2015 ESC guidelines for the management of patients with ventricular arrhythmias and the prevention of sudden cardiac death. Eur Heart J. 2015;36:2793–867.
52. Koruth JS, Lala A, Pinney S, Reddy VY, Dukkipati SR. The clinical use of ivabradine. J Am Coll Cardiol. 2017;70:1777–84.
53. Cappato R, Castelvecchio S, Ricci C, Bianco E, Vitali-Serdoz L, Gnecchi-Ruscone T, et al. Clinical efficacy of ivabradine in patients with inappropriate sinus tachycardia: a prospective, randomized, placebo-controlled, double-blind, crossover evaluation. J Am Coll Cardiol. 2012;60:1323–9.
54. Ptaszynski P, Kaczmarek K, Ruta J, et al. Metoprolol succinate vs. ivabradine in the treatment of inappropriate sinus tachycardia in patients unresponsive to previous pharmacological therapy. Europace. 2013;15:116–21.
55. Sheldon RS, Grubb BP 2nd, Olshansky B, Shen WK, Calkins H, Brignole M, et al. 2015 heart rhythm society expert consensus statement on the diagnosis and treatment of postural tachycar-

dia syndrome, inappropriate sinus tachycardia, and vasovagal syncope. Heart Rhythm. 2015;12:e41–63.
56. Dias da Silva VJ, Tobaldini E, Rocchetti M, Wu MA, Malfatto G, Montano N, et al. Modulation of sympathetic activity and heart rate variability by ivabradine. Cardiovasc Res. 2015;108:31–8.
57. Kleber AG, Rudy Y. Basic mechanisms of cardiac impulse propagation and associated arrhythmias. Physiol Rev. 2004;84:431–88.
58. Noorman M, van der Heyden MA, van Veen TA, Cox MG, Hauer RN, de Bakker JM, et al. Cardiac cell-cell junctions in health and disease: electrical versus mechanical coupling. J Mol Cell Cardiol. 2009;47:23–31.
59. Dhein S, Hagen A, Jozwiak J, Dietze A, Garbade J, Barten M, et al. Improving cardiac gap junction communication as a new antiarrhythmic mechanism: the action of antiarrhythmic peptides. Naunyn Schmiedeberg's Arch Pharmacol. 2010;381:221–34.
60. Shattock MJ, Ottolia M, Bers M, Blaustein MP, Boguslavskyi A, Bossuyt J, et al. $Na^+/Ca^{2+}$ exchange and $Na^+/K^+$-ATPase in the heart. J Physiol. 2015;593:1361–82.
61. Antoons G, Willems R, Sipido KR. Alternative strategies in arrhythmia therapy: evaluation of Na/Ca exchange as an antiarrhythmic target. Pharmacol Ther. 2012;134:26–42.

# Chapter 7
# Antiarrhythmic Properties of Non-Antiarrhythmic Drugs in Atrial Fibrillation: Upstream Therapy

**Alina Scridon and Antoni Martínez-Rubio**

The prevalence of atrial fibrillation (AF), already the most common sustained cardiac arrhythmia encountered in clinical practice, is growing dramatically worldwide [1]. The presence of the arrhythmia is associated with substantial morbidity and mortality, and with significant impairment in the quality of life, causing a heavy economic burden on health care systems around the globe [2]. This epidemiological context has spurred massive interest in developing safe and efficient rhythm control strategies. Yet, despite the more than 100 years of basic and clinical research, currently available antiarrhythmic strategies yield disappointing results over the long-term, as they are often ineffective and have a

A. Scridon (✉)
University of Medicine, Pharmacy, Science and Technology "George Emil Palade" of Târgu Mureş, Târgu Mureş, Romania

A. Martínez-Rubio
Department of Cardiology, University Hospital of Sabadell, Institut d'Investigació i Innovació I3PT, University Autonoma of Barcelona, Sabadell, Spain

 
A. Martínez-Rubio et al. (eds.), *Antiarrhythmic Drugs*, Current Cardiovascular Therapy, https://doi.org/10.1007/978-3-030-34893-9_7

high side-effect profile [3]. This is at least partially due to the complexity of AF pathophysiology and to a still incomplete understanding of the fundamental mechanisms underlying AF.

Mechanistically, AF results from the interaction of three main factors (Fig. 7.1): the *triggers*, most commonly located at the junction between the left atrium and the pulmonary veins; the *substrate*, characterized by interstitial fibrosis, myocyte hypertrophy, chamber dilation, and/or ion channel remodeling; and *modulating factors*, such as autonomic dysfunction, inflammation and oxidative stress, or metabolic imbalance. The triggers are most commonly acute electrical-related events that promote AF initiation, whereas the substrate is responsible for maintaining the arrhythmia. Meanwhile, modulating factors can promote the triggers, the substrate, or both.

Traditionally, antiarrhythmic strategies have focused almost exclusively on atrial electrophysiological alterations, mainly by blocking cardiac ion channels, either to slow intra-atrial conduction (i.e., sodium channel blockers) or to prolong atrial refractoriness (i.e., potassium channel blockers). These interventions have provided very limited success over the long-term, with AF recurring in most patients within the first year of treatment [4]. This has not lowered enthusiasm, however; atrial-specific and/or non-conventional ion channel blockers (e.g., ranolazine) have been studied more recently and several other agents are underway.

→

FIGURE 7.1 The triangle of arrhythmogenesis in atrial fibrillation. In the vast majority of cases, atrial fibrillation (*middle image*) is the result of a combination of three factors: triggers, usually located at the junction between the left atrium and the pulmonary veins (*right upper corner*); substrate, often characterized by atrial fibrosis (*lower image*); and modulating factors, such as an imbalance in the autonomic nervous system (*left upper corner*). At its turn, once installed, atrial fibrillation promotes its own persistence, by inducing electrical, structural, and autonomic remodeling (*red arrows*)

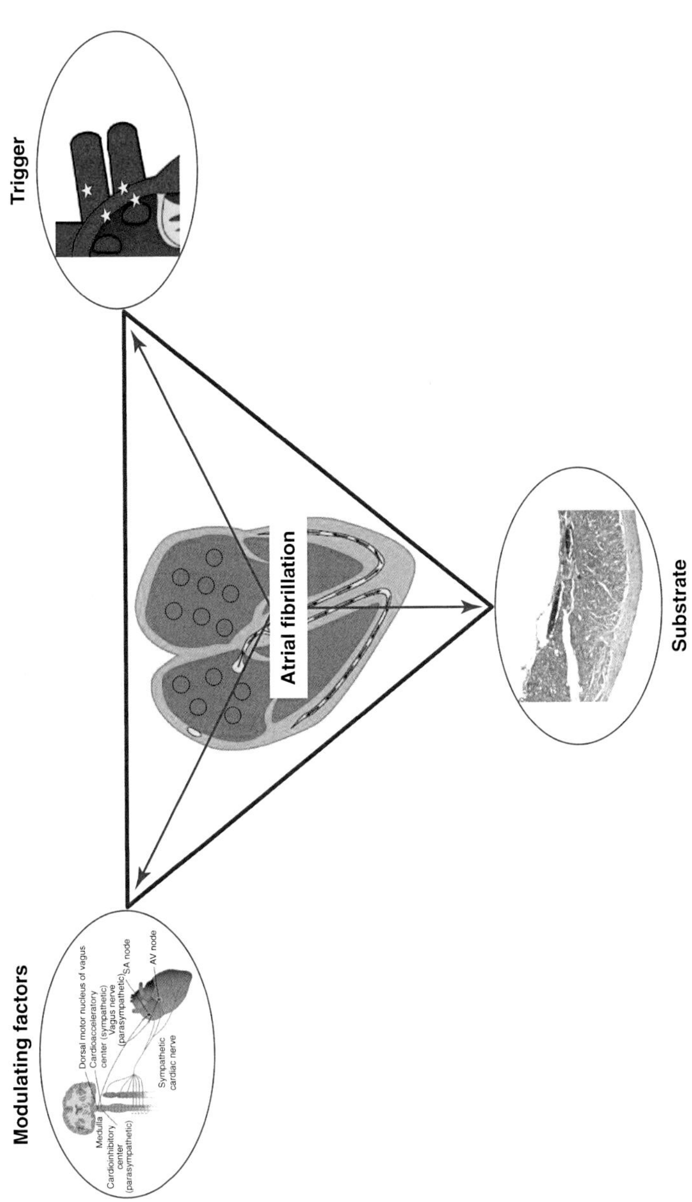
Trigger
Atrial fibrillation
Substrate
Modulating factors
Dorsal motor nucleus of vagus
Cardioacceleratory center (sympathetic)
Vagus nerve (parasympathetic)
SA node
AV node
Medulla
Cardioinhibitory center (parasympathetic)
Sympathetic cardiac nerve

In parallel, a number of 'non-antiarrhythmic' drugs (i.e., whose main effect is not exerted at ion channel level) have gained increasing attention due to their potential to prevent, delay, or even reverse AF-related atrial structural remodeling, while lacking the undesirable effects of ion channel blockers. By modifying the substrate upstream of AF, these new strategies are expected to prevent new-onset AF, to delay AF transition to more persistent forms, and/or to prevent recurrent AF. Such strategies include renin-angiotensin-aldosterone system (RAAS) blockers, 3-hydroxy-3-methyl-glutaryl-coenzyme A reductase inhibitors (statins), long-chain n-3 polyunsaturated fatty acids (PUFAs), steroidal antiinflammatory agents, as well as newer antifibrotic strategies such as matrix metalloproteinase (MMP) inhibitors, and proof-of-concept approaches such as DNA demethylating agents.

## Atrial Structural Remodeling and Atrial Fibrillation

Atrial structural remodeling gathers under its umbrella a potpourri of morphological abnormalities ranging from myocyte hypertrophy, necrosis, and focal or diffuse atrial myocytes rarefaction, to fibroblast proliferation, increased deposition and reduced degradation of collagen, fatty and/or inflammatory infiltration of the atria, and chamber dilation. Most commonly, this proarrhythmic remodeling is the result of long-lasting, pre-existing cardiovascular conditions including, but not restricted to arterial hypertension, heart failure, ischemic heart disease, or diabetes mellitus. In most cases, atrial structural remodeling appears to set in early during the progression of these diseases, although it may take several weeks for atrial enlargement and secondary electrophysiological changes to become apparent [5]. This emphasizes the need for early intervention to prevent atrial proarrhythmic remodeling and new-onset AF. More recent data have demonstrated, however, that structural remodeling is, at least to some extent, reversible [5], suggesting that anti-substrate strategies may be efficient not only for primary AF prophylaxis, but also for preventing AF recurrences in patients with already established arrhythmia.

Among atrial proarrhythmic structural changes, fibrosis has been incriminated as one of the main contributors to AF. Once installed, atrial fibrosis separates physically the myocytes, alters intercellular coupling, causes intra-atrial conduction heterogeneity, and creates a barrier to rapid impulse propagation, thus favoring multiple wavelet reentry [6]. At its turn, AF is also capable of enhancing atrial fibrosis, thus generating a vicious circle in which atrial fibrosis promotes AF persistence, and AF further promotes fibrosis. Indeed, atrial fibrosis is a common finding in the atria of AF patients [7] and the degree of fibrogenic activity has been related with the persistence of AF, as well as with the risk of postoperative AF [8, 9].

## *Atrial Fibrosis: A Consequence of Inflammation and Oxidative Stress*

Atrial fibrosis is often the result of inflammation and increased oxidative stress *via* fibroblast activation and consequent collagen synthesis and deposition, in parallel with decreased collagen degradation (Fig. 7.2). Numerous studies have documented indeed enhanced oxidative stress and increased oxidative damage and reactive oxygen species production in the atria of AF patients [10–12], whereas antioxidant agents such as glutathione or ascorbic acid have been shown to attenuate atrial remodeling and to decrease the AF risk in different experimental models [13, 14]. An inflammatory contribution to AF occurrence is strongly supported by the high AF incidence rates seen in settings with increased inflammatory status, such as myocarditis and pericarditis, as well as after cardiac surgery [15, 16]. Higher levels of inflammatory markers have been observed in the plasma of AF patients compared with controls, and in patients with persistent AF compared with those with paroxysmal AF [17–19]. The role of inflammation in atrial fibrosis and AF pathogenesis is further

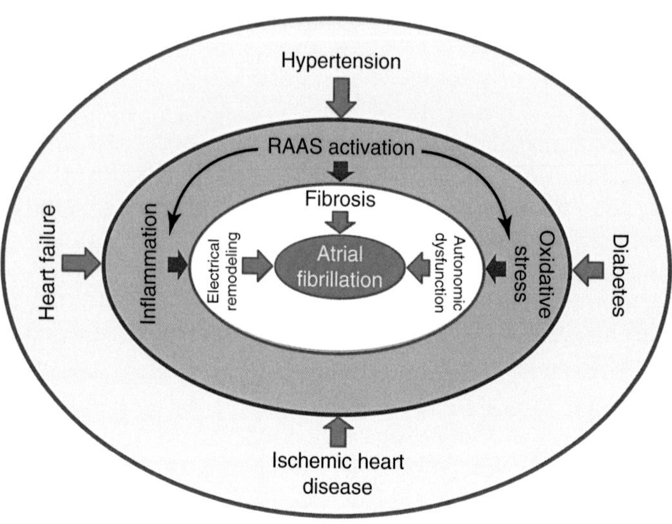


FIGURE 7.2 Pathophysiological pathways linking some of the most common atrial fibrillation risk factors with the occurrence of the arrhythmia. Some of the most common atrial fibrillation risk factors (*yellow circle*) are associated with renin-angiotensin-aldosterone system (RAAS) activation, and promote, directly and/or *via* the RAAS, inflammation and oxidative stress (*red circle*). At their turn, RAAS activation, inflammation, and oxidative stress favor atrial fibrosis and promote electrical and autonomic remodeling (*white circle*), which stand at the basis of atrial fibrillation occurrence (*blue circle*). The concept of 'upstream atrial fibrillation therapy' is based on the hypothesis that preventing, halting, and/or reversing one or several of these pathophysiological pathways will be able to prevent the onset and/or the recurrence of the arrhythmia

supported by the presence of inflammatory infiltrates, myocyte necrosis, and extensive interstitial fibrosis in atrial biopsy specimens from AF patients, but not from sinus rhythm controls [7]. Meanwhile, drugs with known antiinflammatory effects, including glucocorticoids, PUFAs, statins, or RAAS blockers have been shown to alleviate the AF burden [20, 21], with a reduction in AF prevalence seemingly proportional with the degree of decline in inflammatory markers levels [21]. It has even been suggested that part of the antiarrhythmic effect of amiodarone and carvedilol may be due to the antiinflammatory effects that these drugs appear to exhibit [22, 23].

The role of inflammation and oxidative stress in AF pathogenesis extends, however, far beyond the development of atrial fibrosis (Fig. 7.2). Reactive oxygen species and inflammatory cytokines have been shown to promote trigger activity *via* a direct effect on atrial electrophysiology and to modulate the intrinsic autonomic nervous system of the heart, whereas large inflammatory infiltrates may act themselves as a physical barrier to intra-atrial impulse propagation and increase the dispersion of atrial action potentials duration, thus creating the optimal substrate for reentry [24]. The benefit of targeting inflammation and/or oxidative stress may thus extend beyond its antifibrotic effects.

## *The Renin-Angiotensin-Aldosterone System: A Common Denominator of Atrial Inflammation, Oxidative Stress, and Fibrosis*

One of the common denominators of these closely interrelated proarrhythmic processes (i.e., inflammation, oxidative stress, and fibrosis) is the RAAS (Fig. 7.2) [25]. Indeed, the atria of patients with chronic AF have been shown to present increased expression of angiotensin converting enzyme (ACE) and of angiotensin II type 1 and mineralocorticoid receptors, as well as enhanced angiotensin II-dependent activation of fibrogenic pathways [26, 27]. Increased circulating, but not atrial, aldosterone levels have been reported in patients with persistent AF [27, 28], although some studies failed to show an association between AF and aldosterone levels when the model was adjusted for diuretic usage [29]. Finally, ACE polymorphisms have been associated with increased risk of new-onset AF [30] and of post-ablation AF recurrence [31], whereas the aldosterone synthase (CYP11B2) T-344C gene polymorphism has been linked to an increased risk of AF in patients with symptomatic heart failure [32], providing a direct link between RAAS activation and AF.

Angiotensin II has been shown to promote fibrosis *via* numerous inflammatory and oxidative stress pathways including stimulation of fibroblast-derived cytokines such as transforming growth factor *beta* (TGFβ), interleukin (IL) 6, or fibroblast growth factor 2, increased fibroblast secretion of fibrillar and non-fibrillar collagens [33], stimulation of mitogen-activated protein (MAP) kinases [9], and modulation of MMPs [34]. Aldosterone appears to have an even more pro-fibrotic role [35], at least partially mediated by TGFβ, connective tissue growth factor, IL-6, collagen, MMPs, and NADPH oxidase pathways [36, 37], although the exact signaling pathways involved in aldosterone-related atrial fibrosis remain to date unknown [38].

Meanwhile, ACE inhibitors (ACEIs), angiotensin II receptor blockers (ARBs), and mineralocorticoid receptor blockers have been shown to reduce the synthesis of profibrotic cytokines, growth factors, adhesion molecules, and type I collagen, as well as to increase the degradation of type I collagen, and to attenuate the development of cardiac fibrosis, to reduce atrial inflammation and oxidative stress, to limit myocyte apoptosis, and to positively affect intra-atrial conduction times [39–46]. Although all RAAS blockers appear to exhibit such beneficial effects, in a study comparing spironolactone with ACEIs and with a combination of both, only mineralocorticoid receptor blockade attenuated atrial fibrosis, suggesting that specific aldosterone antagonization may be more useful for reversing atrial fibrosis [47]. In aldosterone-treated hypertensive rats, mineralocorticoid receptor blockade also suppressed all inflammatory changes, whereas angiotensin II receptor blockade was only partially effective [43]. Indeed, as both cardiomyocytes and fibroblasts express high-affinity mineralocorticoid receptors and studies have provided evidence for local, myocardial aldosterone synthesis, mineralocorticoid receptor blockade may be of particular interest [48]. The issue of cardiac aldosterone synthesis remains, however, controversial. Particularly, the question remains whether aldosterone is synthetized locally in the *atrial* tissue [27] and whether the amount of aldosterone produced in the heart is high enough to have a significant impact on cardiac pathology [49, 50]. In addition, mineralocorticoid receptor activation is amongst the most important mechanisms incriminated in cardiac oxidative damage [51], whereas eplerenone and spironolactone administration has been shown to reduce circulating levels of oxidants, inflammatory, fibrotic, and neurohormonal factors [52–54], and to suppress cardiac fibrosis and diastolic dysfunction [55, 56].

In addition to its proinflammatory, prooxidant, and profibrotic effects, RAAS activation has also been shown to promote atrial electrical remodeling by increasing the density of cardiac $Ca^{2+}$ currents and the mRNA expression of cardiac Cav1.2 channels subunits [57, 58], decreasing outward potassium channels activity [59], and promoting gap junctions uncoupling [60]. Meanwhile, ARBs have been shown to modify the cardiac delayed rectifying currents [61]. Aldosterone has also been shown to cause dose-dependent increase in inward T- and L-type calcium current activity [62], to promote sarcoplasmic reticulum calcium overload and to increase sarcoplasmic reticulum calcium release *via* abnormally long ryanodine receptor channels opening [63], to alter the density of potassium currents [64], and to inhibit the $Na^+$/$K^+$-dependent ATPase [65]. Meanwhile, mineralocorticoid receptor blockade efficiently reduced potassium channels activities [66], decreased the activity and accelerated the inactivation of the L-type calcium current [67]. In a rat model of heart failure, spironolactone has also been shown to prevent gap junction remodeling, to reverse the down-regulation and to induce phosphorylation of connexin-43, as well as to reverse the progressive slowing of electrical impulse propagation [68]. However, in other experimental models of persistent AF, eplerenone failed to prevent electrical remodeling during AF progression, suggesting that mineralocorticoid receptor blockade might not modify persistent AF-related electrical remodeling [69]. *In vitro* experiments also suggest that in addition to favoring atrial fibrosis, fibroblasts also contribute to atrial electrical remodeling (Fig. 7.2) *via* direct physical contact, but also *via* release of platelet derived growth factor and TGFβ [70]. Indeed, TGFβ1 released by myofibroblast has been shown to alter sodium channel and potassium transient outward current activities, further contributing to atrial proarrhythmic remodeling [71]. Finally, accumulating data demonstrate that RAAS activation also interferes with cardiac autonomic modulation (Fig. 7.2). Meanwhile, ACEIs/ARBs have the ability to inhibit sympathetic nervous system activity [72] and to reduce circulating levels of norepinephrine and of angiotensin II, a facilitator of adrenergic neurotransmission [73].

## Upstream Therapies for Atrial Fibrillation Prevention

### *Renin-Angiotensin-Aldosterone System Blockers*

Given the critical role that the RAAS plays in atrial structural, electrophysiological, and autonomic remodeling, it seemed highly plausible that targeting the RAAS would be an effective additive antiarrhythmic intervention for AF prophylaxis. Thus, it is not surprising that RAAS blockers were amongst the first studied upstream therapies in AF and that the literature on the use of ACEIs, ARBs, and mineralocorticoid receptor blockers as antiarrhythmic strategies is particularly rich.

Numerous experimental studies, using various animal models, have provided extremely promising results; blockade of the RAAS has been shown to prevent or delay atrial electrical and structural remodeling and to decrease the AF burden [59, 61, 74, 75]. In dogs, enalapril and irbesartan both prevented atrial action potential shortening, suppressed the decrease in potassium channels activity, attenuated atrial fibrosis, and reduced AF inducibility and duration [76], whereas valsartan administration efficiently prevented pacing-induced AF [77]. In sheep, eplerenone administration mitigated cardiac structural remodeling during transition to persistent AF, reduced atrial size, myocyte hypertrophy, and atrial fibrosis, significantly reduced AF complexity, inducibility, and burden, and delayed the onset of persistent AF, although it had little effect on atrial electrophysiology [69]. In Dahl salt-sensitive rats, eplerenone reduced AF inducibility [78], whereas in dogs with tachycardia-induced heart failure, it attenuated the inducibility of sustained AF [79]. Spironolactone was also showed to reduce the duration of AF episodes, although it did not result in a complete preventative effect [80].

These promising results have been replicated in several clinical studies, secondary analyses of large clinical trials, and meta-analyses, which associated ACEIs and/or ARBs treatment with an overall 20–30% reduction in AF recurrence following cardioversion or pulmonary vein isolation [20, 81–83], particularly when co-administered with amiodarone [84–87]. A dose- and time-dependent effect of ACEIs and ARBs on AF prophylaxis has been suggested by several studies [88–91]. Several meta-analyses also support these data, indicating RAAS inhibition with either ACEIs or ARBs as an efficient approach for both primary and secondary AF prophylaxis [92, 93]. Spironolactone has also been associated with a reduction in AF burden following cardioversion [94], whereas eplerenone markedly improved sinus rhythm maintenance following catheter ablation for long-standing persistent AF [95], and has been shown to reduce new-onset and recurrent AF in heart failure patients [96]. Data from meta-analyses also indicate that mineralocorticoid receptor blockade may protect against new-onset and recurrent AF in different clinical settings [97, 98].

However, unlike the experimental studies, which strongly support RAAS blockade as a highly effective upstream AF therapy, clinical studies have not been so clear-cut. Clinical studies have provided conflicting results, with several studies showing no benefit of RAAS blockers on AF risk [99–104]. In patients with multiple cardiovascular risk factors, neither ramipril nor telmisartan were able to reduce the incidence of

AF [101, 104]; ACEIs/ARBs also failed to prevent new-onset AF in hypertensive patients [20, 92, 105–107]. The same was seen for secondary AF prevention with olmesartan in patients without structural heart disease [108], and with irbesartan in patients with heart failure and preserved ejection fraction [109]. In several other studies, RAAS antagonism was not effective in preventing AF recurrence following catheter ablation [110–112]. In the Candesartan in the Prevention of Relapsing Atrial Fibrillation (CAPRAF) trial, candesartan also failed to prevent post-cardioversion AF recurrence [113]. Several other large-scale prospective trials also failed to demonstrate a benefit from ACEIs and ARBs for AF prophylaxis [114, 115]. The results of the Gruppo Italiano per lo Studio della Sopravvivenza neII'Infarto Miocardico-Atrial Fibrillation (GISSI AF) trial, a rigorously designed, prospective, large-scale study, were particularly disappointing, showing no significant difference between the active drug (i.e., valsartan) and the placebo arms in preventing AF recurrence in individuals with cardiovascular disease, diabetes, or left atrial enlargement [114]. In the Treatment of Preserved Cardiac Function Heart Failure with an Aldosterone Antagonist (TOPCAT) trial, spironolactone also failed to reduce the risk of AF in patients with heart failure and preserved ejection fraction [116].

Although mechanistically RAAS blockade appears as a promising tool for AF prevention in the cardiac surgery setting, data on postoperative AF are highly conflicting. Several observational studies have even associated RAAS blockade with higher AF incidence following coronary artery bypass grafting (CABG), probably related to a higher incidence of hypotension and of renal dysfunction [117, 118]. In the randomized, double-blind, placebo-controlled study by Pretorius et al., ACE inhibition or mineralocorticoid receptors blockade had no effect on the risk of postoperative AF [119]. Other studies demonstrated, however, a significant reduction in the odds of developing postoperative AF in patients receiving ACEIs or ARBs prior to surgery [120, 121], with further reduction being obtained with combined usage of ACEIs and ARBs [121]. Mineralocorticoid receptor blockade failed to reduce postoperative AF in the study by Pretorius et al., as well as in subsequent meta-analyses [119].

Taken together, these studies appear to point RAAS inhibition as a potentially valuable strategy for preventing AF in patients with hypertension and congestive heart failure that exhibit considerable structural and/or functional abnormalities [86, 103, 122, 123], in which ACEIs/ARBs blockade may reduce the relative risk of new-onset AF with as much as 40% [20, 82, 103]. Meanwhile, the benefit of ACEIs/ARBs in post-myocardial infarction patients without signs of heart failure and in patients with stable coronary artery disease remains questionable [20, 124]. Data are also less clear for secondary AF prevention [92], as well as in patients without [108] or with only mild-to-moderate structural heart disease [20, 84, 85, 87, 92, 114, 125], and in those with heart failure with preserved systolic function [126]. However, even among studies restricted to patients with hypertension or heart failure, there is substantial heterogeneity [93], with several large studies having found no difference in the risk of new-onset AF between patients treated with ACEIs/ARBs and control patients [99, 100, 127, 128]. This was also the case for the GISSI AF trial, although in that study there was a positive trend in patients with heart failure [114]. Overall, these data appear to highlight the 'beneficial' effects of underlying structural heart disease on patients' response to ACEIs/ARBs blockade; a direct relation has been suggested to exist between the extent of cardiac dysfunction and the degree of benefit from RAAS blockade [92, 124]. The disappointing results in secondary AF prevention suggest, however, that in patients with long AF and/or underlying heart disease history, atrial remodeling may reach a point of no return.

Studies have also suggested that ARBs may provide greater benefit than ACEIs [83–85, 91, 107, 110], at least in certain patient categories, although the results are likely to have been affected by the overall longer duration of ARBs than of ACEIs trials [93]. The opposite has also been suggested by at least two independent studies, in which ACEIs appeared to show more benefit than ARBs for new-onset AF prophylaxis [93, 107]. Meanwhile, in the only study providing a direct comparison between ACEIs and ARBs, the risk for new-onset AF was similar in patients who received telmisartan, ramipril, or a combination of both, suggesting that ACEIs and ARBs are more likely to be equally potent in reducing AF risk and that combining them does not offer any additional benefit [129]. Data are much scarcer when it comes to mineralocorticoid receptor blockers. In one of the largest meta-analyses, evaluating over 90,000 patients, ARBs were associated with a clear reduction in new-onset AF, the benefit of ACEIs was less obvious, and mineralocorticoid receptor blockers failed to provide any benefit [101]. In the study by Ito et al., eplerenone reduced however the risk of recurrent AF following catheter ablation, whereas both ACEIs and ARBs failed to provide such a benefit [95]. In the meta-analysis by Neefs et al. mineralocorticoid receptor blockade significantly lowered the risk of both new-onset and recurrent AF, particularly in patients with heart failure, although it failed to prevent postoperative AF [98]. Finally, it has been suggested that ACEIs and ARBs might be more beneficial for primary [130] than for secondary [108, 131, 132] AF prevention, while the mineralocorticoid receptor blockers may provide more benefit for secondary AF prevention [6, 133]. Mechanistically, ACEIs, ARBs, and mineralocorticoid receptor blockers may indeed provide different benefit in AF prophylaxis. By blocking angiotensin II receptors, ARBs are effective on both ACE-dependent and ACE-independent pathways, whereas ACEIs are obviously not [134, 135]. Moreover, selective inhibition of angiotensin II type 1 receptors by the ARBs could lead to a reactive increase in angiotensin II concentration, which would then bind to angiotensin II type 2 receptors [135, 136], whose stimulation has been shown to increase nitric oxide synthesis [137]. Since after several months of treatment ACEIs/ARBs may increase plasma aldosterone levels *via* an 'aldosterone escape' mechanism [138], mineralocorticoid receptor blockade could theoretically provide even more benefit than the ARBs. However, at this point, there is insufficient data to conclude on the superiority of one drug class over the others. Further studies will have to address this issue. Future studies will also have to assess the potential of other drugs that interfere with the RAAS to positively impact on the risk of AF. Downstream RAAS blockers (i.e., ACEIs, ARBs, and mineralocorticoid receptor blockers) have been shown to cause reflex increase in renin, which may then lead to 'RAAS escape' [139]. Direct renin inhibition may thus become particularly appealing for AF prophylaxis. In a dog model of pacing-induced AF, the direct renin inhibitor aliskiren suppressed atrial electrophysiological and structural remodeling, reduced atrial fibrosis, and shortened the duration of AF [140]. However, this was not the case in a rabbit AF model, in which acute aliskiren administration was highly proarrhythmic [141]. In patients with permanent AF, aliskiren efficiently reduced oxidative stress and MMP-2 levels [142]. The ongoing Role of ALiskiren, a Direct Renin Inhibitor, in Preventing Atrial Fibrillation in Patients with a Pacemaker (RALF) trial is expected to provide the first data on the potential antiarrhythmic effect of aliskiren in clinical settings. Novel ARBs (e.g., azilsartan medoxomil), aldosterone synthase blockers, the currently in development third- and fourth-generation mineralocorticoid receptor blockers, and angiotensin converting enzyme 2 (an ACE homolog with protective effects in heart failure [143]) stimulators also deserve to be studied in this setting.

In the meantime, based on the currently available data, European guidelines recommend the use of ACEIs/ARBs inhibitors for primary AF prevention in patients with chronic heart failure and reduced ejection fraction (class IIa, level of evidence A) or with hypertension, especially with left ventricular hypertrophy (class IIa, level of evidence B), but do not recommend these drugs for secondary prevention of paroxysmal AF in patients with little or no underlying heart disease (class III, level of evidence B). However, ACEIs/ARBs use might be reasonable in addition to antiarrhythmic drugs to reduce AF recurrences after cardioversion (class IIb, level of evidence B) [144]. Although promising, data on mineralocorticoid receptor blockade remain rather scarce, precluding at this point any definitive conclusion.

## *3-Hydroxy-3-Methyl-Glutaryl-Coenzyme A Reductase Inhibitors (Statins)*

Statins are already widely used in clinical practice for their lipid-lowering and anti-atherosclerotic effects. However, the 'pleiotropic' effects of statins extend far beyond their impact on lipid metabolism. Statins have been shown to modulate the sympathetic activity, to improve endothelial function, to prevent neurohormonal activation, to exert antiinflammatory, antioxidant, and antifibrotic effects, and even to influence atrial electrophysiology by modifying membrane fluidity and ion channel conduction [145–150]. In experimental settings, simvastatin has also been shown to inhibit myocardial Rac1-GTPase activity and thus to regulate the NADPH pathway, to decrease myocardial production of reactive oxygen species [151], and to reduce atrial myofibroblast proliferation [152] and collagen synthesis [9]. It has also been suggested that statins may antagonize the arrhythmogenic effects of angiotensin II by regulating MMPs pathways and modulating the RAAS-induced increase in sympathetic activity [153]. Taken together, these 'pleiotropic' effects point statins as a potentially promising upstream approach to AF.

Indeed, statins have been shown to decrease AF inducibility in different animal models [151, 154, 155]. Similar antiarrhythmic effects have also been reported in several clinical studies and meta-analyses. Statin administration has been associated with a 61% reduction in the relative risk of incident or recurrent AF in different clinical settings [148]. In the AdvancedSM registry, statin usage was also associated with a 31% relative risk reduction of new-onset AF in patients with reduced ejection fraction [156]. The Sudden Cardiac Death in Heart Failure Trial (SCD-HeFT) showed a similar 28% reduction in the relative risk of AF in heart failure patients with statin therapy [157], whereas in the GISSI Heart Failure (GISSI-HF) study, rosuvastatin reduced the occurrence of new-onset AF in heart failure patients, although it did not reduce AF recurrence [149]. Of note, in GISSI-HF, the difference between the rosuvastatin and placebo arms on new-onset AF occurrence was only statistically significant after adjusting for a number of clinical and laboratory confounders [149]. Several meta-analyses reported however a potential benefit of statin therapy in lowering the risk of AF recurrence as well [158–160]. Atorvastatin usage has been shown to reduce paroxysmal AF recurrences [161], and was also associated with a significant reduction in postoperative AF occurrence in several randomized controlled trials [162–164]. In the Valsartan and Fluvastatin on Hypertensive patients with non-permanent Atrial Fibrillation (VF-HT-AF) study, fluvastatin was similarly shown to reduce the recurrence rate of paroxysmal AF and the incidence of persistent AF when added to conventional antiarrhythmic therapy. Several studies and meta-analyses have also suggested that statin therapy may be useful for preventing recurrences following electrical cardioversion for persistent AF [148, 150, 161, 165].

However, the issue of statin therapy for AF prophylaxis is far from having reached a consensus. In the Antihypertensive and Lipid-Lowering Treatment to Prevent Heart Attack Trial (ALLHAT), pravastatin failed to demonstrate a benefit in preventing incident AF in hypertensive patients [166], whereas in the meta-analysis by Fauchier et al. patients treated with statins displayed only a nonsignificant trend towards fewer AF events [148]. In the Sustained Treatment of Paroxysmal Atrial Fibrillation (STOP AF) trial, high-dose atorvastatin did not reduce AF recurrence following cardioversion, although it did reduce inflammatory markers levels and total cholesterol [150]. In patients with already established AF, statin therapy has also failed to lower the risk of long-standing persistent AF [167].

One could hypothesize that, as it has already been suggested for the RAAS blockers, the benefit of statin therapy may vary depending on the clinical scenario. Oxidative stress is recognized as a major factor in AF occurrence [168] and NADPH activity has been shown to be up-regulated in patients with postoperative AF, as well as in patients with paroxysmal and persistent AF, but not in those with permanent AF [169, 170]. Meanwhile, statins have been shown to inhibit reactive oxygen species production by interfering with the NADPH pathway [169, 171]. Thus, one may suggest that statin therapy may be more efficient in preventing postoperative AF and for reducing AF recurrences in patients with paroxysmal AF or with persistent AF following cardioversion (i.e., for secondary AF prevention) than for primary AF prevention [165]. Although some studies support indeed such a hypothesis [148, 172], this is not the case for the vast majority of studies, which yielded highly discordant results in all clinical settings. It has also been suggested that the intensity of statin treatment may play a role, and that high-dose statins may be more efficient in preventing AF than lower doses [167]. However, this was also not confirmed by all studies [148]. The short duration of clinical studies has also been incriminated as a potential cause for the disappointing results obtained with statins, particularly in primary AF prevention. However, a meta-analysis that compared studies with long *versus* short follow-up found no additional benefit of statins in the trials with longer follow-ups [173]. Finally, given that some statins are lipophilic (e.g., atorvastatin) while others are hydrophilic (e.g., pravastatin) and may thus have different affinity for cardiac cell membranes [174], and that different statins may differ in their antiinflammatory [175], antioxidant [176], and anti-proliferative [177] potency, one cannot exclude that different statins may have different antiarrhythmic effects. Indeed, Komatsu et al. have found that atorvastatin was superior to pravastatin in combination with antiarrhythmic drug therapy for preventing recurrent AF and progression to permanent AF in patients with paroxysmal AF and dyslipidemia [174]. In a retrospective study, atorvastatin has also been shown to be superior to simvastatin in preventing post-cardioversion recurrences in paroxysmal AF patients [178]. Meanwhile, in the meta-analysis of Fang et al. the authors associated atorvastatin and simvastatin, but not pravastatin and rosuvastatin usage with a decreased risk of AF [172]. It has also been suggested that males and females may respond differently to different statins, male AF patients appearing to benefit more from high-potency statins (i.e., rosuvastatin and atorvastatin), whereas female AF patients might benefit more from statins such as simvastatin or lovastatin [179]. At this point, it remains impossible, however, to draw definitive conclusions on the role of statins in primary or secondary AF prevention and there is insufficient evidence to support their use solely to prevent incident or recurrent AF [144].

## *Long-Chain n-3 Polyunsaturated Fatty Acids*

Long-chain n-3 polyunsaturated fatty acids (PUFAs) are contained in large amounts in fish oil and represent crucial constituents of cells membranes. Two PUFAs, the eicosapentaenoic acid (EPA) and the docosahexaenoic acid (DHA), have been particularly shown to possess several properties that may positively affect the AF substrate. These two PUFAs have been shown to exert antiinflammatory, antioxidant, and antifibrotic effects [180, 181], mainly by decreasing the conversion of arachidonic acid into potent inflammatory cytokines such as IL-6, IL-1β, and tumor necrosis factor *alpha* (TNFα) [182], but also to modulate connexins [183] and sodium ($I_{Na}$), potassium ($I_{Kur}$, $I_{K\text{-}Ach}$, $I_{to}$), and calcium ($I_{Ca\text{-}L}$) currents, ion exchangers and pumps [184–187], to cause hyperpolarization and increase the action potential threshold [131, 188], to mitigate endothelial dysfunction, and to augment the vagal and lower the sympathetic tone [188]. In experimental heart failure and ischemia-reperfusion models, PUFAs have also been shown to attenuate phosphorylation of the MAP kinases [9, 181, 189, 190], to regulate the profibrotic activity of MMPs [191], and to countervail the proarrhythmic effects of atrial stretch [192]. PUFAs could further exhibit antiarrhythmic effects by stabilizing atrial myocytes membranes, causing vasodilation and reducing the blood pressure, and improving myocardial contractility [193] and oxygen use [194]. In human studies, fish oil consumption was associated with reduced heart rate, longer atrial refractoriness, and less atrial mechanical stunning following cardioversion [195]. Additional data supporting the potential antiarrhythmic effects of PUFAs emerge from several studies that have associated higher plasma PUFA levels with lower AF risk [196, 197]. Although the effect of PUFAs in reducing inflammatory and oxidative stress markers levels has not been confirmed in all studies [198, 199], taken together, these 'pleiotropic' effects made PUFAs an attractive candidate for AF management.

Studies in animal models of sterile pericarditis have indeed associated PUFAs administration with a significant reduction in AF inducibility [200]. Fish oil extracts have also shown potent antifibrotic effects in experimental heart failure [181] and significantly decreased AF inducibility in animal cardiac surgery models [201]. In isolated Langendorf-perfused rabbit hearts, PUFAs significantly reduced stretch-induced AF vulnerability [192], whereas in dogs with pacing-induced heart failure PUFA administration reduced the duration of AF [181].

Positive data also emerge from several clinical studies and meta-analyses. Administration of PUFAs has been associated with reduced AF risk in post-myocardial infarction patients [202]. Among elderly individuals, consumption of tuna or other broiled or backed fish was also associated with significant AF risk reduction [203]. In the study by Biscione et al., 1 g/day of PUFAs for 4 months reduced paroxysmal AF recurrences in several patient categories with implanted pacemaker [204]. In that study, AF relapses rapidly raised following withdrawal of PUFA administration, further supporting a causal link between PUFAs and decreased AF risk [204]. A reduction in arrhythmia recurrence was also seen in patients treated with 655 mg/day of PUFAs for at least 1 month prior to catheter ablation [205]. Similarly, in the double-blind, placebo-controlled trial by Nodari et al., 1 g/

day of PUFAs significantly reduced AF recurrence following electrical or pharmacological cardioversion in persistent AF patients who were also treated with amiodarone [206]. In the open-label, randomized, prospective study by Kumar et al., diet supplementation with PUFAs has also reduced recurrent AF after cardioversion and significantly prolonged the mean time to AF recurrence [207].

Despite these positive initial data, the issue of using PUFAs as a potential upstream therapy for AF prevention remains controversial. Contrary to the study by Mozzafarian et al., suggesting a potential benefit of boiled or baked fish on AF risk, fish intake failed to provide a benefit in the Rotterdam study [208], whereas in the Danish Diet, Cancer, and Health study, fish intake was associated with augmented AF risk [209]. Administration of 3 g/day of PUFAs on top of antiarrhythmic therapy for at least 1 week prior to electrical cardioversion and continued, at a dose of 2 g/day, for up to 6 months following cardioversion, also failed to prevent AF recurrences and did not facilitate conversion to sinus rhythm in a multicenter randomized controlled trial, despite the suitably increased EPA and DHA levels obtained in the active group [210]. Therapy with 4 g/day of PUFAs also failed to prevent AF recurrences in the 663 symptomatic AF patients included in the double-blind, placebo-controlled Prescription of OMega-3 fatty ethyl esters for prevention of recurrent symptomatic atrial fibrillation (P-OM3) study. The randomized, double-blind, placebo-controlled Fish Oil Research With Omega-3 for Atrial Fibrillation Recurrence Delaying (FORWARD) trial also found no difference between PUFAs supplementation and placebo in preventing recurrent AF in patients with paroxysmal or persistent AF [211]. Similar results emerge from a recent meta-analysis of four randomized controlled trials including more than 1200 patients, which also showed no beneficial effect of PUFAs on AF recurrence, regardless if the patients have or have not been treated with conventional antiarrhythmics [212]. Several other meta-analyses [213–217], as well as a number of cohort studies [209, 218] and randomized controlled trials [198, 199, 219], some of them with relatively large sample sizes, reported similarly disappointing results.

Similarly to statins, PUFAs also appeared to provide better results in the cardiac surgery setting, at least in the early, smaller-scale studies. Intravenous administration of PUFAs from admission to discharge from the intensive care unit reduced the AF risk in patients undergoing CABG [220]. One g/day of PUFA administered orally for a median duration of 5 days was also associated with a significant reduction in early, but not in late postoperative AF [221]. A dose of 2 g/day of PUFAs started before CABG and continued until hospital discharge also reduced the risk of postoperative AF in the study by Calò et al. [222, 223]. However, the same PUFA dose and time of administration was ineffective in the study by Saravanan et al., despite high serum and right atrial appendage tissue PUFA content [224]. In the large, multinational, double-blind, placebo-controlled, randomized Omega-3 Fatty Acids for Prevention of Post-operative Atrial Fibrillation (OPERA) trial, short-term PUFA supplementation also showed no benefit in reducing postoperative AF [225]. These results are in line with other placebo-controlled trials and meta-analyses, which also failed to show an effect of PUFAs on the risk of postoperative AF [213, 220, 226–230].

These highly discordant results obtained with PUFAs suggest that, similarly to RAAS blockers and statins, patients' response to PUFAs may be affected by patient characteristics, PUFAs doses, or composition of PUFAs. Indeed, it has been suggested that the response to PUFAs may depend on the age of the studied population, with elderly patients being more likely to benefit from PUFAs than younger patients, in which PUFAs-related increase in parasympathetic tone could theoretically be proarrhythmic [231]. The different results obtained in animal models of atrial pacing- *versus* heart failure-induced AF also suggest that the underlying AF substrate may cause an impact on patients' response to PUFAs [181]. In addition, PUFA inclusion in cell membrane composition may be gender-dependent, with women requiring higher PUFA doses and combination with multivitamins in order to obtain the same increase in PUFA composition as males [232]. The fact that PUFAs have also been shown to exhibit anti-ischemic properties in certain populations [233] may explain their apparently larger benefit reported in patients undergoing cardiac surgery or following myocardial infarction. The effects of sustained oral dietary PUFA ingestion, which leads to increased membrane PUFA content, may also be considerably different than those of acute PUFA exposure, which produces a higher extracellular-to-membrane PUFA ratio [181]. Given the slow kinetics of incorporation of PUFAs into the cells membranes and the time it may take for PUFAs to affect atrial structural remodeling, it has been suggested that a long duration of administration is probably required for PUFAs to exert antiarrhythmic effects and that short-term PUFAs administration is unlikely to bring substantial benefits in patients with extensively remodeled atria [234, 235]. In patients without severely remodeled atria who develop AF in acute settings such as cardiac surgery, acute PUFA exposure may bring more benefit [236]. Many of the studies that failed to demonstrate a benefit of PUFAs have used formulations containing a 1.24 EPA:DHA ratio [225, 226, 228], whereas an EPA:DHA ratio of 1:2 may be more beneficial [230, 237]. Indeed, due to its stringer effects on $I_{Na}$, DHA may provide better protection from AF than EPA [186]. This hypothesis is also supported by several clinical studies, which have associated higher DHA, but not EPA concentrations with lower AF risk [196, 203, 238]. Meanwhile, the finding by Metcalf et al. that patients within the forth quintile of red blood cell DHA presented the lowest incidence of postoperative AF suggested that a U-shaped relationship may exist between PUFA intake and postoperative AF [239]. Several studies have reported indeed a strong trend towards higher AF risk in individuals consuming more than five fish meals per week [240, 241], suggesting that both low- and high-levels of fatty fish or individual PUFAs consumption may be associated with increased AF risk. Finally, differences may also exist depending on how the fish is cooked; in the Cardiovascular Health Study cohort, although consumption of baked or broiled tuna was associated with lower AF incidence, this was not the case for fried fish or fish sandwiches [203].

Due to their favorable safety profile, relatively low financial costs, and wide availability for oral intake, PUFAs remain an attractive approach for AF prevention. However, although the mechanistic background, experimental evidence, and initial clinical data have pointed PUFAs as a potential tool for AF prophylaxis, to date, there is no compelling argument to support the routine use of PUFAs for either primary or secondary AF prevention [144]. Further studies are needed to clearly establish whether there is a place for PUFAs in AF prevention. The populations of patients that are most likely to benefit from this approach will also have to be identified, taking into consideration that individual ability to incorporate PUFAs, which is likely affected by age, gender, vitamin administration, and genetic background, may affect patients' response to PUFAs. Blood measures of the PUFA status, such as the omega-3 index (i.e., the combined percentage of EPA and DHA of total fatty acids in red blood cell membranes), may be useful for assessing the individual response to PUFAs intake and for guiding PUFAs usage.

## *Glucocorticoids*

Glucocorticoids have been shown to exert antiinflammatory and antioxidant effects [242–247], to suppress vascular endothelial growth factor expression, to inhibit fibroblast proliferation [248], and to modulate atrial electrophysiology [249], and have thus been regarded as a potential upstream therapy for AF, particularly in settings associated with high inflammatory burst such as post-cardiac surgery. In addition, although the aldosterone/mineralocorticoid receptor complex is considerably more stable and more efficient for transactivation than the glucocorticoid/mineralocorticoid receptor complex [250], cardiomyocyte mineralocorticoid receptors have been shown to bind mineralo- and glucocorticoids with equal affinity [251], suggesting that, at least in certain conditions, glucocorticoids may also exhibit proarrhythmic effects *via* mineralocorticoid receptor activation [252].

In animal models of cardiac surgery, sterile pericarditis, and atrial pacing, glucocorticoid administration attenuated the inflammatory response, prevented proarrhythmic atrial electrical remodeling, and reduced atrial tachyarrhythmias inducibility [242, 243, 253]. Similarly to experimental studies, several randomized controlled trials showed that preoperative administration of methylprednisolone [254, 255], hydrocortisone [256], and dexamethasone [257] significantly decreased postoperative AF occurrence. In the meta-analysis by Ho and Tan including 50 randomized controlled trials, intravenous corticosteroid therapy before and/or after cardiopulmonary bypass significantly reduced the risk of postoperative AF [258]. In three other meta-analyses, intermediate-dose glucocorticoids reduced the risk of postoperative AF compared with placebo with as much as 50% [259], although corticosteroids use was also associated with increased risk of postoperative pneumonia, gastrointestinal bleeding, and urinary tract infections [259–261]. In the more recent meta-analysis by Liu et al., both low- and medium-dose glucocorticoids significantly reduced the incidence of postoperative AF, as well as the rate of postoperative infections, and significantly shortened the length of intensive care unit and total hospital stay [262]. Low-dose methylprednisolone (i.e., 16 mg for 4 weeks, tapered to 4 mg for 4 months) has also demonstrated benefits in secondary AF prevention following cardioversion [263]. Glucocorticoid administration during and after catheter ablation has also been associated with reduced AF recurrence rates, particularly in the period immediately following AF ablation; however, early (i.e., 1 month) recurrence rates were not different compared with placebo [264]. In addition, corticosteroid administration was associated with significantly lower late AF recurrences, at 14 months after ablation, in the absence of any conventional antiarrhythmic therapy [264]. The potential benefit of glucocorticoids in patients undergoing AF ablation and their possible time-dependent antiarrhythmic effect have also been suggested by the meta-analysis by Lei et al., which associated corticoids usage with a decrease in early (i.e., 3 months) and late (i.e., 12–14 months), but not in immediate (i.e., 2–3 days) and very late (i.e., 24 months) AF recurrences [265]. Similar findings were also reported in the recent meta-analysis by Jaiswal et al. [266].

In other clinical studies, however, dexamethasone failed to prevent postoperative AF [267–269]. Intravenous and oral corticosteroid administration in various doses also failed to prevent early and/or late AF recurrence in patients undergoing AF ablation [247, 264, 270, 271], despite inducing a significant decrease in inflammatory markers levels [272]. A recent meta-analysis including two randomized controlled trials and three cohort studies also failed to demonstrate any benefit of perioperative corticosteroid administration on the risk of late AF recurrence following catheter ablation, although it did show a reduction in early AF recurrence [266]. This is in line with the results of the prospective, randomized, single-blind study by Kim et al., in which methylprednisolone also failed to reduce late AF recurrence following ablation [273]. Moreover, several case reports, case-control, and cohort studies suggested that glucocorticoid therapy could even precipitate AF in different clinical settings, particularly when administered for the first time [274, 275] and/or at high doses [274, 276–283]. In the population-based, case-control study by Christiansen et al., systemic glucocorticoid administration almost doubled the risk of atrial tachyarrhythmias; the risk was 4 times higher for new users of glucocorticoids compared with never users, irrespective of the presence or absence of asthma, chronic obstructive pulmonary disease, or cardiovascular disease [274]. A trend towards higher incidence of AF recurrence with administration of steroids, likely related to higher pulmonary veins reconnection rate and higher prevalence of dormant conduction, has also been reported in patients undergoing catheter ablation for AF [270, 272]. Several hypotheses have been proposed to explain the proarrhythmic effects of glucocorticoid pulse therapy, including the associated hypertensive effect of high-dose corticosteroids, or the severe underlying conditions (e.g., asthma, pulmonary inflammation, chronic systemic inflammatory diseases) that required high-dose glucocorticoids administration [231]. In addition, high-dose corticosteroids could mediate the local potassium efflux *via* a direct effect on cells membranes [284], but could also promote AF due to the mineralocorticoid effects that high glucocorticoid doses are known to exhibit, including sodium and fluid retention, leading to arterial hypertension, left atrial dilation, and congestive heart failure, in addition to their potential local effects on atrial mineralocorticoid receptors. The electrolyte shift across myocardial cells membranes and the increased potassium loss at the renal level induced by high-dose corticoid therapy could be particularly important in patients receiving concomitant diuretic therapy, in those who have previously received high-dose corticoids, as well as in those with liver dysfunction, in which the half-life or corticoids may be considerably prolonged [285]. Over the long term, glucocorticoid use also increases the risk of several well-known AF risk factors, including atherosclerosis, diabetes mellitus, arterial hypertension, ischemic heart disease, and heart failure, which could further increase the AF risk in these patients [274].

Glucocorticoid therapy thus appears to exhibit both pro- and antiarrhythmic effects, depending on a number of variables. Different compounds may exert different effects; whereas methylprednisolone and hydrocortisone appear to be rather antiarrhythmic [254–256], dexamethasone does not seem to provide such a benefit [267, 268], at least in the perioperative setting. The potential side effects associated with the use of corticosteroids with longer half-lives, such as dexamethasone, could indeed cancel their potential beneficial effects [231]. The risk of proarrhythmia also appears to be higher in new users and in those who have used corticosteroids before, compared with those with chronic, low-dose (e.g. inhalation) corticosteroid therapy [275, 277]. However, the dose of corticosteroids appears to be amongst the most important factors that dictate the effects of glucocorticoid therapy, with high, but not low or intermediate doses being associated with potential proarrhythmic effects [275, 277]. Oppositely, intermediate doses may be rather protective against AF, at least in patients undergoing cardiac surgery [258–261], whereas low doses may be more useful for secondary AF prophylaxis [263]. Other studies, however, failed to show any difference between low, medium, and high glucocorticoid doses in patients undergoing cardiac surgery [262].

Taken together, the currently available data is insufficient to support the use of glucocorticoids for AF prophylaxis. Future studies, including in the already heavily studied perioperative setting, will have to clarify whether steroids have a true merit for AF prophylaxis. If this is the case, further studies will also have to establish which drug, at which dose, and for what duration is most likely to prevent AF occurrence and/or recurrence.

## *Colchicine*

Colchicine, a potentially poisonous natural product and secondary metabolite, is mainly known for its beneficial effects in treating and preventing gouty attacks, and, more recently, for primary and secondary prophylaxis of pericarditis [286]. In addition, colchicine has been shown to prevent early and late arrhythmia recurrences following AF ablation, *via* its antiinflammatory properties [287, 288] including attenuation of neutrophil activation, endothelial cell adhesion, and inflammatory cells migration [289], in addition to potential direct effects on atrial myocytes and on cardiac autonomic balance [290]. In patients undergoing cardiac surgery, low-dose colchicine has also been shown to reduce the incidence of postoperative AF [291], although this effect was not confirmed in the double-blind, randomized, Colchicine for Prevention of Postpericardiotomy Syndrome and Postoperative Atrial Fibrillation (COPPS-2) trial [292].

## *Antidiabetic Agents*

Although stringent glycemic control does not appear to affect the rate of new-onset AF [293] in the diabetic population, metformin use has been associated with a decreased risk of AF in patients with type 2 diabetes, probably by attenuating myolysis and oxidative stress [294]. The antiarrhythmic effect of metformin appeared to fade, however, after about three years, probably due to the progression of atrial structural remodeling with increased duration of diabetes [294]. Thiazolidindiones, insulin sensitizing agents with peroxisome proliferator-activated receptor $\gamma$ activation effects, have also been shown to prevent atrial electrical and structural remodeling *via* their antioxidant and antiinflammatory properties [295–299]. In animal studies, pioglitazone reduced TGF$\beta$, TNF$\alpha$, and MAP kinases, attenuated atrial structural remodeling, and decreased AF inducibility [9], whereas in clinical settings pioglitazone administration was associated with marked improvement in sinus rhythm maintenance and reduced reintervention rates following catheter ablation for paroxysmal AF [300]. A remarkable improvement of paroxysmal AF has been reported in two patients with type 2 diabetes mellitus treated with rosiglitazone [301], whereas in the study by Chao et al. thiazolidindione administration was associated with a 31% reduction in the relative risk of new-onset AF [302].

## *Other Agents with Antioxidant Properties*

In experimental settings, probucol, a lipid-lowering agent with potent antioxidant effects, has been shown to favorably affect atrial proarrhythmic remodeling [303] by reducing left atrial interstitial fibrosis [304] and apoptosis [305], to decrease inflammatory markers levels and atrial oxidative stress [306], to attenuate atrial nerve sprouting and heterogeneous sympathetic hyperinnervation [306], as well as to reduce AF inducibility and duration [304, 306]. Different other antioxidant agents, including vitamins C and E, N-acetylcysteine, and xanthine oxidase inhibitors have also been proposed as potential therapeutic interventions in AF patients [307, 308], but data concerning these agents remain insufficient to allow any definitive conclusions.

## *Novel Approaches*

### Matrix Metalloproteinase Inhibitors

Interstitial fibrosis, resulting from long-term imbalance between collagen deposition and degradation is recognized as the hallmark of proarrhythmic atrial structural remodeling [309]. This observation has encouraged the development of direct antifibrotic strategies. Among them, MMP inhibitors have gained increasing attention over the past years. Indeed, MMP activation, together with down-regulation of tissue inhibitors of metalloproteinases (TIMPs), has been incriminated in the development of extensive atrial fibrosis [310] and in AF occurrence [311]. Matrix metalloproteinases, a multigene family of proteolytic enzymes, together with their tissue inhibitors, regulate the extracellular matrix turnover [312, 313]. Although theoretically higher activity of MMPs should results in higher extracellular matrix degradation, and not in fibrosis, in addition to their role in breaking down the extracellular matrix [314], proteases such as MMP-9 and MMP-2 have been shown to activate the TGF$\beta$, TNF$\alpha$, IL-1b, angiotensin II, endothelin-1, and vascular endothelial growth factor pathways, and thus to stimulate the synthesis of extracellular matrix, as well as to inhibit extracellular matrix degradation by increasing TIMP expression [315–319].

Studies have associated the presence of AF with increased MMP-2 [8] and MMP-9 levels [320–322], and a gradual increase in plasma and atrial MMP-9 levels has been shown with progression from sinus rhythm to paroxysmal, persistent, and permanent AF [320, 321, 323]. This latter finding is in complete agreement with histology studies showing more extensive atrial fibrosis in persistent *versus* paroxysmal AF, and in permanent *versus* persistent AF [324–329]. The active form of MMP-9, but not of MMP-1, MMP-2, or TIMP-1, was also significantly increased in the atria of AF patients compared with sinus rhythm controls [321], although the exact mechanisms responsible for these changes remain to date unknown. Increased MMP-2 and decreased TIMP-2 activities have been reported, however, in association with AF in the study by Xu et al. [8]. In a canine model of pacing-induced AF, MMP-9 activity in the atrial matrix was 50% higher and TIMP levels were 50% lower than in sinus rhythm controls [330]. However, no changes in MMP-2, MMP-3, and MMP-7 activities were observed in that study [330]. Increased MMP activity, with a predominant increase in MMP-9 expression, was also reported in pigs with pacing-induced AF [331]. Oppositely, a decreased expression of MMP-1 and MMP-9 has been reported in patients with chronic non-rheumatic AF [332] and in those with mitral valve disease and AF [333]. These discrepancies have been related to potential time-dependent changes in MMP expression [334, 335], as well as to the different features of the studied populations, with different cardiac pathologies leading to different MMPs activation patterns (i.e., heart failure has been associated with increased MMP-9 expression, whereas MMP-9 was decreased in patients with hypertension) [336]. In the Atherosclerosis Risk in Communities (ARIC) cohort, elevated MMP-9 levels were also independently associated with an increased risk of incident AF [337], whereas in patients with persistent AF high baseline MMP-9 levels have been associated with increased AF maintenance [322], as well as with increased AF recurrence rates following catheter ablation [338]. Elevated MMP-2 levels at baseline have also been associated with increased AF recurrence following pharmacological or electrical cardioversion [339].

Given the accumulating evidence that links MMPs with AF, it has been assumed that long-term MMP inhibition could suppress atrial fibrosis and exert antiarrhythmic effects [340]. In animal models, gene deletion and pharmacological inhibition of MMP activity have been shown to reduce myocyte hypertrophy and atrial fibrosis, and to decrease AF inducibility [331, 341], suggesting that MMP inhibition may indeed emerge as a promising new tool for AF prophylaxis. To date, no clinical trial has tested the use of MMP inhibitors for AF therapy and/or prophylaxis. However, in the Early short-term doxycycline therapy in patients with acute myocardial infarction and left ventricular dysfunction and the ominous progression to adverse remodeling (TIPTOP) trial, short-term use of the MMP inhibitor doxycycline significantly reduced the infarct size and the severity of left ventricular dilation in patients with acute myocardial infarction [342], demonstrating a potential benefit of MMP inhibition in patients with established cardiovascular disease.

## Galectin-3 Inhibition

Galectin-3 is a β-galactosidase-binding protein that contains a collagenase domain cleavable by MMPs such as MMP-9 and MMP-2 [343, 344]. In the extracellular space, galectin-3 can bind to different extracellular matrix glycans and cells surfaces, leading to pro-apoptotic effects, whereas in the intracellular space galectin-3 favors anti-apoptotic processes [345]. Together, these effects contribute to angiogenesis, inflammation, fibroblast proliferation, and collagen deposition, probably mediated by TGFβ pathway activation [346]. Recent studies have linked galectin-3 with atrial remodeling in AF patients [323]. In a large cohort from the general population, higher galectin-3 levels were associated with an increased risk of incident AF, although the association was lost after accounting for various known AF risk factors [347]. Similar results were also reported by van der Velde et al. [348]. However, in the large, prospective, population-based ARIC study, high galectin-3 plasma levels were associated with an increased risk of AF independently of baseline AF risk factors [349]. Galectin-3 levels were also reported to be higher in patients with persistent, non-self-terminating AF, than in those with paroxysmal AF [350, 351], and were also independently correlated with the extent of left atrial fibrosis detected by cardiac magnetic resonance imaging [352]. It has also been suggested that paroxysmal AF patients that present higher galectin-3 levels may require more extensive intervention in addition to pulmonary vein isolation [353]. In patients with persistent AF, galectin-3 levels independently predicted AF recurrence following catheter ablation [351, 354, 355], although this was not the case in the study by Kornej et al. [356].

Meanwhile, galectin-3 inhibition has been shown to interfere with cardiac fibrogenesis and to reduce the AF burden [357]. In a sheep model of persistent AF, inhibition of galectin-3 using a relatively low intravenous dose of the galactomannan GM-CT-01 (GMCT) attenuated both atrial structural and electrical remodeling, significantly reduced the AF burden, and increased the probability of spontaneous conversion to sinus rhythm, although it did not maintain the sinus rhythm over the long term [351]. These promising initial results suggest that one of the several recently described types of galectin-3 inhibitors [358] may be useful for preventing AF progression and perpetuation and/or as an adjunctive therapy for improving the outcomes of AF catheter ablation.

## Molecular Targets: A New Paradigm in Atrial Fibrillation Therapy?

Recent studies have demonstrated that altered regulation of gene expression plays major roles in AF initiation and/or maintenance [359–364]. Particularly, Pitx2 (paired-like homeodomain transcription factor 2) has been identified as the most altered transcription factor in the left atria of AF patients [365, 366], and reduced left atrial Pitx2 expression has been proposed as a potential AF diagnostic marker [367], although increased [368] and unaltered [369] Pitx2 have also been reported in atrial biopsy specimens from AF patients. Given that PITX2 regulates the activities of half of the genes with left-sided enrichment [370], the impact of altered left atrial Pitx2 expression on atrial remodeling is probably related to its positioning at the crossroad of several arrhythmogenic pathways [371], including pathways related to fibrosis, $Ca^{2+}$ handling, gap junctions, and ion channels [372]. Animal and human studies have recently demonstrated that AF is associated with DNA hypermethylation of the Pitx2 promoter region [366]. In rats with spontaneous AF, chronic administration of decitabine, a DNA methylation inhibitor currently used in clinical practice for cancer therapy, reduced perivascular myocardial fibrosis, increased superoxid dismutase activity, and significantly decreased the AF burden [366], suggesting that hypomethylating agents may emerge as a tool for reducing the AF burden.

Abnormal levels of several microARNs have also been associated with the presence of AF. Studies have demonstrated elevated miR-21 levels in the left atria of AF patients and this was associated with decreased expression of Sprouty, an endogenous inhibitor of the MAP kinases pathway, with increased expression of fibrogenic factors and with increased collagen synthesis, as well as with myocardial hypertrophy, reduced inotropy, and left atrial enlargement [373, 374]. Meanwhile, in experimental models, anti-miR-21 administration decreased atrial fibrosis, attenuated inhomogeneous conduction, and reduced AF duration [374, 375]. However, as microARNs are highly dynamic, act collectively on gene expression, interact at multiple levels, and regulate many overlapping pathways at the same time, it is questionable whether selectively targeting unique microRNAs, either by up-regulating them using adenovirus transfection or by down-regulating them using antagomirs, will be useful for treating AF patients [376]. As research in this area continues, molecular studies are expected to significantly contribute to a better understanding of the AF pathophysiology and to identify novel therapeutic targets.

## Gaps in Knowledge and Future Research

Overall, strategies aiming to prevent, halt, and/or reverse atrial proarrhythmic structural remodeling have demonstrated very promising effects in experimental settings. The initial clinical results, mainly derived from hypothesis-generating small clinical trials and retrospective analyses of studies that did not have AF as prespecified endpoint, were also rather encouraging. However, with the advent of larger, randomized controlled trials, human data have proved rather unconvincing.

Despite the numerous similarities between laboratory animals and humans, there are obvious interspecies differences that mandate caution when extrapolating data from animal studies to human medicine. However, other factors may play an even more important role in the discordances observed between animal and human studies. Animal studies have often used drug doses higher than those used in clinical practice. The timing of drug administration may have also been considerably different in animal *versus* human studies; the tested therapeutic strategies are very likely to be applied in healthy animals, prior to AF onset, whereas in clinical practice upstream therapies are expected to be initiated after the first clinical event or, at the earliest, once established AF risk factors have been identified. One of the main issues, however, is likely to be related to the features of the currently used animal AF models, which, with very few exceptions [377], have limited ability to mimic the human condition. Whereas in clinical practice AF is generally a disease of the elderly with numerous concomitant cardiovascular conditions that increase propensity to AF (such as hypertension, heart failure, coronary artery disease, diabetes mellitus, etc.) and who are already on numerous other medications that may affect the AF risk (including RAAS blockers, statins, *beta*-blockers, etc.), most of the experimental data arises from juvenile, healthy animals, without concomitant conditions or drug therapies. Additionally, whereas in clinical practice AF arises spontaneously, usually on a background of factors that modify the structural substrate, in experimental settings AF is most often induced by rapid atrial pacing, in otherwise structurally normal hearts. Finally, whereas negative clinical trials have a good chance of being published, due to their potential immediate clinical impact, negative animal studies are much less likely to become visible, thus creating a publication bias.

Taken together, these factors may considerably limit the translational value of the data obtained in animal models and may explain why experimentally promising strategies have often failed when applied in clinical settings. Future studies will thus have to employ more clinically-relevant AF models, also taking into account comorbidities and comedication relevant to the AF population.

In the same time, however, data from clinical studies are also far from being concordant, with some studies showing an impressive benefit, while others showed no change, or even an increased AF risk, even when using similar therapies. Discrepancies are probably largely due to different study design, inclusion criteria, and study populations, different concomitant drugs usage and underlying pathologies, different severity of structural atrial remodeling, different duration of follow-up, different sample sizes, and different criteria used to diagnose AF. Whereas some strategies might be highly efficient in certain patients, they could be futile in many other settings. Upstream therapies may be of interest as adjuvant therapy in addition to conventional antiarrhythmic therapy, but they may be insufficient as unique therapy for secondary AF prevention, in patients in whom the atria is already severely remodeled. In addition, studies have used different agents, with different 'pleiotropic' properties, and in various doses. Since AF recurrences are known to be highly variable [108] and often asymptomatic [378], subjective symptoms assessment and non-systematic, intermittent ECG or Holter monitoring, which were used in the vast majority of studies for detecting AF relapses, may not be the most adequate means for assessing the true AF burden or the time to first AF recurrence. Also, whereas short-term studies may be adequate for assessing the impact of AF occurrence in acute settings, such as post-cardiac surgery, in the vast majority of studies on secondary AF prevention, follow-ups may have been too short to capture the entire benefit of these strategies. Contrary to conventional antiarrhythmic drugs, which act on the rapidly reversible electrical AF substrate, agents targeting the structural substrate may take a longer time to attain their full antiarrhythmic potential. Even if studies with longer-term follow-ups have been made, AF was usually not a prespecified endpoint in those studies, and this may have led to underestimation of the true AF burden [379].

The reality remains, however, that currently available antiarrhythmic strategies, which target the AF-related electrophysiological changes, are far from being ideal [380]. Meanwhile, given the mechanisms underlying AF occurrence and persistence, the concept of upstream AF therapy, which has moved us out of our well-established way of approaching AF, remains, at least theoretically, highly appealing. More should be made in the near future to successfully bring this concept into clinical practice. A number of novel drugs have showed promising results in experimental studies and now await confirmation in clinical settings. In parallel, researchers will have to continue to elucidate the intimate pathophysiological mechanisms of AF, which are very unlikely to have been fully unraveled, and to identify new therapeutic targets, including those that may very well deviate from our classical concepts of AF pathophysiology.

Despite the highly controversial results, the older, already widely tested upstream AF therapies remain of great interest. There are strong, at least theoretical, reasons to believe that statins, glucocorticoids, PUFAs, and especially RAAS blockers [381], may find their place in AF prophylaxis, at least in selected categories of patients. Their antiarrhythmic effects are likely to depend on the degree of atrial structural remodeling, as well as on the dominant underlying mechanisms of the arrhythmia. Future larger-scale, prospective, randomized controlled studies, specifically designed to assess the impact of these drugs on AF occurrence and/or recurrence, using newer, more sophisticated methods for detecting AF, such as telemonitoring or implantable loop recorders, will have to provide a definitive answer regarding the antiarrhythmic potential of these 'non-antiarrhythmic' drugs. These studies will have to confirm the role of each of these agents in AF primary and/or secondary prevention, and to identify in which patient, what single drug, in which dose, and at which moment could be of benefit against AF. Studies will also have to establish the potential impact of the genetic profile on patients' response to upstream therapies. After these goals have been reached, it is expected that these data will set the basis for a tailored approach for each individual patient.

While awaiting answers to these questions and/or clinical confirmation for the newer upstream therapies, the solution could reside in a much wider approach, that targets several substrate-modifying pathways, rather than in one single type of upstream therapy. In the randomized Routine vs. Aggressive upstream rhythm Control for prevention of Early persistent atrial fibrillation in heart failure (RACE3) study, an aggressive approach including ACEIs and/or ARBs, mineralocorticoid receptor antagonists, statins, cardiac rehabilitation therapy, and intensive counseling on dietary restrictions, exercise maintenance, and drug adherence significantly increased sinus rhythm maintenance compared with conventional rhythm control alone in mild-to-moderate heart failure patients with early persistent AF [382]. A combination of ARB and statin was also more efficient than a calcium channel blocker or an ARB alone in reducing the recurrence rate of non-permanent AF and delaying the progression from non-permanent to permanent AF in the hypertensive patients included in the VF-HT-AF study [383].

## Conclusions

Currently available antiarrhythmic drugs have obvious limitations with regard to their efficacy and safety. Increasing knowledge concerning the major role of atrial structural remodeling in AF onset and persistence clarifies, at least partially, the failure of conventional antiarrhythmic drugs, and opens the way for a different therapeutic approach, upstream of AF. If proved efficient, such an approach could prevent or at least postpone the need for conventional antiarrhythmic drugs, and would considerably lower the adverse effects. To date, with the exception of ACEIs/ARBs, which should be considered in certain patient subgroups (i.e., with heart failure and reduced ejection fraction or with arterial hypertension, especially with left ventricular hypertrophy), there is insufficient evidence to support the wide use of non-conventional antiarrhythmic drugs for AF prophylaxis in clinical practice. It still remains to be established whether this approach is truly effective, by itself or at least in addition to conventional rhythm control strategies. Clarification of the most adequate target population, of the most suitable drug, dose, and timing to intervene is also required. This endeavor obviously mandates sustained, coordinated efforts from basic and clinical scientists, and implies considerable financial costs. However, if proved efficient, novel and/or already established upstream AF therapies are expected to considerably decrease AF-related hospitalization rates, morbidity, and mortality, and thus to have a major social and economic impact.

## References


1. Lip GY, Tse HF, Lane DA. Atrial fibrillation. Lancet. 2012;379:648–61.
2. Reynolds MR, Essebag V, Zimetbaum P, et al. Healthcare resource utilization and costs associated with recurrent episodes of atrial fibrillation: the FRACTAL registry. J Cardiovasc Electrophysiol. 2007;18:628–33.
3. Ehrlich JR, Nattel S. Novel approaches for pharmacological management of atrial fibrillation. Drugs. 2009;69:757–74.
4. Aviles RJ, Martin DO, Apperson-Hansen C, et al. Inflammation as a risk factor for atrial fibrillation. Circulation. 2003;108:3006–10.
5. Disertori M, Latini R, Maggioni AP. Role of renin–angiotensin system inhibitors in atrial fibrillation. J Cardiovasc Med. 2010;11:912–8.
6. Mayyas F, Alzoubi KH, Van Wagoner DR. Impact of aldosterone antagonists on the substrate for atrial fibrillation: aldosterone promotes oxidative stress and atrial structural/electrical remodeling. Int J Cardiol. 2013;168:5135–42.
7. Frustaci A, Chimenti C, Bellocci F, et al. Histological substrate of atrial biopsies in patients with lone atrial fibrillation. Circulation. 1997;96:1180–4.

8. Xu J, Cui G, Esmailian F, et al. Atrial extracellular matrix remodeling and the maintenance of atrial fibrillation. Circulation. 2004;109:363–8.
9. Schotten U, Verheule S, Kirchhof P, et al. Pathophysiological mechanisms of atrial fibrillation: a translational appraisal. Physiol Rev. 2011;91:265–325.
10. Mihm MJ, Coyle CM, Schanbacher BL, et al. Peroxynitrite induced nitration and inactivation of myofibrillar creatine kinase in experimental heart failure. Cardiovasc Res. 2001;49:798–807.
11. Kim YM, Guzik TJ, Zhang YH, et al. A myocardial Nox2 containing NAD(P)H oxidase contributes to oxidative stress in human atrial fibrillation. Circ Res. 2005;97:629–36.
12. Briggs LE, Takeda M, Cuadra AE, et al. Perinatal loss of Nkx2-5 results in rapid conduction and contraction defects. Circ Res. 2008;103:580–90.
13. Babu GJ, Bhupathy P, Carnes CA, et al. Differential expression of sarcolipin protein during muscle development and cardiac pathophysiology. J Mol Cell Cardiol. 2007;43:215–22.
14. Carnes CA, Chung MK, Nakayama T, et al. Ascorbate attenuates atrial pacing-induced peroxynitrite formation and electrical remodeling and decreases the incidence of postoperative atrial fibrillation. Circ Res. 2001;89:E32–8.
15. Morgera T, Di Lenarda A, Dreas L, et al. Electrocardiography of myocarditis revisited: clinical and prognostic significance of electrocardiographic changes. Am Heart J. 1992;124:455–67.
16. Bruins P, te Velthuis H, Yazdanbakhs AP, et al. Activation of the complement system during and after cardiopulmonary bypass surgery: post-surgery activation involves C-reactive protein and is associated with postoperative arrhythmia. Circulation. 1997;96:3542–8.
17. Dernellis J, Panaretou M. C-reactive protein and paroxysmal atrial fibrillation: evidence of the implication of an inflammatory process in paroxysmal atrial fibrillation. Acta Cardiol. 2001;56:375–80.
18. Gedikli O, Dogan A, Altuntas I, et al. Inflammatory markers according to types of atrial fibrillation. Int J Cardiol. 2007;120:193–7.
19. Scridon A, Girerd N, Rugeri L, et al. Progressive endothelial damage revealed by multilevel von Willebrand factor plasma concentrations in atrial fibrillation patients. Europace. 2013;15:1562–6.

20. Healey JS, Baranchuk A, Crystal E, et al. Prevention of atrial fibrillation with angiotensin converting enzyme inhibitors and angiotensin receptor blockers: a meta-analysis. J Am Coll Cardiol. 2005;45:1832–9.
21. Siu CW, Lau CP, Tse HF. Prevention of atrial fibrillation recurrence by statin therapy in patients with lone atrial fibrillation after successful cardioversion. Am J Cardiol. 2003;92:1343–5.
22. Ito H, Ono K, Nishio R, et al. Amiodarone inhibits interleukin 6 production and attenuates myocardial injury induced by viral myocarditis in mice. Cytokine. 2002;17:197–202.
23. Merritt JC, Niebauer M, Tarakji K, et al. Comparison of effectiveness of carvedilol versus metoprolol or atenolol for atrial fibrillation appearing after coronary artery bypass grafting or cardiac valve operation. Am J Cardiol. 2003;92:735–6.
24. Scridon A, Dobreanu D, Chevalier P, et al. Inflammation, a link between obesity and atrial fibrillation. Inflamm Res. 2015;64:383–93.
25. Lendeckel UDD, Goette A. Aldosterone-receptor antagonism as a potential therapeutic option for atrial fibrillation. Br J Pharmacol. 2010;159:1581–3.
26. Boldt A, Wetzel U, Weigl J, et al. Expression of angiotensin II receptors in human left and right atrial tissue in atrial fibrillation with and without underlying mitral valve disease. J Am Coll Cardiol. 2003;42:1785–92.
27. Tsai CT, Chiang FT, Tseng CD, et al. Increased expression of mineralocorticoid receptor in human atrial fibrillation and a cellular model of atrial fibrillation. J Am Coll Cardiol. 2010;55:758–70.
28. Goette A, Hoffmanns P, Enayati W, et al. Effect of successful electrical cardioversion on serum aldosterone in patients with persistent atrial fibrillation. Am J Cardiol. 2001;88:906–9.
29. Dixen U, Ravn L, Soeby-Rasmussen C, et al. Raised plasma aldosterone and natriuretic peptides in atrial fibrillation. Cardiology. 2007;108:35–9.
30. Liu T, Korantzopoulos P, Xu G, et al. Association between angiotensin-converting enzyme insertion/deletion gene polymorphism and atrial fibrillation: a meta-analysis. Europace. 2011;13:346–54.
31. Ueberham L, Bollmann A, Shoemaker MB, et al. Genetic ACE I/D polymorphism and recurrence of atrial fibrillation after catheter ablation. Circ Arrhythm Electrophysiol. 2013;6:732–7.

32. Amir O, Amir RE, Paz H, et al. Aldosterone synthase gene polymorphism as a determinant of atrial fibrillation in patients with heart failure. Am J Cardiol. 2008;102:326–9.
33. Dobaczewski M, Bujak M, Li N, et al. SMAD3 signaling critically regulates fibroblast phenotype and function in healing myocardial infarction. Circ Res. 2010;107:418–28.
34. Brilla CG, Zhou G, Matsubara L, et al. Collagen metabolism in cultured adult rat cardiac fibroblasts: response to angiotensin II and aldosterone. J Mol Cell Cardiol. 1994;26:809–20.
35. Weber KT. Aldosterone and spironolactone in heart failure. N Engl J Med. 1999;341:753–5.
36. Marney AM, Brown NJ. Aldosterone and end-organ damage. Clin Sci (Lond). 2007;113:267–78.
37. Johar S, Cave AC, Narayanapanicker A, et al. Aldosterone mediates angiotensin II-induced interstitial cardiac fibrosis via a Nox2-containing NADPH oxidase. FASEB J. 2006;20:1546–8.
38. Gekle M, Mildenberger S, Freudinger R, et al. Altered collagen homeostasis in human aortic smooth muscle cells (HAoSMCs) induced by aldosterone. Pflugers Arch. 2007;454:403–13.
39. Brilla CG, Funck RC, Rupp H. Lisinopril-mediated regression of myocardial fibrosis in patients with hypertensive heart disease. Circulation. 2000;102:1388–93.
40. Pitt B, Zannad F, Remme WJ, et al. The effect of spironolactone on morbidity and mortality in patients with severe heart failure. Randomized Aldactone Evaluation Study Investigators. N Engl J Med. 1999;341:709–17.
41. Cardin S, Li D, Thorin-Trescases N, et al. Evolution of the atrial fibrillation substrate in experimental congestive heart failure: angiotensin dependent and independent pathways. Cardiovasc Res. 2003;60:315–25.
42. Burniston JG, Saini A, Tan LB, et al. Aldosterone induces myocyte apoptosis in the heart and skeletal muscles of rats in vivo. J Mol Cell Cardiol. 2005;39:395–9.
43. Hirono Y, Yoshimoto T, Suzuki N, et al. Angiotensin II receptor type 1-mediated vascular oxidative stress and proinflammatory gene expression in aldosterone-induced hypertension: the possible role of local renin-angiotensin system. Endocrinology. 2007;148:1688–96.
44. Kobayashi N, Yoshida K, Nakano S, et al. Cardioprotective mechanisms of eplerenone on cardiac performance and remodeling in failing rat hearts. Hypertension. 2006;47:671–9.

45. Klanke B, Cordasic N, Hartner A, et al. Blood pressure versus direct mineralocorticoid effects on kidney inflammation and fibrosis in DOCA-salt hypertension. Nephrol Dial Transplant. 2008;23:3456–63.
46. López B, Querejeta R, Varo N, et al. Usefulness of serum carboxy-terminal propeptide of procollagen type I in assessment of the cardioreparative ability of antihypertensive treatment in hypertensive patients. Circulation. 2001;104:286–91.
47. Milliez P, Deangelis N, Rucker-Martin C, et al. Spironolactone reduces fibrosis of dilated atria during heart failure in rats with myocardial infarction. Eur Heart J. 2005;26:2193–9.
48. Funder JW. Mineralocorticoid receptors: distribution and activation. Heart Fail Rev. 2005;10:15–22.
49. Schmidt BM, Schmieder RE. Aldosterone-induced cardiac damage: focus on blood pressure independent effects. Am J Hypertens. 2003;16:80–6.
50. Rocha R, Stier CT Jr, Kifor I, et al. Aldosterone: a mediator of myocardial necrosis and renal arteriopathy. Endocrinology. 2000;141:3871–8.
51. Cooper SA, Whaley-Connell A, Habibi J, et al. Renin–angiotensin-aldosterone system and oxidative stress in cardiovascular insulin resistance. Am J Physiol Heart Circ Physiol. 2007;293:H2009–23.
52. Kobayashi N, Fukushima H, Takeshima H, et al. Effect of eplerenone on endothelial progenitor cells and oxidative stress in ischemic hindlimb. Am J Hypertens. 2010;23:1007–13.
53. Bayorh MA, Mann G, Walton M, et al. Effects of enalapril, tempol, and eplerenone on saltinduced hypertension in Dahl salt-sensitive rats. Clin Exp Hypertens. 2006;28:121–32.
54. Ceron CS, Castro MM, Rizzi E, et al. Spironolactone and hydrochlorothiazide exert antioxidant effects and reduce vascular matrix metalloproteinase-2 activity and expression in a model of renovascular hypertension. Br J Pharmacol. 2010;160:77–87.
55. Habibi J, DeMarco VG, Ma L, et al. Mineralocorticoid receptor blockade improves diastolic function independent of blood pressure reduction in a transgenic model of RAAS overexpression. Am J Physiol Heart Circ Physiol. 2011;300:H1484–91.
56. Lastra G, Whaley-Connell A, Manrique C, et al. Low-dose spironolactone reduces reactive oxygen species generation and improves insulin-stimulated glucose transport in skeletal muscle in the TG(mRen2)27 rat. Am J Physiol Endocrinol Metab. 2008;295:E110–6.

57. Benitah JP, Vassort G. Aldosterone upregulates Ca(2+) current in adult rat cardiomyocytes. Circ Res. 1999;85:1139–45.
58. Lalevee N, Rebsamen MC, Barrere-Lemaire S, et al. Aldosterone increases T-type calcium channel expression and in vitro beating frequency in neonatal rat cardiomyocytes. Cardiovasc Res. 2005;67:216–24.
59. Chen YJ, Chen YC, Tai CT, et al. Angiotensin II and angiotensin II receptor blocker modulate the arrhythmogenic activity of pulmonary veins. Br J Pharmacol. 2006;147:12–22.
60. Goette A, Lendeckel U. Electrophysiological effects of angiotensin II. Part I: signal transduction and basic electrophysiological mechanisms. Europace. 2008;10:238–41.
61. Nakashima H, Kumagai K, Urata H, et al. Angiotensin II antagonist prevents electrical remodeling in atrial fibrillation. Circulation. 2000;101:2612–7.
62. Perrier R, Richard S, Sainte-Marie Y, et al. A direct relationship between plasma aldosterone and cardiac L-type Ca2+ current in mice. J Physiol. 2005;569:153–62.
63. Gómez AM, Rueda A, Sainte-Marie Y, et al. Mineralocorticoid modulation of cardiac ryanodine receptor activity is associated with downregulation of FK506-binding proteins. Circulation. 2009;119:2179–87.
64. Lammers C, Dartsch T, Brandt MC, et al. Spironolactone prevents aldosterone induced increased duration of atrial fibrillation in rat. Cell Physiol Biochem. 2012;29:833–40.
65. Mihailidou AS, Bundgaard H, Mardini M, et al. Hyperaldosteronemia in rabbits inhibits the cardiac sarcolemmal Na(+)-K(+). Circ Res. 2000;86:37–42.
66. Benitah JP, Perrier E, Gomez AM, et al. Effects of aldosterone on transient outward K+ current density in rat ventricular myocytes. J Physiol. 2001;537:151–60.
67. Laszlo R, Bentz K, Konior A, et al. Effects of selective mineralocorticoid receptor antagonism on atrial ion currents and early ionic tachycardia-induced electrical remodelling in rabbits. Naunyn Schmiedeberg's Arch Pharmacol. 2010;382:347–56.
68. Qu J, Volpicelli FM, Garcia LI, et al. Gap junction remodeling and spironolactone-dependent reverse remodeling in the hypertrophied heart. Circ Res. 2009;104:365–71.
69. Takemoto Y, Ramirez RJ, Kaur K, et al. Eplerenone reduces atrial fibrillation burden without preventing atrial electrical remodeling. J Am Coll Cardiol. 2017;70:2893–905.

70. Musa H, Kaur K, O'Connell R, et al. Inhibition of platelet-derived growth factor-AB signaling prevents electromechanical remodeling of adult atrial myocytes that contact myofibroblasts. Heart Rhythm. 2013;10:1044–51.
71. Kaur K, Zarzoso M, Ponce-Balbuena D, et al. TGF-β1, released by myofibroblasts, differentially regulates transcription and function of sodium and potassium channels in adult rat ventricular myocytes. PLoS One. 2013;8:e55391.
72. Konno S, Hirooka Y, Kishi T, et al. Sympathoinhibitory effects of telmisartan through the reduction of oxidative stress in the rostral ventrolateral medulla of obesity-induced hypertensive rats. J Hypertens. 2012;30:1992–9.
73. Lewandowski J, Abramczyk P, Dobosiewicz A, et al. The effect of enalapril and telmisartan on clinical and biochemical indices of sympathetic activity in hypertensive patients. Clin Exp Hypertens. 2008;30:423–32.
74. Zhao J, Li J, Li W, et al. Effects of spironolactone on atrial structural remodelling in a canine model of atrial fibrillation produced by prolonged atrial pacing. Br J Pharmacol. 2010;159:1584–94.
75. Li D, Shinagawa K, Pang L, et al. Effects of angiotensin-converting enzyme inhibition on the development of the atrial fibrillation substrate in dogs with ventricular tachypacing-induced congestive heart failure. Circulation. 2001;104:2608–14.
76. Liu E, Xu Z, Li J, et al. Enalapril, irbesartan, and angiotensin-(1–7) prevent atrial tachycardia-induced ionic remodeling. Int J Cardiol. 2011;146:364–70.
77. Li Y, Li WM, Gong YT, et al. The effects of cilazapril and valsartan on the mRNA and protein expressions of atrial calpains and atrial structural remodeling in atrial fibrillation dogs. Basic Res Cardiol. 2007;102:245–56.
78. Kimura S, Ito M, Tomita M, et al. Role of mineralocorticoid receptor on atrial structural remodeling and inducibility of atrial fibrillation in hypertensive rats. Hypertens Res. 2011;34:584–91.
79. Shroff SC, Ryu K, Martovitz NL, et al. Selective aldosterone blockade suppresses atrial tachyarrhythmias in heart failure. J Cardiovasc Electrophysiol. 2006;17:534–41.
80. Yang SS, Han W, Zhou HY, et al. Effects of spironolactone on electrical and structural remodeling of atrium in congestive heart failure dogs. Chin Med J. 2008;121:38–42.

81. Birnie DH, Gollob M, Healey JS. Clinical trials, the renin angiotensin system and atrial fibrillation. Curr Opin Cardiol. 2006;21:368–75.
82. Maggioni AP, Latini R, Carson PE, et al. Valsartan reduces the incidence of atrial fibrillation in patients with heart failure: results from the Valsartan Heart Failure Trial (Val-HeFT). Am Heart J. 2005;149:548–57.
83. Ishikawa K, Yamada T, Yoshida Y, et al. Renin-angiotensin system blocker use may be associated with suppression of atrial fibrillation recurrence after pulmonary vein isolation. Pacing Clin Electrophysiol. 2011;34:296–303.
84. Madrid AH, Bueno MG, Rebollo JM, et al. Use of irbesartan to maintain sinus rhythm in patients with long lasting persistent atrial fibrillation: a prospective and randomized study. Circulation. 2002;106:331–6.
85. Ueng KC, Tsai TP, Yu WC, et al. Use of enalapril to facilitate sinus rhythm maintenance after external cardioversion of long standing persistent atrial fibrillation. Results of a prospective and controlled study. Eur Heart J. 2003;24:2090–8.
86. Fogari R, Mugellini A, Destro M, et al. Losartan and prevention of atrial fibrillation recurrence in hypertensive patients. J Cardiovasc Pharmacol. 2006;47:46–50.
87. Yin Y, Dalal D, Liu Z, et al. Prospective randomized study comparing amiodarone vs. amiodarone plus losartan vs. amiodarone plus perindopril for prevention of atrial fibrillation recurrence in patients with lone paroxysmal atrial fibrillation. Eur Heart J. 2006;27:1841–6.
88. Cui Y, Ma C, Long D, et al. Effect of valsartan on atrial fibrillation recurrence following pulmonary vein isolation in patients. Exp Ther Med. 2015;9:631–5.
89. Madrid AH, Marín IM, Cervantes CE, et al. Prevention of recurrences in patients with lone atrial fibrillation. The dose-dependent effect of angiotensin II receptor blockers. J Renin-Angiotensin-Aldosterone Syst. 2004;5:114–20.
90. Huang CY, Yang YH, Lin LY, et al. Renin-angiotensin-aldosterone blockade reduces atrial fibrillation in hypertrophic cardiomyopathy. Heart. 2018;104:1276–83.
91. Hsieh YC, Hung CY, Li CH, et al. Angiotensin-receptor blocker, angiotensin-converting enzyme inhibitor, and risks of atrial fibrillation: a nationwide cohort study. Medicine (Baltimore). 2016;95:e3721.

92. Schneider MP, Hua TA, Böhm M, et al. Prevention of atrial fibrillation by renin-angiotensin system inhibition: a meta-analysis. J Am Coll Cardiol. 2010;55:2299–307.
93. Huang G, Xu JB, Liu JX, et al. Angiotensin-converting enzyme inhibitors and angiotensin receptor blockers decrease the incidence of atrial fibrillation: a meta-analysis. Eur J Clin Investig. 2011;41:719–33.
94. Williams RS, Delemos JA, Dimas V, et al. Effect of spironolactone on patients with atrial fibrillation and structural heart disease. Clin Cardiol. 2011;34:415–9.
95. Ito Y, Yamasaki H, Naruse Y, et al. Effect of eplerenone on maintenance of sinus rhythm after catheter ablation in patients with long-standing persistent atrial fibrillation. Am J Cardiol. 2013;111:1012–8.
96. Swedberg K, Zannad F, McMurray JJ, et al. Eplerenone and atrial fibrillation in mild systolic heart failure: results from the EMPHASIS-HF (Eplerenone in Mild Patients Hospitalization And SurvIval Study in Heart Failure) study. J Am Coll Cardiol. 2012;59:1598–603.
97. Liu T, Korantzopoulos P, Shao Q, et al. Mineralocorticoid receptor antagonists and atrial fibrillation: a meta-analysis. Europace. 2016;18:672–8.
98. Neefs J, van den Berg NW, Limpens J, et al. Aldosterone pathway blockade to prevent atrial fibrillation: a systematic review and meta-analysis. Int J Cardiol. 2017;231:155–61.
99. Hansson L, Lindholm LH, Niskanen L, et al. Effect of angiotensin-converting-enzyme inhibition compared with conventional therapy on cardiovascular morbidity and mortality in hypertension: the Captopril Prevention Project (CAPPP) randomised trial. Lancet. 1999;353:611–6.
100. Hansson L, Lindholm LH, Ekbom T, et al. Randomised trial of old and new antihypertensive drugs in elderly patients: cardiovascular mortality and morbidity the Swedish Trial in Old Patients with Hypertension-2 study. Lancet. 1999;354:1751–6.
101. Salehian O, Healey J, Stambler B, et al. Impact of ramipril on the incidence of atrial fibrillation: results of the Heart Outcomes Prevention Evaluation study. Am Heart J. 2007;154:448–53.
102. Schmieder RE, Kjeldsen SE, Julius S, et al. Reduced incidence of new-onset atrial fibrillation with angiotensin II receptor blockade: the VALUE trial. J Hypertens. 2008;26:403–11.

103. Wachtell K, Lehto M, Gerdts E, et al. Angiotensin II receptor blockade reduces new-onset atrial fibrillation and subsequent stroke compared to atenolol: the Losartan Intervention for End Point Reduction in Hypertension (LIFE) study. J Am Coll Cardiol. 2005;45:712–9.
104. Yusuf S, Teo K, Anderson C, et al. Effects of the angiotensin-receptor blocker telmisartan on cardiovascular events in high-risk patients intolerant to angiotensin-converting enzyme inhibitors: a randomised controlled trial. Lancet. 2008;372:1174–83.
105. Zhao D, Wang ZM, Wang LS. Prevention of atrial fibrillation with renin-angiotensin system inhibitors on essential hypertensive patients: a meta-analysis of randomized controlled trials. J Biomed Res. 2015;29:475–85.
106. Dewland TA, Soliman EZ, Yamal JM, et al. Pharmacologic prevention of incident atrial fibrillation: long-term results from the ALLHAT (Antihypertensive and Lipid-Lowering Treatment to Prevent Heart Attack Trial). Circ Arrhythm Electrophysiol. 2017;10:e005463.
107. Anand K, Mooss AN, Hee TT, et al. Meta-analysis: inhibition of renin-angiotensin system prevents new-onset atrial fibrillation. Am Heart J. 2006;152:217–22.
108. Goette A, Schon N, Kirchhof P, et al. Angiotensin II-antagonist in paroxysmal atrial fibrillation (ANTIPAF) trial. Circ Arrhythm Electrophysiol. 2012;5:43–51.
109. Massie BM, Carson PE, McMurray JJ, et al. Irbesartan in patients with heart failure and preserved ejection fraction. N Engl J Med. 2008;359:2456–67.
110. Al Chekakie MO, Akar JG, Wang F, et al. The effects of statins and renin-angiotensin system blockers on atrial fibrillation recurrence following antral pulmonary vein isolation. J Cardiovasc Electrophysiol. 2007;18:942–6.
111. Zheng B, Kang J, Tian Y, et al. Angiotensin-converting enzyme inhibitors and angiotensin II receptor blockers have no beneficial effect on ablation outcome in chronic persistent atrial fibrillation. Acta Cardiol. 2009;64:335–40.
112. Patel D, Mohanty P, Di Biase L, et al. The impact of statins and renin-angiotensin-aldosterone system blockers on pulmonary vein antrum isolation outcomes in post-menopausal females. Europace. 2010;12:322–30.
113. Tveit A, Grundvold I, Olufsen M, et al. Candesartan in the prevention of relapsing atrial fibrillation. Int J Cardiol. 2007;120:85–91.

114. Disertori M, Latini R, Barlera S, et al. Valsartan for prevention of recurrent atrial fibrillation. N Engl J Med. 2009;360:1606–17.
115. Yusuf S, Healey JS, Pogue J, et al. Irbesartan in patients with atrial fibrillation. N Engl J Med. 2011;364:928–38.
116. Cikes M, Claggett B, Shah AM, et al. Atrial fibrillation in heart failure with preserved ejection fraction: the TOPCAT trial. JACC Heart Fail. 2018;6(8):689–97.
117. Carrel T, Englberger L, Mohacsi P, et al. Low systemic vascular resistance after cardiopulmonary bypass: incidence, etiology, and clinical importance. J Card Surg. 2000;15:347–53.
118. Arora P, Rajagopalam S, Ranjan R, et al. Preoperative use of angiotensin converting enzyme inhibitors/angiotensin receptor blockers is associated with increased risk for acute kidney injury after cardiovascular surgery. Clin J Am Soc Nephrol. 2008;3:1266–73.
119. Pretorius M, Murray KT, Yu C, et al. Angiotensin-converting enzyme inhibition or mineralocorticoid receptor blockade do not affect prevalence of atrial fibrillation in patients undergoing cardiac surgery. Crit Care Med. 2012;40:2805–12.
120. El-Haddad MA, Zalawadiya SK, Awdallah H, et al. Role of irbesartan in prevention of post-coronary artery bypass graft atrial fibrillation. Am J Cardiovasc Drugs. 2011;11:277–84.
121. Ozaydin M, Dede O, Varol E, et al. Effect of renin-angiotensin aldosteron system blockers on postoperative atrial fibrillation. Int J Cardiol. 2008;127:362–7.
122. Shi Y, Li D, Tardif JC, et al. Enalapril effects on atrial remodeling and atrial fibrillation in experimental congestive heart failure. Cardiovasc Res. 2002;54:456–61.
123. Vermes E, Tardif JC, Bourassa MG, et al. Enalapril decreases the incidence of atrial fibrillation in patients with left ventricular dysfunction: insight from the Studies Of Left Ventricular Dysfunction (SOLVD) trials. Circulation. 2003;107:2926–31.
124. Singh JP, Kulik A, Levin R, et al. Renin-angiotensin-system modulators and the incidence of atrial fibrillation following hospitalization for coronary artery disease. Europace. 2012;14:1287–93.
125. Belluzzi F, Sernesi L, Preti P, et al. Prevention of recurrent lone atrial fibrillation by the angiotensin-II converting enzyme inhibitor ramipril in normotensive patients. J Am Coll Cardiol. 2009;53:24–9.
126. Ducharme A, Swedberg K, Pfeffer MA, et al. Prevention of atrial fibrillation in patients with symptomatic chronic

heart failure by candesartan in the Candesartan in Heart failure: assessment of Reduction in Mortality and morbidity (CHARM) program. Am Heart J. 2006;152:86–92.
127. Pizzetti F, Turazza FM, Franzosi MG, et al. Incidence and prognostic significance of atrial fibrillation in acute myocardial infarction: the GISSI 3 data. Heart. 2001;86:527–32.
128. Salchian O, Healey J, Stambler B, et al. Impact of ramipril on the incidence of atrial fibrillation: results of the Heart Outcomes Prevention Evaluation study. Am Heart J. 2007;154:448–53.
129. Yusuf S, Teo KK, Pogue J, et al. Telmisartan, ramipril, or both in patients at high risk for vascular events. N Engl J Med. 2008;358:1547–59.
130. Aksnes TA, Flaa A, Strand A, et al. Prevention of new-onset atrial fibrillation and its predictors with angiotensin II-receptor blockers in the treatment of hypertension and heart failure. J Hypertens. 2007;25:15–23.
131. Savelieva I, Kakouros N, Kourliouros A, et al. Upstream therapies for management of atrial fibrillation: review of clinical evidence and implications for European Society of Cardiology guidelines. Part I: primary prevention. Europace. 2011;13:308–28.
132. Yamashita T, Inoue H, Okumura K, et al. Randomized trial of angiotensin II-receptor blocker vs. dihydropiridine calcium channel blocker in the treatment of paroxysmal atrial fibrillation with hypertension (J-RHYTHM II study). Europace. 2011;13:473–9.
133. Dabrowski R, Borowiec A, Smolis-Bak E, et al. Effect of combined spironolactone-β-blocker ± enalapril treatment on occurrence of symptomatic atrial fibrillation episodes in patients with a history of paroxysmal atrial fibrillation (SPIR-AF study). Am J Cardiol. 2010;106:1609–14.
134. Han M, Zhang Y, Sun S, et al. Renin-angiotensin system inhibitors prevent the recurrence of atrial fibrillation: a meta-analysis of randomized controlled trials. J Cardiovasc Pharmacol. 2013;62:405–15.
135. Strauss MH, Hall AS. Angiotensin receptor blockers may increase risk of myocardial infarction: unraveling the ARB-MI paradox. Circulation. 2006;114:838–54.
136. Chrysant SG, Chrysant GS. The pleiotropic effects of angiotensin receptor blockers. J Clin Hypertens (Greenwich). 2006;8:261–8.

137. Siragy HM, Carey RM. The subtype 2 (AT2) angiotensin receptor mediates renal production of nitric oxide in conscious rats. J Clin Invest. 1997;100:264–9.
138. Pitt B. "Escape" of aldosterone production in patients with left ventricular dysfunction treated with an angiotensin converting enzyme inhibitor: implications for therapy. Cardiovasc Drugs Ther. 1995;9:145–9.
139. Mentz RJ, Bakris GL, Waeber B, et al. The past, present and future of renin-angiotensin aldosterone system inhibition. Int J Cardiol. 2013;167:1677–87.
140. Satoh A, Niwano S, Niwano H, et al. Aliskiren suppresses atrial electrical and structural remodeling in a canine model of atrial fibrillation. Heart Vessel. 2017;32:90–100.
141. Ellermann C, Mittelstedt A, Güner F, et al. Acute proarrhythmic effect of aliskiren in an experimental model of atrial fibrillation. Clin Res Cardiol. 2018;107. (Abstract).
142. Takei Y, Ichikawa M, Kijima Y. Oral direct renin inhibitor aliskiren reduces in vivo oxidative stress and serum matrix metalloproteinase-2 levels in patients with permanent atrial fibrillation. J Arrhythm. 2015;31:76–7.
143. Der Sarkissian S, Huentelman MJ, Stewart J, et al. ACE2: a novel therapeutic target for cardiovascular diseases. Prog Biophys Mol Biol. 2006;91:163–98.
144. Kirchhof P, Benussi S, Kotecha D, et al. 2016 ESC Guidelines for the management of atrial fibrillation developed in collaboration with EACTS. Eur Heart J. 2016;37:2893–962.
145. Savelieva I, Kourliouros A, Camm J. Primary and secondary prevention of atrial fibrillation with statins and polyunsaturated fatty acids: review of evidence and clinical relevance. Naunyn Schmiedeberg's Arch Pharmacol. 2010;381:1–13.
146. Riesen WF, Engler H, Risch M, et al. Short-term effects of atorvastatin on C-reactive protein. Eur Heart J. 2002;23:794–9.
147. Lefer DJ. Statins as potent antiinflammatory drugs. Circulation. 2002;106:2041–2.
148. Fauchier L, Pierre B, de Labriolle A, et al. Antiarrhythmic effect of statin therapy and atrial fibrillation a meta-analysis of randomized controlled trials. J Am Coll Cardiol. 2008;51:828–35.
149. Imazio M. Primary prevention of atrial fibrillation where are we in 2012? J Atr Fibrillation. 2012;5:608.
150. Maggioni AP, Fabbri G, Lucci D, et al. Effect of rosuvastatin on atrial fibrillation: ancillary results of the GISSI-HF trial. Eur Heart J. 2009;30:2327–36.

151. Shiroshita-Takeshita A, Brundel BJ, et al. Effects of simvastatin on the development of the atrial fibrillation substrate in dogs with congestive heart failure. Cardiovasc Res. 2007;74:75–84.
152. Porter KE, O'Regan DJ, Balmforth AJ, et al. Simvastatin reduces human atrial myofibroblast proliferation independently of cholesterol lowering via inhibition of RhoA. Cardiovasc Res. 2004;61:745–55.
153. Negi S, Shukrullah I, Veledar E, et al. Statin therapy for the prevention of atrial fibrillation trial (SToP AF trial). J Cardiovasc Electrophysiol. 2011;22:414–9.
154. Kumagai K, Nakashima H, Saku K. The HMG-CoA reductase inhibitor atorvastatin prevents atrial fibrillation by inhibiting inflammation in a canine sterile pericarditis model. Cardiovasc Res. 2004;62:105–11.
155. Shiroshita-Takeshita A, Schram G, Lavoie J, et al. The effect of simvastatin and antioxidant vitamins on atrial fibrillation—promotion by atrial tachycardia remodeling in dogs. Circulation. 2004;110:2313–9.
156. Hanna IR, Heeke B, Bush H, et al. Lipid-lowering drug use is associated with reduced prevalence of atrial fibrillation in patients with left ventricular systolic dysfunction. Heart Rhythm. 2006;3:881–6.
157. Dickinson MG, Hellkamp AS, Ip JH, et al. Statin therapy was associated with reduced atrial fibrillation and flutter in heart failure patients in SCD-HEFT. Heart Rhythm. 2006;3:S49. (Abstract).
158. Liu T, Li L, Korantzopoulos P, et al. Statin use and development of atrial fibrillation: a systematic review and meta-analysis of randomized clinical trials and observational studies. Int J Cardiol. 2008;126:160–70.
159. Bang CN, Greve AM, Abdulla J, et al. The preventive effect of statin therapy on new-onset and recurrent atrial fibrillation in patients not undergoing invasive cardiac interventions: a systematic review and meta-analysis. Int J Cardiol. 2013;167:624–30.
160. Fauchier L, Clementy N, Babuty D. Statin therapy and atrial fibrillation: systematic review and updated meta-analysis of published randomized controlled trials. Curr Opin Cardiol. 2013;28:7–18.
161. Dernellis J, Panaretou M. Effect of C-reactive protein reduction on paroxysmal atrial fibrillation. Am Heart J. 2005;150:1064.

162. Song YB, On YK, Kim JH, et al. The effects of atorvastatin on the occurrence of postoperative atrial fibrillation after off-pump coronary artery bypass grafting surgery. Am Heart J. 2008;156:373.
163. Patti G, Chello M, Candura D, et al. Randomized trial of atorvastatin for reduction of postoperative atrial fibrillation in patients undergoing cardiac surgery: results of the ARMYDA-3 (Atorvastatin for Reduction of MYocardial Dysrhythmia After cardiac surgery) study. Circulation. 2006;114:1455–61.
164. Ji Q, Mei Y, Wang X, et al. Effect of preoperative atorvastatin therapy on atrial fibrillation following off-pump coronary artery bypass grafting. Circ J. 2009;73:2244–9.
165. Loffredo L, Angelico F, Perri L, et al. Upstream therapy with statin and recurrence of atrial fibrillation after electrical cardioversion. Review of the literature and meta-analysis. BMC Cardiovasc Disord. 2012;12:107.
166. Haywood LJ, Ford CE, Crow RS, ALLHAT Collaborative Research Group, et al. Atrial fibrillation at baseline and during follow-up in ALLHAT (Antihypertensive and lipid-lowering treatment to prevent heart attack trial). J Am Coll Cardiol. 2009;54:2023–31.
167. Thacker EL, Jensen PN, Psaty BM, et al. Use of statins and antihypertensive medications in relation to risk of long-standing persistent atrial fibrillation. Ann Pharmacother. 2015;49:378–86.
168. Neuman RB, Bloom HL, Shukrullah I, et al. Oxidative stress markers are associated with persistent atrial fibrillation. Clin Chem. 2007;53:1652–7.
169. Reilly SN, Jayaram R, Nahar K, et al. Atrial sources of reactive oxygen species vary with the duration and substrate of atrial fibrillation: implications for the antiarrhythmic effect of statins. Circulation. 2011;124:1107–17.
170. Cangemi R, Celestini A, Calvieri C, et al. Different behaviour of NOX2 activation in patients with paroxysmal/persistent or permanent atrial fibrillation. Heart. 2012;98:1063–6.
171. Antoniades C, Demosthenous M, Reilly S, et al. Myocardial redox state predicts in-hospital clinical outcome after cardiac surgery effects of short-term pre-operative statin treatment. J Am Coll Cardiol. 2012;59:60–70.
172. Fang WT, Li HJ, Zhang H, et al. The role of statin therapy in the prevention of atrial fibrillation: a meta-analysis of randomized controlled trials. Br J Clin Pharmacol. 2012;74:744–56.

173. Rahimi K, Emberson J, McGale P, et al. Effect of statins on atrial fibrillation: collaborative meta-analysis of published and unpublished evidence from randomised controlled trials. BMJ. 2011;342:d1250.
174. Komatsu T, Tachibana H, Sato Y, et al. Long-term efficacy of upstream therapy with lipophilic or hydrophilic statins on anti-arrhythmic drugs in patients with paroxysmal atrial fibrillation: comparison between atorvastatin and pravastatin. Int Heart J. 2011;52:359–65.
175. Hognestad A, Aukrust P, Wergeland R, et al. Effects of conventional and aggressive statin treatment on markers of endothelial function and inflammation. Clin Cardiol. 2004;27:199–203.
176. Mason RP. Molecular basis of differences among statins and a comparison with antioxidant vitamins. Am J Cardiol. 2006;98:34P–41P.
177. Turner NA, Midgley L, O'Regan DJ, et al. Comparison of the efficacies of five different statins on inhibition of human saphenous vein smooth muscle cell proliferation and invasion. J Cardiovasc Pharmacol. 2007;50:458–61.
178. Naji F, Suran D, Kanic V, et al. Comparison of atorvastatin and simvastatin in prevention of atrial fibrillation after successful cardioversion. Int Heart J. 2009;50:153–60.
179. Hung CY, Hsieh YC, Wang KY, et al. Efficacy of different statins for primary prevention of atrial fibrillation in male and female patients: a nationwide population-based cohort study. Int J Cardiol. 2013;168:4367–9.
180. Savelieva I, Camm J. Statins and polyunsaturated fatty acids for treatment of atrial fibrillation. Nat Clin Pract Cardiovasc Med. 2008;5:30–41.
181. Sakabe M, Shiroshita-Takeshita A, Maguy A, et al. Omega-3 polyunsaturated fatty acids prevent atrial fibrillation associated with heart failure but not atrial tachycardia remodeling. Circulation. 2007;116:2101–9.
182. Yashodhara BM, Umakanth S, Pappachan JM, et al. Omega-3 fatty acids: a comprehensive review of their role in health and disease. Postgrad Med J. 2009;85:84–90.
183. Sarrazin JF, Comeau G, Daleau P, et al. Reduced incidence of vagally induced atrial fibrillation and expression levels of connexins by n-3 polyunsaturated fatty acids in dogs. J Am Coll Cardiol. 2007;50:1505–12.
184. Li GR, Sun HY, Zhang XH, et al. Omega-3 polyunsaturated fatty acids inhibit transient outward and ultra-rapid delayed

rectifier K+currents and Na+current in human atrial myocytes. Cardiovasc Res. 2009;81:286–93.
185. Boland LM, Drzewiecki MM. Polyunsaturated fatty acid modulation of voltage-gated ion channels. Cell Biochem Biophys. 2008;52:59–84.
186. Dhein S, Michaelis B, Mohr FW. Antiarrhythmic and electrophysiological effects of long-chain omega-3 polyunsaturated fatty acids. Naunyn Schmiedeberg's Arch Pharmacol. 2005;371:202–11.
187. Xiao Y-F, Ke Q, Chen Y, et al. Inhibitory effect of n-3 fish oil fatty acids on cardiac Na+/Ca2+ exchange currents in HEK293t cells. Biochem Biophys Res Commun. 2004;321:116–23.
188. Naccarelli GV, Wolbrette DL, Samii S, et al. New anti-arrhythmic treatment of atrial fibrillation. Expert Rev Cardiovasc Ther. 2007;5:707–14.
189. Chen H, Li D, Roberts GJ, et al. Eicosapentanoic acid inhibits hypoxia-reoxygenation-induced injury by attenuating upregulation of MMP-1 in adult rat myocytes. Cardiovasc Res. 2003;59:7–13.
190. Engelbrecht AM, Engelbrecht P, Genade S, et al. Long-chain polyunsaturated fatty acids protect the heart against ischemia/reperfusion-induced injury via a MAPK dependent pathway. J Mol Cell Cardiol. 2005;39:940–54.
191. Kourliouros A, Savelieva I, Kiotsekoglou A, et al. Current concepts in the pathogenesis of atrial fibrillation. Am Heart J. 2009;157:243–52.
192. Ninio DM, Murphy KJ, Howe PR, et al. Dietary fish oil protects against stretch-induced vulnerability to atrial fibrillation in a rabbit model. J Cardiovasc Electrophysiol. 2005;16:1189–94.
193. Savelieva I, Camm AJ. Polyunsaturated fatty acids for prevention of atrial fibrillation: a 'fishy' story. Europace. 2011;13:149–52.
194. Mozaffarian D, Wu JH. Omega-3 fatty acids and cardiovascular disease: effects on risk factors, molecular pathways, and clinical events. J Am Coll Cardiol. 2011;58:2047–67.
195. Kumar S, Sutherland F, Rosso R, et al. Effects of chronic omega-3 polyunsaturated fatty acid supplementation on human atrial electrophysiology. Heart Rhythm. 2011;8:562–8.
196. Virtanen JK, Mursu J, Voutilainen S, et al. Serum long-chain n-3 polyunsaturated fatty acids and risk of hospital diagnosis of atrial fibrillation in men. Circulation. 2009;120:2315–21.

197. Kirkegaard E, Svensson M, Strandhave C, et al. Marine n-3 fatty acids, atrial fibrillation and QT interval in haemodialysis patients. Br J Nutr. 2012;107:903–9.
198. Darghosian L, Free M, Li J, Gebretsadik T, et al. Effect of omega-three polyunsaturated fatty acids on inflammation, oxidative stress, and recurrence of atrial fibrillation. Am J Cardiol. 2015;115:196–201.
199. Nigam A, Talajic M, Roy D, et al. Fish oil for the reduction of atrial fibrillation recurrence, inflammation, and oxidative stress. J Am Coll Cardiol. 2014;64:1441–8.
200. Zhang Z, Zhang C, Wang H, et al. n-3 polyunsaturated fatty acids prevents atrial fibrillation by inhibiting inflammation in a canine sterile pericarditis model. Int J Cardiol. 2011;153:14–20.
201. Mayyas F, Sakurai S, Ram R, et al. Dietary ω3 fatty acids modulate the substrate for post-operative atrial fibrillation in a canine cardiac surgery model. Cardiovasc Res. 2011;89:852–61.
202. Macchia A, Monte S, Pellegrini F, et al. Omega-3 fatty acid supplementation reduces one-year risk of atrial fibrillation in patients hospitalized with myocardial infarction. Eur J Clin Pharmacol. 2008;64:627–34.
203. Mozaffarian D, Psaty BM, Rimm EB, et al. Fish intake and risk of incident atrial fibrillation. Circulation. 2004;110:368–73.
204. Biscione F, Totteri A, De Vita A, et al. Effetti degli acidi grassi omega-3 nella prevenzione delle aritmie atriali. Ital Heart J Suppl. 2005;6:53–9.
205. Patel D, Shaheen M, Venkatraman P, et al. Omega-3 polyunsaturated fatty acid supplementation reduced atrial fibrillation recurrence after pulmonary vein antrum isolation. Indian Pacing Electrophysiol J. 2009;9:292–8.
206. Nodari S, Triggiani M, Foresti A, et al. Use of n-3 polyunsaturated fatty acids to maintain sinus rhythm after conversion from persistent atrial fibrillation: a prospective randomized study. J Am Coll Cardiol. 2010;55:10A. (Abstract).
207. Kumar S, Sutherland F, Morton JB, et al. Long-term omega-3 polyunsaturated fatty acid supplementation reduces the recurrence of persistent atrial fibrillation after electrical cardioversion. Heart Rhythm. 2012;9:483–91.
208. Brouwer IA, Heeringa J, Geleijnse JM, et al. Intake of very long-chain n-3 fatty acids from fish and incidence of atrial fibrillation. The Rotterdam study. Am Heart J. 2006;151:857–62.

209. Frost L, Vestergaard P. N-3 fatty acids consumed from fish and risk of atrial fibrillation or flutter: the Danish Diet, Cancer, and Health study. Am J Clin Nutr. 2005;81:50–4.
210. Bianconi L, Calò L, Mennuni S, et al. N-3 poly-unsaturated fatty acids for the prevention of atrial fibrillation recurrence after electrical cardioversion of chronic persistent atrial fibrillation. A randomized, double-blind, mlticentre study. Europace. 2011;13:174–81.
211. Macchia A, Varini S, Grancelli H, et al. The rationale and design of the FORomegaARD Trial: a randomized, double-blind, placebo-controlled, independent study to test the efficacy of n-3 PUFA for the maintenance of normal sinus rhythm in patients with previous atrial fibrillation. Am Heart J. 2009;157:423–7.
212. Jiang Y, Tan HC, Tam WWS, et al. A meta-analysis on Omega-3 supplements in preventing recurrence of atrial fibrillation. Oncotarget. 2017;9:6586–94.
213. Mariani J, Doval HC, Nul D, et al. N-3 polyunsaturated fatty acids to prevent atrial fibrillation: updated systematic review and meta-analysis of randomized controlled trials. J Am Heart Assoc. 2013;2:e005033.
214. He Z, Yang L, Tian J, et al. Efficacy and safety of omega-3 fatty acids for the prevention of atrial fibrillation: a meta-analysis. Can J Cardiol. 2013;29:196–203.
215. Cao H, Wang X, Huang H, et al. Omega-3 fatty acids in the prevention of atrial fibrillation recurrences after cardioversion: a meta-analysis of randomized controlled trials. Intern Med. 2012;51:2503–8.
216. Liu T, Korantzopoulos P, Shehata M, et al. Prevention of atrial fibrillation with omega-3 fatty acids: a meta-analysis of randomised clinical trials. Heart. 2011;97:1034–40.
217. Khawaja O, Gaziano JM, Djoussé L. A meta-analysis of omega-3 fatty acids and incidence of atrial fibrillation. J Am Coll Nutr. 2012;31:4–13.
218. Berry JD, Prineas RJ, van Horn L, et al. Dietary fish intake and incident atrial fibrillation (from the Women's Health Initiative). Am J Cardiol. 2010;105:844–8.
219. Aleksova A, Masson S, Maggioni AP, et al. n-3 polyunsaturated fatty acids and atrial fibrillation in patients with chronic heart failure: the GISSI-HF trial. Eur J Heart Fail. 2013;15:1289–95.
220. Heidt MC, Vician M, Stracke SK, et al. Beneficial effects of intravenously administered N-3 fatty acids for the prevention of atrial fibrillation after coronary artery bypass surgery:

a prospective randomized study. Thorac Cardiovasc Surg. 2009;57:276–80.
221. Mariscalco G, Sarzi Braga S, Banach M, et al. Preoperative n-3 polyunsaturated fatty acids are associated with a decrease in the incidence of early atrial fibrillation following cardiac surgery. Angiology. 2010;61:643–50.
222. Calò L, Bianconi L, Colivicchi F, et al. N-3 fatty acids for the prevention of atrial fibrillation after coronary artery bypass surgery. A randomized, controlled trial. J Am Coll Cardiol. 2005;45:1723–8.
223. Sorice M, Tritto FP, Sordelli C, et al. N-3 polyunsaturated fatty acids reduces post-operative atrial fibrillation incidence in patients undergoing "on-pump" coronary artery bypass graft surgery. Monaldi Arch Chest Dis. 2011;76:93–8.
224. Saravanan P, Bridgewater B, West AL, et al. Omega-3 fatty acid supplementation does not reduce risk of atrial fibrillation after coronary artery bypass surgery: a randomized, double blind, placebo controlled clinical trial. Circ Arrhythm Electrophysiol. 2010;3:46–53.
225. Mozaffarian D, Marchioli R, Macchia A, et al. Fish oil and postoperative atrial fibrillation: the Omega-3 Fatty Acids for Prevention of Post-operative Atrial Fibrillation (OPERA) randomized trial. JAMA. 2012;308:2001–11.
226. Heidarsdottir R, Arnar DO, Skuladottir GV, et al. Does treatment with n-3 polyunsaturated fatty acids prevent atrial fibrillation after open heart surgery? Europace. 2010;12:356–63.
227. Farquharson AL, Metcalf RG, Sanders P, et al. Effect of dietary fish oil on atrial fibrillation after cardiac surgery. Am J Cardiol. 2011;108:851–6.
228. Sandesara CM, Chung MK, Van Wagoner DR, et al. A randomized, placebo-controlled trial of omega-3 fatty acids for inhibition of supraventricular arrhythmias after cardiac surgery: the FISH trial. J Am Heart Assoc. 2012;1:e000547.
229. Armaganijan L, Lopes RD, Healey JS, et al. Do omega-3 fatty acids prevent atrial fibrillation after open heart surgery? A meta-analysis of randomized controlled trials. Clinics (Sao Paulo). 2011;66:1923–8.
230. Benedetto U, Angeloni E, Melina G, et al. n-3 Polyunsaturated fatty acids for the prevention of postoperative atrial fibrillation: a meta-analysis of randomized controlled trials. J Cardiovasc Med (Hagerstown). 2013;14:104–9.

231. Calò L, Martino A, Sciarra L, et al. Upstream effect for atrial fibrillation: still a dilemma? Pacing Clin Electrophysiol. 2011;34:111–28.
232. Pipingas A, Cockerell R, Grima N, et al. Randomized controlled trial examining the effects of fish oil and multivitamin supplementation on the incorporation of n-3 and n-6 fatty acids into red blood cells. Nutrients. 2014;6:1956–70.
233. Yokoyama M, Origasa H, Matsuzaki M, et al. Effects of eicosapentaenoic acid on major coronary events in hypercholesterolaemic patients (JELIS): a randomised open-label, blinded endpoint analysis. Lancet. 2007;369:1090–8.
234. Owen AJ, Peter-Przyborowska BA, Hoy AJ, et al. Dietary fish oil dose- and time-response effects on cardiac phospholipid fatty acid composition. Lipids. 2004;39:955–61.
235. Sullivan RM, Olshansky B. Using omega-3 fatty acids to treat persistent atrial fibrillation: time to fish or cut bait? Heart Rhythm. 2012;9:492–3.
236. Den Ruijter HM, Berecki G, Opthof T, et al. Pro- and antiarrhythmic properties of a diet rich in fish oil. Cardiovasc Res. 2007;73:316–25.
237. Rodrigo R, Korantzopoulos P, Cereceda M, et al. A randomized controlled trial to prevent post-operative atrial fibrillation by antioxidant reinforcement. J Am Coll Cardiol. 2013;62:1457–65.
238. Kumar S, Sutherland F, Rosso R, et al. Chronic fish oil ingestion in humans prevents atrial electrical remodeling and reduces susceptibility to atrial fibrillation. Heart Rhythm. 2010;7:S108. (Abstract).
239. Metcalf RG, Skuladottir GV, Indridason OS, et al. U-shaped relationship between tissue docosahexaenoic acid and atrial fibrillation following cardiac surgery. Eur J Clin Nutr. 2014;68:114–8.
240. Aizer A, Gaziano JM, Manson JE, et al. Relationship between fish consumption and the development of atrial fibrillation in men. Heart Rhythm. 2006;3:S5. (Abstract).
241. Rix TA, Joensen AM, Riahi S, et al. A U-shaped association between consumption of marine n-3 fatty acids and development of atrial fibrillation/atrial flutter-a Danish cohort study. Europace. 2014;16:1554–61.
242. Goldstein RN, Ryu K, Khrestian C, et al. Prednisone prevents inducible atrial flutter in the canine sterile pericarditis model. J Cardiovasc Electrophysiol. 2008;19:74–81.

243. Shiroshita-Takeshita A, Brundel BJ, Lavoie J, et al. Prednisone prevents atrial fibrillation promotion by atrial tachycardia remodeling in dogs. Cardiovasc Res. 2006;69:865–75.
244. Bourbon A, Vionnet M, Leprince P, et al. The effect of methylprednisolone treatment on the cardiopulmonary bypass-induced systemic inflammatory response. Eur J Cardiothorac Surg. 2004;26:932–8.
245. Kilger E, Weis F, Briegel J, et al. Stress doses of hydrocortisone reduce severe systemic inflammatory response syndrome and improve early outcome in a risk group of patients after cardiac surgery. Crit Care Med. 2003;31:1068–74.
246. Liakopoulos OJ, Schmitto JJD, Kazmaier S, et al. Cardiopulmonary and systemic effects of methylprednisolone in patients undergoing cardiac surgery. Ann Thorac Surg. 2007;84:110–8.
247. Won H, Kim JY, Shim J, et al. Effect of a single bolus injection of low-dose hydrocortisone for prevention of atrial fibrillation recurrence after radiofrequency catheter ablation. Circ J. 2013;77:53–9.
248. Andrade JG, Khairy P, Verma A, et al. Early recurrence of atrial tachyarrhythmias following radiofrequency catheter ablation of atrial fibrillation. Pacing Clin Electrophysiol. 2012;35:106–16.
249. Tse G, Yeo JM. Conduction abnormalities and ventricular arrhythmogenesis: the roles of sodium channels and gap junctions. Int J Cardiol Heart Vasc. 2015;9:75–82.
250. Farman N, Rafestin-Oblin ME. Multiple aspects of mineralocorticoid selectivity. Am J Physiol Renal Physiol. 2001;280:F181–92.
251. Nguyen Dinh Cat A, Griol-Charhbili V, Loufrani L, et al. The endothelial mineralocorticoid receptor regulates vasoconstrictor tone and blood pressure. FASEB J. 2010;24:2454–63.
252. Gravez B, Tarjus A, Jaisser F. Mineralocorticoid receptor and cardiac arrhythmia. Clin Exp Pharmacol Physiol. 2013;40:910–5.
253. Ishii Y, Schuessler RB, Gaynor SL, et al. Inflammation of atrium after cardiac surgery is associated with inhomogeneity of atrial conduction and atrial fibrillation. Circulation. 2005;111:2881–8.
254. Rubens FD, Nathan H, Labow R, et al. Effects of methylprednisolone and a biocompatible copolymer circuit on blood

activation during cardiopulmonary bypass. Ann Thorac Surg. 2005;79:655–65.

255. Prasongsukarn K, Abel JG, Jamieson WR, et al. The effects of steroids on the occurrence of postoperative atrial fibrillation after coronary artery bypass grafting surgery: a prospective randomized trial. J Thorac Cardiovasc Surg. 2005;130:93–8.
256. Halonen J, Halonen P, Järvinen O, et al. Corticosteroids for the prevention of atrial fibrillation after cardiac surgery: a randomized controlled trial. JAMA. 2007;297:1562–7.
257. Abbaszadeh M, Khan ZH, Mehrani F, et al. Perioperative intravenous corticosteroids reduce incidence of atrial fibrillation following cardiac surgery: a randomized study. Rev Bras Cir Cardiovasc. 2012;27:18–23.
258. Ho KM, Tan JA. Benefits and risks of corticosteroid prophylaxis in adult cardiac surgery: a dose-response meta-analysis. Circulation. 2009;119:1853–66.
259. Marik PE, Fromm R. The efficacy and dosage effect of corticosteroids for the prevention of atrial fibrillation after cardiac surgery: a systematic review. J Crit Care. 2009;24:458–63.
260. Whitlock RP, Chan S, Devereaux PJ, et al. Clinical benefit of steroid use in patients undergoing cardiopulmonary bypass: a meta-analysis of randomized trials. Eur Heart J. 2008;29:2592–600.
261. Baker WL, White CM, Kluger J, et al. Effect of perioperative corticosteroid use on the incidence of postcardiothoracic surgery atrial fibrillation and length of stay. Heart Rhythm. 2007;4:461–8.
262. Liu C, Wang J, Yiu D, et al. The efficacy of glucocorticoids for the prevention of atrial fibrillation, or length of intensive care unite or hospital stay after cardiac surgery: a meta-analysis. Cardiovasc Ther. 2014;32:89–96.
263. Dernellis J, Panaretou M. Relationship between C-reactive protein concentrations during glucocorticoid therapy and recurrent atrial fibrillation. Eur Heart J. 2004;25:1100–7.
264. Koyama T, Tada H, Sekiguchi Y, et al. Prevention of atrial fibrillation recurrence with corticosteroids after radiofrequency catheter ablation: a randomized controlled trial. J Am Coll Cardiol. 2010;56:1463–72.
265. Lei M, Gong M, Bazoukis G, et al. Steroids prevent early recurrence of atrial fibrillation following catheter ablation: a systematic review and meta-analysis. Biosci Rep. 2018;38:BSR20180462.

266. Jaiswal S, Liu XB, Wei QC, et al. Effect of corticosteroids on atrial fibrillation after catheter ablation: a meta-analysis. J Zhejiang Univ Sci B. 2018;19:57–64.
267. Yared JP, Bakri MH, Erzurum SC, et al. Effect of dexamethasone on atrial fibrillation after cardiac surgery: prospective, randomized, double-blind, placebo-controlled trial. J Cardiothorac Vasc Anesth. 2007;21:68–75.
268. Halvorsen P, Raeder J, White PF, et al. The effect of dexamethasone on side effects after coronary revascularization procedures. Anesth Analg. 2003;96:1578–83.
269. van Osch D, Dieleman JM, van Dijk D, et al. Dexamethasone for the prevention of postoperative atrial fibrillation. Int J Cardiol. 2015;182:431–7.
270. Andrade JG, Khairy P, Nattel S, et al. Corticosteroid use during pulmonary vein isolation is associated with a higher prevalence of dormant pulmonary vein conduction. Heart Rhythm. 2013;10:1569–75.
271. Kim DR, Won H, Uhm JS, et al. Comparison of two different doses of single bolus steroid injection to prevent atrial fibrillation recurrence after radiofrequency catheter ablation. Yonsei Med J. 2015;56:324–31.
272. Iskandar S, Reddy M, Afzal MR, et al. Use of oral steroid and its effects on atrial fibrillation recurrence and inflammatory cytokines post ablation - the steroid AF study. J Atr Fibrillation. 2017;9:1604.
273. Kim YR, Nam GB, Han S, et al. Effect of short-term steroid therapy on early recurrence during the blanking period after catheter ablation of atrial fibrillation. Circ Arrhythm Electrophysiol. 2015;8:1366–72.
274. Christiansen CF, Christiansen S, Mehnert F, et al. Glucocorticoi use and risk of atrial fibrillation or flutter: a population-based, case-control study. Arch Intern Med. 2009;169:1677–83.
275. Huerta C, Lanes SF, García Rodríguez LA. Respiratory medications and the risk of cardiac arrhythmias. Epidemiology. 2005;16:360–6.
276. Moretti R, Torre P, Antonello RM, et al. Recurrent atrial fibrillation associated with pulse administration of high doses of methylprednysolone: a possible prophylactic treatment. Eur J Neurol. 2000;7:130.
277. Van Der Hooft CS, Heeringa J, Brusselle GG, et al. Corticosteroids and the risk of atrial fibrillation. Arch Intern Med. 2006;166:1016–20.

278. Jahangiri M, Camm AJ. Do corticosteroids prevent atrial fibrillation after cardiac surgery? Nat Clin Pract Cardiovasc Med. 2007;4:592–3.
279. Kumari R, Uppal SS. First report of supraventricular tachycardia after intravenous pulse methylprednisolone therapy, with a brief review of the literature. Rheumatol Int. 2005;26:70–3.
280. Ueda N, Yoshikawa T, Chihara M, et al. Atrial fibrillation following methylprednisolone pulse therapy. Pediatr Nephrol. 1988;2:29–31.
281. Aslam AK, Vasavada BC, Sacchi TJ, et al. Atrial fibrillation associated with systemic lupus erythematosus and use of methylprednisolone. Am J Ther. 2001;8:303–5.
282. McLuckie AE, Savage RW. Atrial fibrillation following pulse methylprednisolone therapy in an adult. Chest. 1993;104:622–3.
283. Chikanza C, Fernandes L. Arrhythmia after pulse methylprednisolone therapy. Br J Rheumatol. 1991;30:392–3.
284. Fujimoto S, Kondoh H, Yamamoto Y, et al. Holter electrocardiogram monitoring in nephrotic patients during methylprednisolone pulse therapy. Am J Nephrol. 1990;10:231–6.
285. Chiappini B, El Khoury G. Risk of atrial fibrillation with high-dose corticosteroids. Expert Opin Drug Saf. 2006;5:811–4.
286. Imazio M, Brucato A, Forno D, et al. Efficacy and safety of colchicine for pericarditis prevention. Systematic review and meta-analysis. Heart. 2012;98:1078–82.
287. Deftereos S, Giannopoulos G, Kossyvakis C, et al. Colchicine for prevention of early atrial fibrillation recurrence after pulmonary vein isolation: a randomized controlled study. J Am Coll Cardiol. 2012;60:1790–6.
288. Deftereos S, Giannopoulos G, Efremidis M, et al. Colchicine for prevention of atrial fibrillation recurrence after pulmonary vein isolation: mid-term efficacy and effect on quality of life. Heart Rhythm. 2014;11:620–8.
289. Head BP, Patel HH, Roth DM, et al. Microtubules and actin microfilaments regulate lipid raft/caveolae localization of adenylyl cyclase signaling components. J Biol Chem. 2006;281:26391–9.
290. Van Wagoner DR. Colchicine for the prevention of postoperative atrial fibrillation: a new indication for a very old drug? Circulation. 2011;124:2281–2.
291. Imazio M, Brucato A, Ferrazzi P, et al. Colchicine reduces postoperative atrial fibrillation: results of the Colchicine for the Prevention of the Postpericardiotomy Syndrome (COPPS) atrial fibrillation substudy. Circulation. 2011;124:2290–5.

292. Imazio M, Brucato A, Ferrazzi P, et al. Colchicine for prevention of postpericardiotomy syndrome and postoperative atrial fibrillation: the COPPS-2 randomized clinical trial. JAMA. 2014;312:1016–23.
293. Fatemi O, Yuriditsky E, Tsioufis C, et al. Impact of intensive glycemic control on the incidence of atrial fibrillation and associated cardiovascular outcomes in patients with type 2 diabetes mellitus (from the action to control cardiovascular risk in diabetes study). Am J Cardiol. 2014;114:1217–22.
294. Chang SH, Wu LS, Chiou MJ, et al. Association of metformin with lower atrial fibrillation risk among patients with type 2 diabetes mellitus: a population-based dynamic cohort and in vitro studies. Cardiovasc Diabetol. 2014;13:123.
295. Shimano M, Tsuji Y, Inden Y, et al. Pioglitazone, a peroxisome proliferator-activated receptor-gamma activator, attenuates atrial fibrosis and atrial fibrillation promotion in rabbits with congestive heart failure. Heart Rhythm. 2008;5:451–9.
296. Kume O, Takahashi N, Wakisaka O, et al. Pioglitazone attenuates inflammatory atrial fibrosis and vulnerability to atrial fibrillation induced by pressure overload in rats. Heart Rhythm. 2011;8:278–85.
297. Xu D, Murakoshi N, Igarashi M, et al. Ppar-gamma activator pioglitazone prevents age-related atrial fibrillation susceptibility by improving antioxidant capacity and reducing apoptosis in a rat model. J Cardiovasc Electrophysiol. 2012;23:209–17.
298. Nakajima T, Iwasawa K, Oonuma H, et al. Troglitazone inhibits voltage-dependent calcium currents in guinea pig cardiac myocytes. Circulation. 1999;99:2942–50.
299. Liu T, Zhao H, Li J, et al. Rosiglitazone attenuates atrial structural remodeling and atrial fibrillation promotion in alloxan-induced diabetic rabbits. Cardiovasc Ther. 2014;32:178–83.
300. Gu J, Liu X, Wang X, et al. Beneficial effect of pioglitazone on the outcome of catheter ablation in patients with paroxysmal atrial fibrillation and type 2 diabetes mellitus. Europace. 2011;13:1256–61.
301. Korantzopoulos P, Kokkoris S, Kountouris E, et al. Regression of paroxysmal atrial fibrillation associated with thiazolidinedione therapy. Int J Cardiol. 2008;125:e51–3.
302. Chao TF, Leu HB, Huang CC, et al. Thiazolidinediones can prevent new onset atrial fibrillation in patients with noninsulin dependent diabetes. Int J Cardiol. 2012;156:199–202.

303. Liu T, Li G. Probucol and succinobucol in atrial fibrillation: pros and cons. Int J Cardiol. 2010;144:295–6.
304. Fu H, Li G, Liu C, et al. Probucol prevents atrial remodeling by inhibiting oxidative stress and TNF-α/NF-κB/TGF-β signal transduction pathway in alloxan-induced diabetic rabbits. J Cardiovasc Electrophysiol. 2015;26:211–22.
305. Li Y, Sheng L, Li W, et al. Probucol attenuates atrial structural remodeling in prolonged pacing-induced atrial fibrillation in dogs. Biochem Biophys Res Commun. 2009;381:198–203.
306. Gong YT, Li WM, Li Y, et al. Probucol attenuates atrial autonomic remodeling in a caninemodel of atrial fibrillation produced by prolonged atrial pacing. Chin Med J. 2009;122:74–82.
307. Liu T, Korantzopoulos P, Li G. Antioxidant therapies for the management of atrial fibrillation. Cardiovasc Diagn Ther. 2012;2:298–307.
308. Sovari AA, Dudley SC Jr. Reactive oxygen species-targeted therapeutic interventions for atrial fibrillation. Front Physiol. 2012;3:311.
309. Burstein B, Nattel S. Atrial fibrosis: mechanisms and clinical relevance in atrial fibrillation. J Am Coll Cardiol. 2008;51:802–9.
310. Spinale FG. Myocardial matrix remodeling and the matrix metalloproteinases: influence on cardiac form and function. Physiol Rev. 2007;87:1285–342.
311. Mukherjee R, Herron AR, Lowry AS, et al. Selective induction of matrix metalloproteinases and tissue inhibitor of metalloproteinases in atrial and ventricular myocardium in patients with atrial fibrillation. Am J Cardiol. 2006;97:532–7.
312. Li YY, Feldman AM, Sun Y, et al. Differential expression of tissue inhibitors of metalloproteinases in the failing human heart. Circulation. 1998;98:1728–34.
313. Thomas CV, Coker ML, Zellner JL, et al. Increased matrix metalloproteinase activity and selective upregulation in LV myocardium from patients with end-stage dilated cardiomyopathy. Circulation. 1998;97:1708–15.
314. Spinale FG. Matrix metalloproteinases: regulation and dysregulation in the failing heart. Circ Res. 2002;90:520–30.
315. Schiller M, Javelaud D, Mauviel A. TGF-beta-induced SMAD signaling and gene regulation: consequences for extracellular matrix remodeling and wound healing. J Dermatol Sci. 2004;35:83–92.
316. Flesch M, Höper A, Dell'Italia L, et al. Activation and functional significance of the renin-angiotensin system in mice

with cardiac restricted overexpression of tumor necrosis factor. Circulation. 2003;108:598–604.

317. Diwan A, Dibbs Z, Nemoto S, et al. Targeted overexpression of noncleavable and secreted forms of tumor necrosis factor provokes disparate cardiac phenotypes. Circulation. 2004;109:262–8.
318. Dell'Italia LJ, Meng QC, Balcells E, et al. Compartmentalization of angiotensin II generation in the dog heart. Evidence for independent mechanisms in intravascular and interstitial spaces. J Clin Invest. 1997;100:253–8.
319. Multani MM, Ikonomidis JS, Kim PY, et al. Dynamic and differential changes in myocardial and plasma endothelin in patients undergoing cardiopulmonary bypass. J Thorac Cardiovasc Surg. 2005;129:584–90.
320. Li M, Yang G, Xie B, et al. Changes in matrix metalloproteinase-9 levels during progression of atrial fibrillation. J Int Med Res. 2014;42:224–30.
321. Nakano Y, Niida S, Dote K, et al. Matrix metalloproteinase-9 contributes to human atrial remodeling during atrial fibrillation. J Am Coll Cardiol. 2004;43:818–25.
322. Lewkowicz J, Knapp M, Tankiewicz-Kwedlo A, et al. MMP-9 in atrial remodeling in patients with atrial fibrillation. Ann Cardiol Angeiol (Paris). 2015;64:285–91.
323. Sonmez O, Ertem FU, Vatankulu MA, et al. Novel fibro-inflammation markers in assessing left atrial remodeling in non-valvular atrial fibrillation. Med Sci Monit. 2014;20:463–70.
324. Hirsh BJ, Copeland-Halperin RS, Halperin JL. Fibrotic atrial cardiomyopathy, atrial fibrillation, and thromboembolism: mechanistic links and clinical inferences. J Am Coll Cardiol. 2015;65:2239–51.
325. Boldt A, Wetzel U, Lauschke J, et al. Fibrosis in left atrial tissue of patients with atrial fibrillation with and without underlying mitral valve disease. Heart. 2004;90:400–5.
326. Kottkamp H. Human atrial fibrillation substrate: towards a specific fibrotic atrial cardiomyopathy. Eur Heart J. 2013;34:2731–8.
327. Platonov PG, Mitrofanova LB, Orshanskaya V, et al. Structural abnormalities in atrial walls are associated with presence and persistency of atrial fibrillation but not with age. J Am Coll Cardiol. 2011;58:2225–32.
328. Teh AW, Kistler PM, Lee G, et al. Electroanatomic remodeling of the left atrium in paroxysmal and persistent atrial fibrillation patients without structural heart disease. J Cardiovasc Electrophysiol. 2012;23:232–8.

329. Oakes RS, Badger TJ, Kholmovski EG, et al. Detection and quantification of left atrial structural remodeling with delayed-enhancement magnetic resonance imaging in patients with atrial fibrillation. Circulation. 2009;119:1758–67.
330. Hoit BD, Takeishi Y, Cox MJ, et al. Remodeling of the left atrium in pacing-induced atrial cardiomyopathy. Mol Cell Biochem. 2002;238:145–50.
331. Chen CL, Huang SK, Lin JL, et al. Upregulation of matrix metalloproteinase-9 and tissue inhibitors of metalloproteinases in rapid atrial pacing-induced atrial fibrillation. J Mol Cell Cardiol. 2008;45:742–53.
332. Marin F, Roldan V, Climent V, et al. Is thrombogenesis in atrial fibrillation related to matrix metalloproteinase-1 and its inhibitor, TIMP-1? Stroke. 2003;34:1181–6.
333. Anné W, Willems R, Roskams T, et al. Matrix metalloproteinases and atrial remodeling in patients with mitral valve disease and atrial fibrillation. Cardiovasc Res. 2005;67:655–66.
334. Nagatomo Y, Carabello BA, Coker ML, et al. Differential effects of pressure or volume overload on myocardial MMP levels and inhibitory control. Am J Physiol Heart Circ Physiol. 2000;278:H151–61.
335. Khan A, Moe GW, Nili N, et al. The cardiac atria are chambers of active remodeling and dynamic collagen turnover during evolving heart failure. J Am Coll Cardiol. 2004;43:68–76.
336. Zervoudaki A, Economou E, Stefanadis C, et al. Plasma levels of active extracellular matrix metalloproteinases 2 and 9 in patients with essential hypertension before and after antihypertensive treatment. J Hum Hypertens. 2003;17:119–24.
337. Huxley RR, Lopez FL, MacLehose RF, et al. Novel association between plasma matrix metalloproteinase-9 and risk of incident atrial fibrillation in a case-cohort study: the Atherosclerosis Risk in Communities study. PLoS One. 2013;8:e59052.
338. Wu G, Wang S, Cheng M, et al. The serum matrix metalloproteinase-9 level is an independent predictor of recurrence after ablation of persistent atrial fibrillation. Clinics (Sao Paulo). 2016;71:251–6.
339. Kato K, Fujimaki T, Yoshida T, et al. Impact of matrix metalloproteinase-2 levels on long-term outcome following pharmacological or electricalcardioversion in patients with atrial fibrillation. Europace. 2009;11:332–7.
340. Nattel S, Shiroshita-Takeshita A, Cardin S, et al. Mechanisms of atrial remodeling and clinical relevance. Curr Opin Cardiol. 2005;20:21–5.

341. Moe GW, Laurent G, Doumanovskaia L, et al. Matrix metalloproteinase inhibition attenuates atrial remodeling and vulnerability to atrial fibrillation in a canine model of heart failure. J Card Fail. 2008;14:768–76.
342. Cerisano G, Buonamici P, Gori AM, et al. Matrix metalloproteinases and their tissue inhibitor after reperfused ST-elevation myocardial infarction treated with doxycycline. Insights from the TIPTOP trial. Int J Cardiol. 2015;197:147–53.
343. Hughes RC. Mac-2: a versatile galactose-binding protein of mammalian tissues. Glycobiology. 1994;4:5–12.
344. Barondes SH, Castronovo V, Cooper DN, et al. Galectins: a family of animal beta-galactoside-binding lectins. Cell. 1994;76:597–8.
345. Clementy N, Piver E, Bisson A, et al. Galectin-3 in atrial fibrillation: mechanisms and therapeutic implications. Int J Mol Sci. 2018;19:976.
346. Mackinnon AC, Gibbons MA, Farnworth SL, et al. Regulation of transforming growth factor-β1-driven lung fibrosis by galectin-3. Am J Respir Crit Care Med. 2012;185:537–46.
347. Ho JE, Yin X, Levy D, et al. Galectin 3 and incident atrial fibrillation in the community. Am Heart J. 2014;167:729–34.
348. van der Velde AR, Meijers WC, Ho JE, et al. Serial galectin-3 and future cardiovascular disease in the general population. Heart. 2016;102:1134–41.
349. Fashanu OE, Norby FL, Aguilar D, et al. Galectin-3 and incidence of atrial fibrillation: the Atherosclerosis Risk in Communities (ARIC) study. Am Heart J. 2017;192:19–25.
350. Clementy N, Piver E, Benhenda N, et al. Galectin-3 in patients undergoing ablation of atrial fibrillation. IJC Metabolic Endocrine. 2014;5:56–60.
351. Takemoto Y, Ramirez RJ, Yokokawa M, et al. Galectin-3 regulates atrial fibrillation remodeling and predicts catheter ablation outcomes. JACC Basic Transl Sci. 2016;1:143–54.
352. Yalcin MU, Gurses KM, Kocyigit D, et al. The association of serum galectin-3 levels with atrial electrical and structural remodeling. J Cardiovasc Electrophysiol. 2015;26:635–40.
353. Verma A, Mantovan R, Macle L, et al. Substrate and Trigger Ablation for Reduction of Atrial Fibrillation (STAR AF): a randomized, multicentre, international trial. Eur Heart J. 2010;31:1344–56.
354. Wu XY, Li SN, Wen SN, et al. Plasma galectin-3 predicts clinical outcomes after catheter ablation in persistent atrial fibril-

lation patients without structural heart disease. Europace. 2015;17:1541–7.

355. Clementy N, Benhenda N, Piver E, et al. Serum galectin-3 levels predict recurrences after ablation of atrial fibrillation. Sci Rep. 2016;6:34357.
356. Kornej J, Schmidl J, Ueberham L. Galectin-3 in patients with atrial fibrillation undergoing radiofrequency catheter ablation. PLoS One. 2015;10:e0123574.
357. Yu L, Ruifrok WP, Meissner M, et al. Genetic and pharmacological inhibition of galectin-3 prevents cardiac remodeling by interfering with myocardial fibrogenesis. Circ Heart Fail. 2013;6:107–17.
358. Tellez-Sanz R, Garcia-Fuentes L, Vargas-Berenguel A. Human galectin-3 selective and high affinity inhibitors. Present state and future perspectives. Curr Med Chem. 2013;20:2979–90.
359. Ohki R, Yamamoto K, Ueno S, et al. Gene expression profiling of human atrial myocardium with atrial fibrillation by DNA microarray analysis. Int J Cardiol. 2005;102:233–8.
360. Kim YH, Lim DS, Lee JH, et al. Gene expression profiling of oxidative stress on atrial fibrillation in humans. Exp Mol Med. 2003;35:336–49.
361. Lai LP, Lin JL, Lin CS, et al. Functional genomic study on atrial fibrillation using cDNA microarray and two-dimensional protein electrophoresis techniques and identification of the myosin regulatory light chain isoform reprogramming in atrial fibrillation. J Cardiovasc Electrophysiol. 2004;15:214–23.
362. Kim NH, Ahn Y, Oh SK, et al. Altered patterns of gene expression in response to chronic atrial fibrillation. Int Heart J. 2005;46:383–95.
363. Kharlap MS, Timofeeva AV, Goryunova LE, et al. Atrial appendage transcriptional profile in patients with atrial fibrillation with structural heart diseases. Ann N Y Acad Sci. 2006;1091:205–17.
364. Censi F, Calcagnini G, Bartolini P, et al. A systems biology strategy on differential gene expression data discloses some biological features of atrial fibrillation. PLoS One. 2010;5:e13668.
365. Scridon A, Fouilloux-Meugnier E, Loizon E, et al. Long-standing arterial hypertension is associated with Pitx2 down-regulation in a rat model of spontaneous atrial tachyarrhythmias. Europace. 2015;17:160–5.

366. Doñate Puertas R, Meugnier E, Romestaing C, et al. Atrial fibrillation is associated with hypermethylation in human left atrium, and treatment with decitabine reduces atrial tachyarrhythmias in spontaneously hypertensive rats. Transl Res. 2017;184:57–67.
367. Yao M, Cao Y, Zhu H, et al. Paired-like homeodomain 2: a novel therapeutic target for atrial fibrillation? Front Genet. 2014;5:74.
368. Perez-Hernandez M, Matamoros M, Barana A, et al. Pitx2c increases in atrial myocytes from chronic atrial fibrillation patients enhancing IKs and decreasing ICa,L. Cardiovasc Res. 2016;109:431–41.
369. Gore-Panter SR, Hsu J, Hanna P, et al. Atrial fibrillation associated chromosome 4q25 variants are not associated with PITX2c expression in human adult left atrial appendages. PLoS One. 2014;9:e86245.
370. Kahr PC, Piccini I, Fabritz L, et al. Systematic analysis of gene expression differences between left and right atria in different mouse strains and in human atrial tissue. PLoS One. 2011;6:e26389.
371. Şerban RC, Scridon A. Data linking diabetes mellitus and atrial fibrillation-how strong is the evidence? From epidemiology and pathophysiology to therapeutic implications. Can J Cardiol. 2018;34:1492–502.
372. Kirchhof P, Kahr PC, Kaese S, et al. PITX2c is expressed in the adult left atrium, and reducing Pitx2c expression promotes atrial fibrillation inducibility and complex changes in gene expression. Circ Cardiovasc Genet. 2011;4:123–33.
373. Huang Z, Chen XJ, Qian C, et al. Signal transducer and activator of transcription 3/MicroRNA-21 feedback loop contributes to atrial fibrillation by promoting atrial fibrosis in a rat sterile pericarditis model. Circ Arrhythm Electrophysiol. 2016;9:e003396.
374. Adam O, Löhfelm B, Thum T, et al. Role of miR-21 in the pathogenesis of atrial fibrosis. Basic Res Cardiol. 2012;107:278.
375. Cardin S, Guasch E, Luo X, et al. Role for MicroRNA-21 in atrial profibrillatory fibrotic remodeling associated with experimental postinfarction heart failure. Circ Arrhythm Electrophysiol. 2012;5:1027–35.
376. Doñate Puertas R, Jalabert A, Meugnier E, et al. Analysis of the microRNA signature in left atrium from patients with

valvular heart disease reveals their implications in atrial fibrillation. PLoS One. 2018;13:e0196666.
377. Scridon A, Gallet C, Arisha MM, et al. Unprovoked atrial tachyarrhythmias in aging spontaneously hypertensive rats: the role of the autonomic nervous system. Am J Physiol Heart Circ Physiol. 2012;303:H386–92.
378. Orlov MV, Ghali JK, Araghi-Niknam M, et al. Asymptomatic atrial fibrillation in pacemaker recipients: incidence, progression, and determinants based on the atrial high rate trial. Pacing Clin Electrophysiol. 2007;30:404–11.
379. Ioannidis JP, Evans SJ, Gotzsche PC, et al. Better reporting of harms in randomized trials: an extension of the CONSORT statement. Ann Intern Med. 2004;141:781–8.
380. Dan GA, Martinez-Rubio A, Agewall S, et al. Antiarrhythmic drugs-clinical use and clinical decision making: a consensus document from the European Heart Rhythm Association (EHRA) and European Society of Cardiology (ESC) Working Group on Cardiovascular Pharmacology, endorsed by the Heart Rhythm Society (HRS), Asia-Pacific Heart Rhythm Society (APHRS) and International Society of Cardiovascular Pharmacotherapy (ISCP). Europace. 2018;20:731–2.
381. Iravanian S, Dudley SC Jr. The renin-angiotensin-aldosterone system (RAAS) and cardiac arrhythmias. Heart Rhythm. 2008;5:S12–7.
382. Rienstra M, Hobbelt AH, Alings M, et al. Targeted therapy of underlying conditions improves sinus rhythm maintenance in patients with persistent atrial fibrillation: results of the RACE 3 trial. Eur Heart J. 2018;39:2987–96.
383. Zhao Z, Niu X, Dong Z, et al. Upstream therapeutic strategies of valsartan and fluvastatin on hypertensive patients with non-permanent atrial fibrillation. Cardiovasc Ther. 2018;36:e12478.

# Chapter 8
# Clinical Significance and Management of Arrhythmias

**Antoni Martínez-Rubio and Gheorghe-Andrei Dan**

## Introduction

The human normal heart rhythm occurs when a person has a regular heart beat originated by depolarization of the sinus node, which is normally transmitted through the atria to the AV node, and thereafter normally using the His-Purkinje system to the myocytes of the ventricles. This normal heart beat occurs in a rate which is appropriated to the clinical circumstances of the individual (e.g. faster during exercise than at rest) and is called sinus rhythm. The term arrhythmia com-

A. Martínez-Rubio (✉)
Department of Cardiology, University Hospital of Sabadell, Institut d'Investigació i Innovació I3PT, University Autonoma of Barcelona, Sabadell, Spain

G.-A. Dan
"Carol Davila" University of Medicine, Colentina University Hospital, Bucharest, Romania



A. Martínez-Rubio et al. (eds.), *Antiarrhythmic Drugs*, Current Cardiovascular Therapy, https://doi.org/10.1007/978-3-030-34893-9_8

prises a group of heterogeneous conditions with abnormal electrical activity of the heart in origin, rate or both (absence of sinus rhythm). Arrhythmias may be clinically silent (at least during a period) or cause symptoms and signs (palpitations, syncope or even sudden cardiac death). The terms bradycardia and tachycardia refer to a deficit and to an excess of heart rate (compared to normal), respectively.

This chapter summarizes the recommendations for diagnosis and pharmacological treatment of arrhythmias based in the recent recommendations of major international societies [1–9].

## General Recommendations

For properly treating those patients referring at risk of arrhythmias, it is crucial a detailed clinical history, physical examination and evaluation of the ECG (at rest and during arrhythmia if it has been documented). Echocardiographic or even more sophisticated image explorations (e.g. magnetic resonance tomography) should be performed to exclude significant structural heart disease, if the echocardiographic window is limited. Exercise testing might be useful for detection of arrhythmias related to exertion. Ambulatory Holter or wearable event monitoring is advisable for patients referring frequent transient not documented tachyarrhythmias. Implantable loop recorders are helpful for those patients with rare and severe symptoms (e.g. with hemodynamic instability) whom had no inducible arrhythmias after an invasive electrophysiological testing.

Thus, the first step for correct treatment is to have the correct diagnosis. Thereafter, the best strategy for the person can be decided based on the confirmed individual characteristics. Table 8.1 presents the role of diagnostic tools available for the evaluation of patients with arrhythmias who might be candidate for antiarrhythmic therapy. In summary, the precise identification of the arrhythmia type that the patient presents as well as the individual characteristics are essential for taking the right therapeutic decisions which can be palliative or even curative depending on the type of arrhythmia, clinical presentation and patient comorbidities (Fig. 8.1). The suggested

TABLE 8.1 Role of diagnostic tools for the evaluation of the patient with arrhythmia candidate for antiarrhythmic drug therapy

| Tool | Utility | Limitations | Examples of indications |
|---|---|---|---|
| Clinical history | Always necessary for evaluation of acute and chronic risk profile, symptoms and their evolution | Subjectivity of perception of symptoms and limitations of memory and/or neurological limitations if they exist | All patients |
| Physical examination | Always necessary for evaluation of acute and chronic risk profile, signs and their evolution | Unable to detect very small/focal signs | All patients |
| Electrocardiogram | Always necessary for evaluation of rhythm, heart rate, intraventricular conduction disturbances, PR and QTc intervals and possible presence of arrhythmias or high risk markers (e.g. presence of delta wave or of acute myocardial ischemia). Prognostic value. High availability and low cost | High specificity but low sensitivity for arrhythmias since it evaluates the cardiac electrical activity with high resolution but during a very short period of time | All patients at evaluation, previous to therapy initiation and during follow-up |
| Holter and external loop recorders | High specificity for detection of arrhythmias. Allows prolonged (24 h to 30 days) evaluation of rhythm and heart rate and intervals | Low sensitivity for arrhythmia detection (although higher than with ECG). Higher cost and lower availability than ECG | To evaluate burden of arrhythmia with or without AAD<br>To evaluate proarrhythmic risk |
| Implantable loop recorder | High specificity for detection of arrhythmias | The highest sensitivity for arrhythmia detection. Higher cost and lower availability than Holter. Invasive | To evaluate unapparent arrhythmic cause of syncope |

(continued)

Table 8.1 (continued)

| Tool | Utility | Limitations | Examples of indications |
|---|---|---|---|
| Pacemakers and ICDs | High sensitivity and specificity for detection and treatment of arrhythmias | Only available in those patients with already implanted devices | Interrogation for arrhythmia and to evaluate any antiarrhythmic treatment effect on arrhythmia burden |
| Echocardiogram | Mostly necessary. Detection of structural heart disease, LVEF and other functional parameters. Non-invasive and without radiation | Constitutional limitations of echocardiographic window may limit the sensitivity. Some availability limitations | Evaluate cardiac substrate of arrhythmias and the effect of arrhythmia on cardiac performance |
| Transoesophageal echocardiogram | Higher sensitivity than transthoracic echocardiogram for atrial function, morphology and thrombus detection. Without radiation | Invasive. Lower availability than transthoracic echocardiogram | Evaluation of thrombotic risk |
| Magnetic resonance imaging | Higher sensitivity and specificity for morphological and functional changes than echocardiogram. Includes coronary evaluation | Time-consuming and expensive equipment. Availability limitations | Evaluation of myocardial scars, atrial fibrosis, precise sizes and function of chambers |
| Computed tomography | High sensitivity and specificity for morphological changes and noninvasive coronary angiography. Faster acquisition than MRI | Uses radiation. Expensive equipment limited availability | Evaluation of coronary circulation (noninvasively) and of myocardial substrate |

| | | | |
|---|---|---|---|
| Exercise testing | Useful for detection of myocardial ischemia, exercise-dependent arrhythmias, evaluation of chronotropism, functional capacity and arterial pressure reaction to exercise | Sensitivity limitations (especially if left bundle branch block or pacemaker rhythm is present) | Used by many clinicians before administration of class IC AAD |
| Cardiac nuclear imaging | Similar indications and with higher sensitivity than exercise testing. Useful in presence of advance branch block or pacemakers. Evaluates macro and microcirculation of the heart | Higher cost than exercise testing. Uses radiation. Limited availability | Evaluation of the ischemia when exercise test results are doubtful or exercise test is not recommended |
| Coronary angiography | Evaluates the epicardial coronary arteries and their branches. It is indicated in selected cases based on clinical context (always if significant ventricular arrhythmias are present) | Invasive. Uses radiation. Risk of contrast induced nephropathy. Limited availability | Evaluation of possible amendable arrhythmia triggers (correction of significant irrigation abnormalities) |
| Electrophysiological study | Useful for precise diagnostic of arrhythmia mechanism and therapeutical decision-making | Invasive. Uses (usually) radiation. Limited availability | Evaluation of arrhythmia mechanism, especially in the view of future device implantation or ablation |

*AAD* antiarrhythmic drug, *ECG* electrocardiogram, *LVEF* left ventricular ejection fraction, *MRI* magnetic resonance imaging

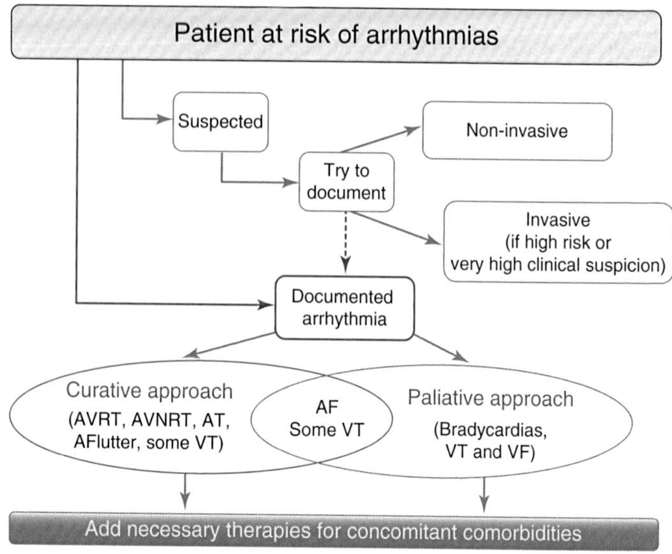


FIGURE 8.1 General approach for patients at risk of arrhythmias. Abbreviations: *AF* atrial fibrillation, *AFlutter* atrial flutter, *AT* atrial tachycardia, *AVNRT* atrioventricular nodal re-entrant tachycardia, *AVRT* atrioventricular reciprocating tachycardia, *VF* ventricular fibrillation, *VT* ventricular tachycardia

algorithm for evaluation of patients referring palpitations which is often the first clinical manifestation of arrhythmias is presented in Fig. 8.2.

## The Rhythm of the Patient

### *Supraventricular Tachyarrhythmias*

Supraventricular tachyarrhythmias (SVT) include those rhythms originated from the sinus node, from atrial or junctional tissue as well as mediated by accessory pathways. Thus,

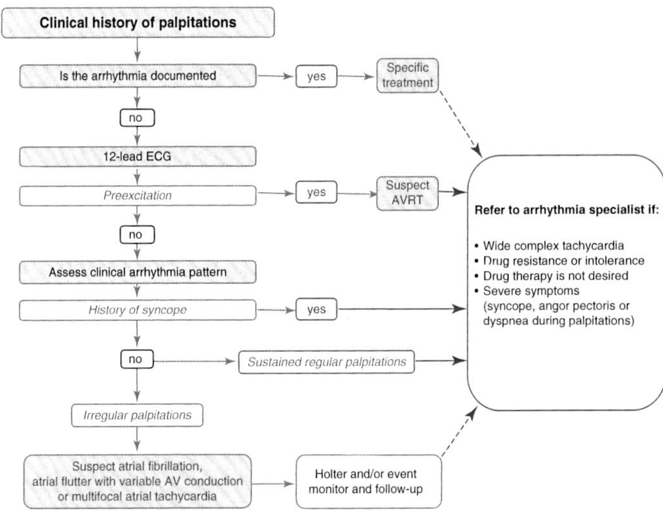


FIGURE 8.2 Sequential evaluation of patients referring palpitations. Abbreviations: *AVRT* atrioventricular reciprocating tachycardia, *ECG* electrocardiogram

the term SVT encloses atrioventricular nodal reciprocating tachycardia (AVNRT), atrial tachycardia (AT) and AV-reciprocating rhythms (AVRT). Atrial fibrillation (AF) and atrial flutter (Aflutter) are also from supraventricular origin.

Figure 8.3 presents the differential diagnosis for narrow (<120 ms) QRS tachycardia, which is the usual morphology of QRS during supraventricular tachyarrhythmias in the absence of (permanent or rate-dependent) bundle branch block or of preexcitation due to an accessory pathway. The differential diagnosis of SVT versus ventricular tachycardia (VT) is crucial for appropriate treatment (Fig. 8.4). The drugs recommended for acute management of hemodynamically stable and regular tachycardia with narrow and broad QRS complex with the levels of evidence are presented in Table 8.2 and Fig. 8.5.

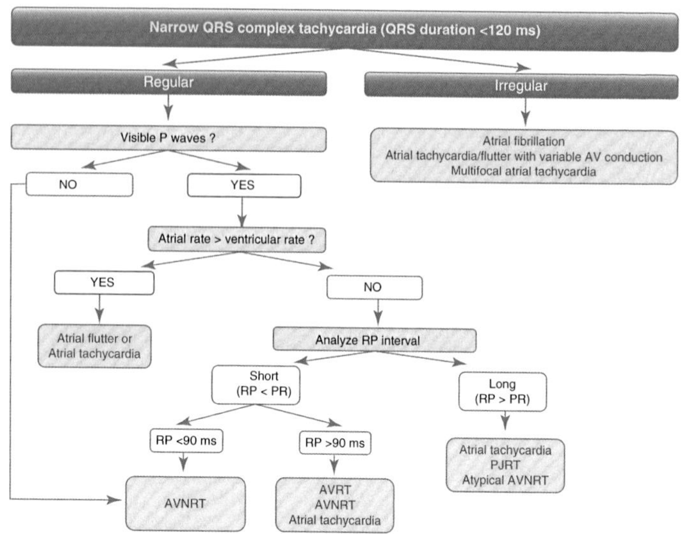


FIGURE 8.3 Differential diagnosis for narrow (<120 ms) QRS tachycardia. Patients with focal junctional tachycardia may mimic the pattern of slow-fast AVNRT and may show AV dissociation and/or market irregularity in the junctional rate. Abbreviations: *AVNRT* atrioventricular nodal re-entrant tachycardia, *AVRT* atrioventricular re-entrant tachycardia, *ms* miliseconds, *PJRT* permanent juctional reciprocating tachycardia, *QRS* ventricular activation on electrocardiogram

The sinus node may be involved in diverse arrhythmias. The *sinus node re-entry tachycardia* may respond to vagal manoeuvers, adenosine, betablockers, nondihydropyridine calcium-channel blockers, amiodarone and to digoxin. In very rare cases it might be necessary a catheter ablation. Table 8.3 presents the recommend strategies for patients presenting *inappropriate sinus tachycardia and postural orthostatic tachycardia syndrome.*

The *AVNRT* and the *AVRT* are usually curable with catheter ablation. Thus, it is usually the most recommended option for the broad majority of those patients. However, till definitive treatment is possible, they may respond to vagal

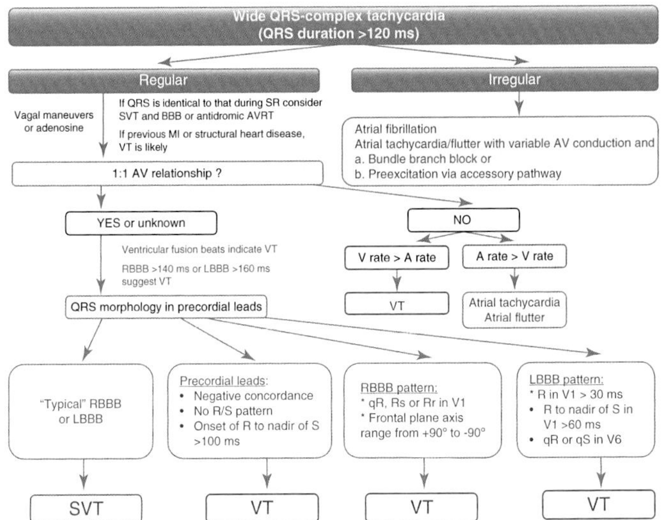


FIGURE 8.4 Differential diagnosis for wide (>120 ms) QRS complex tachycardia. Abbreviations: *A* auricular, *LBBB* left budle branch block, *ms* miliseconds, *QRS* ventricular activation on electrocardiogram, *RBBB* right bundle branch block, *SVT* supraventricular tachycardia, *V* ventricular, *VT* ventricular tachycardia

manoeuvres, carotid massage or adenosine which is helpful for arrhythmia termination and/or for differential diagnosis with other arrhythmias (Fig. 8.6). Importantly, adenosine should be used with caution because it may provoke atrial fibrillation with a rapid ventricular response in presence of preexcitation, and it can also cause myocardial ischemia in territories affected of severe coronary stenosis (because of vasodilatation of normal territories). Alternative options for those patients suffering of *AVNRT* or of *AVRT* are presented in Tables 8.4 and 8.5, respectively. Importantly, drugs that mainly slow the conduction through the AV node (e.g. digoxin, verapamil, betablockers, adenosine, diltiazem) are discouraged in patients with preexcitation because of the risk of AV-nodal blockade and acceleration of ventricular rate if atrial fibrillation occurs. Class Ic drugs (i.e. flecainide, propafe-

Table 8.2 Drugs recommended for acute management of hemodynamically stable and regular tachycardia with the levels of evidence

| ECG | Recommendation | Classification | Level of evidence |
|---|---|---|---|
| Narrow QRS-complex tachycardia (SVT) | Vagal maneuvers | I | B |
| | Adenosine | I | A |
| | Verapamil/diltiazem | IIa | B |
| | Betablockers | IIa | C |
| *Wide QRS-complex tachycardia* | | | |
| • SVT and BBB | See above SVT | | |
| • Preexcited SVT | Flecainide* | I | B |
| | Ibutilide* | I | B |
| | Procainamide* | I | B |
| | DC cardioversion | I | C |
| • Of unknown origin and preserved LV function | Procainamide* | I | B |
| | Sotalol* | I | B |
| | Amiodarone | I | B |
| | DC cardioversion | I | B |
| | Lidocaine | IIb | B |
| | Adenosine** | IIa | C |
| | Betablockers*** | III | C |
| | Verapamil**** | III | B |
| • Of unknown origin and poor LV function | Amiodarone | I | B |
| | DC cardioversion | I | B |
| | Lidocaine | | |

*BBB* bundle branch block, *DC* direct current, *LV* left ventricular, *QRS* ventricular activation on ECG, *SVT* supraventricular tachycardia, * should not be used in patients with depressed left ventricular function, ** adenosine should be used with caution in patients with severe coronary artery disease because it may cause vasodilatation of normal coronaries causing ischemia in stenotic territories. It should only be uses with full resuscitative equipment available, *** betablockers may be used as first-line teherapy for catecholamine-sensitive tachycardia (e.g. right ventricular outflow tract tachycardia), **** verapamil may be used as first-line teherapy for left ventricular fascicular tachycardia

All drugs should be administered intravenously

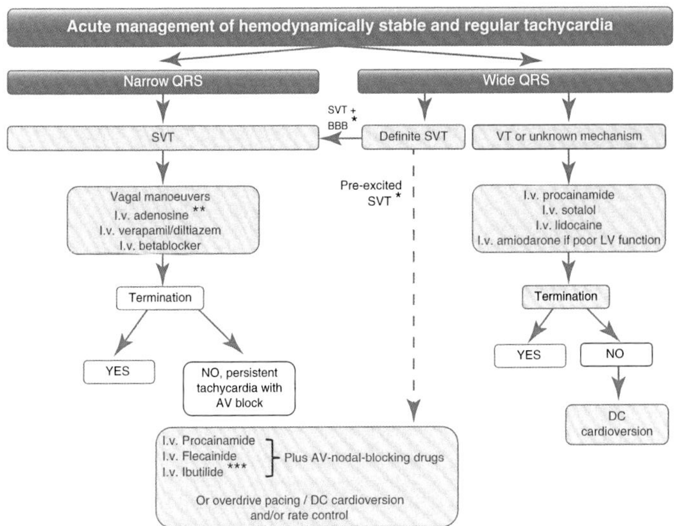


FIGURE 8.5 Acute management of haemodynamically stable and regular tachycardia. Abbreviations: * a 12-lead ECG during sinus rhythm must be available for diagnosis, ** adenosine should be used with caution in patients with severe coronary artery disease and may facilitate atrial fibrillation, *** ibutilide is especially effective for atrial flutter but should not be used in patients with left ventricular ejection fraction <30% due to increased risk of polymorphic VT, *BBB* bundle branch block, *DC* direct current, *ms* miliseconds, *QRS* ventricular activation on electrocardiogram, *SVT* supraventricular tachycardia, *VT* ventricular tachycardia

none) are considered contraindicated in presence of structural heart disease (especially after myocardial infarction). Furthermore, class III drugs are discouraged for the treatment of supraventricular tachyarrhythmias (although they might be effective) because of their toxicities and potential of proarrhythmia (e.g. torsade de pointes).

Table 8.6 presents the recommended therapeutically options for *focal and nonparoxysmal junctional tachycardia* whereas recommendations for treatment of patients with *focal atrial tachycardia* are resumed in Table 8.7. This

TABLE 8.3 Therapies recommended and levels of evidence for management of inappropriate sinus tachycardia and postural orthostatic tachycardia syndrome

| Arrhythmia | Recommendation | Classification | Level of evidence |
|---|---|---|---|
| Inappropriate sinus tachycardia | Betablockers | IIa | C |
| | Verapamil/diltiazem | IIa | C |
| | Ivabradine | IIa | C |
| | Catheter ablation of sinus node modification/ elimination | IIb | C |
| Postural orthostatic tachycardia syndrome | | | |
| • Non-pharmacological | Increase salt/fluid intake | IIb | B |
| | Head-up tilt sleep | IIa | B |
| | Physical maneuvers | IIa | B |
| | Compression stockings | IIa | B |
| | Catheter ablation/ surgery | III | B |
| • Pharmacologic | | | |
| Mineralcorticoids | Fludrocortisone* | IIa | B |
| Betablockers | Bisoprolol | IIa | B |
| Betablockers plus | Bisoprolol plus | IIa | B |
| Mineralcorticoids | Fludrocortisone | | |
| Sympatholytic | Clonidine | IIb | B |
| | Midodrine | IIb | B |
| | Methylphenidate | IIb | C |
| | Fluoxetine | IIb | C |
| Serotonin reuptake inhibitors | Erythropoietin | IIb | B |
| Others | Ergotamine/ octroetide | IIb | B |
| | Phenobarbital** | IIb | C |

* fludrocortisone requires high salt intake and regular monitoring of plasma potassium levels, ** phenobarbital may be useful for the hyperadrenergic form but with the potential hazard of dependence

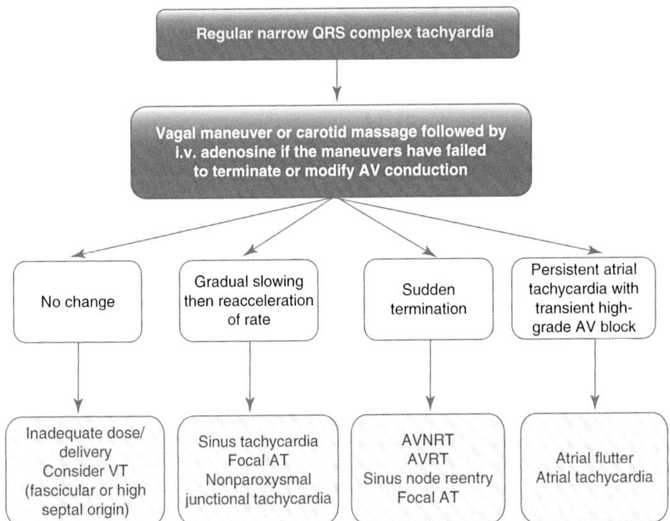


FIGURE 8.6 Usual response of narrow complex tachycardias to vagal maneuvers, carotid massage and adenosine. Abbreviations: *AT* atrial tachycardia, *AVNRT* atrioventricular nodal re-entrant tachycardia; *AVRT* atrioventricular re-entrant tachycardia, *ms* miliseconds, *QRS* ventricular activation on electrocardiogram, *VT* ventricular tachycardia

arrhythmia may be produced by digitalis excess (usually with AV block) and exacerbated by hypokalemia. Very rarely it will be terminated by vagal manoeuvers but adenosine-sensitive will. For patients with automatic AT, pacing, adenosine and DC cardioversion seldom terminates the arrhythmia. However, they may be successful if the mechanism is micro-reentry or triggered automaticity. Multifocal atrial tachycardia is usually associated to severe pulmonary disease and often requires treatment with calcium-channel blockers without any definitive role for other antiarrhythmic drugs, DC cardioversion or ablation.

*Atrial flutter* is based in a macroreentrant circuit (in the broad majority of cases in the right atrium) that usually provokes regular RR-intervals (although variable AV node conduction might cause irregular RR-intervals mimicking

TABLE 8.4 Therapies recommended for long-term treatment of patients with AVNRT

| AVNRT | Recommendation | Classification | Level of evidence |
|---|---|---|---|
| Poorly tolerated with hemodynamic intolerance | Catheter ablation | I | A |
| | Verapamil, diltiazem | IIa | C |
| | Betablockers | IIa | C |
| | Sotalol, amiodarone | IIa | C |
| | Flecainide* | IIa | C |
| | Propafenone* | IIa | C |
| Recurrent symptomatic | Catheter ablation | I | A |
| | Verapamil | I | B |
| | Diltiazem | I | C |
| | Betablockers | I | C |
| | Digoxin** | IIb | C |
| Recurrent unresponsive to betablockers or calcium-channel blockers and patients not desiring RF ablation | Flecainide* | IIa | B |
| | Propafenone* | IIa | B |
| | Sotalol | IIa | B |
| | Amiodarone | IIb | C |
| Infrequent or single episode in patients not desiring long-term drug therapy | Catheter ablation | I | B |

AF) and is usually curable with catheter ablation. However, if atrial flutter cannot be ablated, then a "normal" mean ventricular rate is mandatory and can be achieved with AV nodal conduction modulating drugs (betablocker, non-dihydropyridine calcium channel antagonist and/or digitalis).

TABLE 8.4 (continued)

| AVNRT | Recommendation | Classification | Level of evidence |
|---|---|---|---|
| Documented SVT with only AV-nodal dual pathways or single echo beats demonstrated during electrophysiological study and no other identified cause of arrhythmia | Verapamil, diltiazem | I | C |
| | Betablockers | | |
| | Flecainide∗ | | |
| | Propafenone∗ | | |
| | Catheter ablation | I | B |
| Infrequent, well tolerated | No therapy | I | C |
| | Vagal maneuvers | I | B |
| | "Pill-in-the-pocket" | I | B |
| | Verapamil, diltiazem | I | B |
| | Betablockers | I | B |
| | Catheter ablation | I | B |

*AVNRT* AV nodal re-entrant tachycardia, *SVT* supraventricular tachycardia, ∗ contraindicated for patients with coronary artery disease, left ventricular dysfunction, or other significant heart disease, ∗∗ often ineffective because of enhanced sympathetic tone

In some patients, electrical cardioversion might be necessary for atrial flutter termination. Atrial or transoesophageal pacing might be use for acute termination. In addition, high-rate atrial pacing is recommended for termination of atrial flutter in the presence of an implanted pacemaker or defibrillator. Ibutilide (i.v.) or in-hospital dofetilide administration (oral or i.v.) might be use for conversion of atrial flutter. Importantly, pharmacological rhythm- controlling, as well as rate- controlling, therapies may be far less effective for atrial flutter than for AF, especially in the long term. Thus, if feasible usually the curative approach with ablation is advisable.

Table 8.5 Therapies recommended for long-term treatment of patients with AVRT

| AVRT | Recommendation | Classification | Level of evidence |
|---|---|---|---|
| WPW syndrome (preexcitation and symptomatic arrhythmias) well tolerared | Catheter ablation | I | B |
| | Flecainide, propafenone | IIa | C |
| | Sotalol, amiodarone | IIa | C |
| | Betablockers | IIa | C |
| | Verapamil, diltiazem | III | C |
| | Digoxin | III | C |
| WPW syndrome with AF and rapid conduction or poorly tolerated AVRT | Catheter ablation | I | B |
| AVRT poorly tolerated (without preexcitation) | Catheter ablation | I | B |
| | Flecainide, propafenone | IIa | C |
| | Sotalol, amiodarone | IIa | C |
| | Betablockers | IIb | C |
| | Verapamil, diltiazem | III | C |
| | Digoxin | III | C |
| Single or infrequent AVRT (without preexcitation) | Vagal maneuvers | I | B |
| | "Pill in the pocket" | I | B |
| | Verapamil, diltiazem | | |
| | Betablockers | | |
| | Catheter ablation | IIa | B |
| | Sotalol, amiodarone | IIb | B |
| | Flecainide, propafenone | IIb | C |
| | Digoxin | III | C |
| Preexcitation without symptoms | None | I | C |
| | Catheter ablation | IIa | B |

*AF* atrial fibrillation, *AVRT* atrioventricular re-entrant tachycardia, *WPW* Wolff-Parkinson-White

Table 8.6 Therapies recommended for focal and nonparoxysmal junctional tachycardia

| Arrhythmia | Recommendation | Classification | Level of evidence |
|---|---|---|---|
| Focal junctional tachycardia | Betablockers | IIa | C |
| | Flecainide | IIa | C |
| | Propafenone* | IIa | C |
| | Sotalol* | IIa | C |
| | Amiodarone* | IIa | C |
| | Catheter ablation | IIa | C |
| Non-paroxysmal junctional tachycardia | Reverse digitalis toxicity | I | C |
| | Correct hypokalemia | I | C |
| | Treat myocardial ischemia | I | C |
| | Betablockers | IIa | C |
| | Calcium-channel blockers | IIa | C |

* data available only from pediatric patients

*Atrial fibrillation* occurs when a chaotic atrial activity (depolarization and repolarization) causes irregular RR-intervals by different rotors in the atria. *AF* represents a common electrical phenotype of several mechanisms and risk factors which contribute to modify the atrial substrate. Therefore, not only the arrhythmia has to be prevented and treated but also those risk factors which facilitate the perpetuation of the arrhythmia which diminishes the quality of life, cognitive and ventricular function and increases stroke rate, dementia and mortality. Furthermore, since AF favours thromboembolism in diverse situations (e.g. advanced age), the evaluation of the particular thromboembolic (stroke and peripheral embolism) risk (recommended the use of the CHA2DS2- VASc score) has to be evaluated and treated, if high in an individual. Furthermore, the bleeding risk has to be assessed as it might be necessary to modulate the intensity of the anticoagulant treatment.

TABLE 8.7 Recommendations for treatment of focal atrial tachycardias

| Clinical situation | Recommendation | Classification | Level of evidence |
|---|---|---|---|
| *Acute treatment* | | | |
| ∗*Conversion* | | | |
| Hemodynamically unstable | DC cardioversion | I | B |
| Hemodynamically stable | Adenosine | IIa | C |
| | Betablockers | IIa | C |
| | Verapamil, diltiazem | IIa | C |
| | Flecainide, propafenone | IIb | C |
| | Amiodarone | IIb | C |
| ∗*Rate regulation* | Betablockers | I | C |
| | Verapamil, diltiazem | I | C |
| *Long term treatment* | | | |
| Recurrent symptomatic AT | Catheter ablation | I | B |
| | Betablockers | IIa | C |
| | $Ca^{++}$-channel blockers | IIa | C |
| | Flecainide∗ | IIa | C |
| | Propafenone∗ | IIa | C |
| | Amiodarone | IIa | C |
| Any incessant AT | Catheter ablation | I | B |
| Nonsustained and asymptomatic | No therapy | I | C |
| | Catheter ablation | III | C |

All drugs for acute treatment are to be given intravenously. Excluded are patients with multifocal atrial tachycardia in whom betablockers and sotalol are often contraindicated due to severe pulmonary disease. *AT* atrial tachycardia, *DC* direct current, ∗ should not be used unless they are combined with an AV-nodal blocking agent

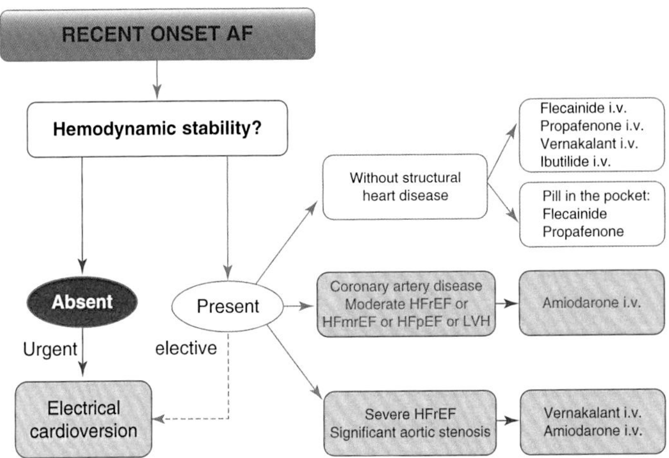


Figure 8.7 Management of recent-onset atrial fibrillation for rhythm restoration with electrical or pharmacological cardioversion. The figure indicates for each drug the level of evidence and recommendation. Abbreviations: *AF* atrial fibrillation, *HFmrEF* heart failure with mid- range ejection fraction, *HFpEF* heart failure with preserved ejection fraction, *HFrEF* heart failure with reduced ejection fraction, *LVH* left ventricular hypertrophy

Figure 8.7 presents the algorithm for management of an episode of recent- onset AF. Importantly, patients with Wolff–Parkinson–White syndrome (manifest atrioventricular accessory pathway) may present with very high ventricular rates (often >200 bpm) and a broad QRS complex with irregular RR-intervals. In this so-called 'pre-excited AF', flecainide is a useful alternative to amiodarone for cardioversion. In contrast, AVN-blocking agents (non- dihydropyridine CCBs, adenosine, and digoxin) should not be used in this situation, as it may lead to increased ventricular rates via uninhibited anterograde accessory pathway conduction. The long-term strategy for rhythm control strategy in AF patients is presented in Fig. 8.8 whereas Fig. 8.9 presents the recommendations for rate control if this strategy is chosen.

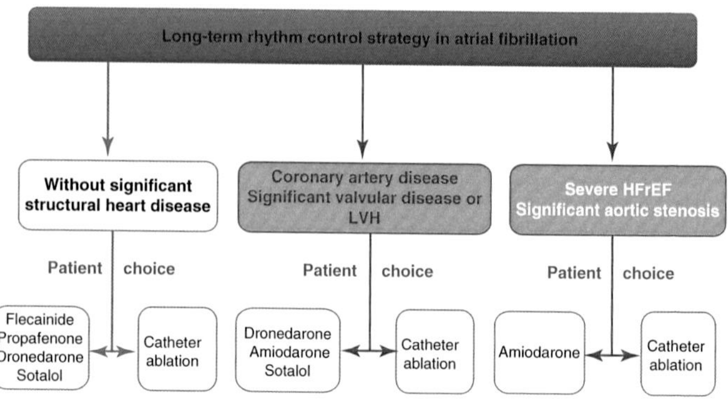


FIGURE 8.8 Recommendation for long term rhythm-control strategy

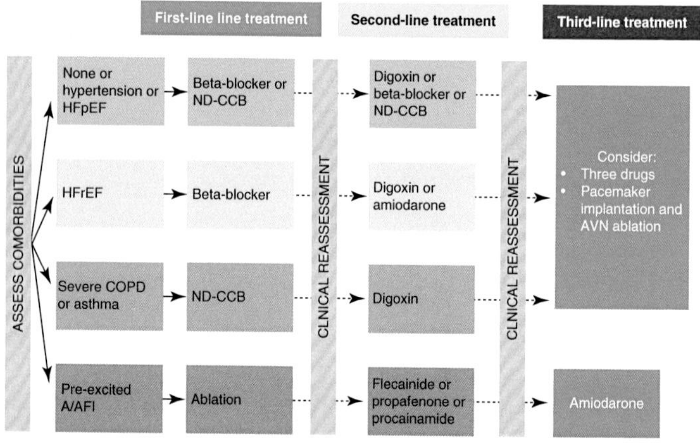


FIGURE 8.9 Recommendation for rate-control strategy. Abbreviations: *AF/AFl* atrial fibrillation/flutter, *COPD* chronic obstructive pulmonary disease, *HFpEF* heart failure with preserved ejection fraction, *HFrEF* heart failure with reduced ejection fraction, *LVH* left ventricular hypertrophy, *ND-CCB* non-dihydropyridine calcium channel antagonist

### *Ventricular Tachyarrhythmias*

Ventricular tachyarrhythmias are abnormal rhythms that originate from below the AV node which include *premature ventricular complexes* (PVC), *ventricular tachycardia* (VT), and *ventricular fibrillation* (VF). VT may be monomorphic or polymorphic. In addition, VT is classified as non-sustained or sustained (if lasts >30 s and/or causes hemodynamic instability (intolerance) and needs urgent termination because it is life-threatening). VF occurs from disorganized (chaotic) electrical activity irregular resulting in uncoordinated ventricular contractions which are ineffective for blood pumping. These arrhythmias may occur in patients with structural heart disease (e.g. ischaemic heart disease, cardiomyopathies like dilated, hypertrophic or arrhythmogenic right ventricular cardiomyopathy, etc.) or in patients with structurally normal hearts (genetic arrhythmia syndromes like long QT syndrome, Brugada syndrome, catecholaminergic polymorphic ventricular tachycardia (CPVT), or as idiopathic VTs). Symptoms depend on the haemodynamic effects of the arrhythmia and they range from asymptomatic to cardiac arrest.

## Management of Cardiac Arrest

Cardiac arrest refers to an abrupt loss of cardiac output caused by ventricular arrhythmias (VT or VF), pulseless electrical activity (PEA), or asystole. The cardiac arrest algorithm (Fig. 8.10) is based on the 2015 European Resuscitation Council guidelines [3]. Cardiac arrest due to VT or VF requires urgent cardioversion or defibrillation.

Antiarrhythmic drug therapy is recommended in patients with cardiac arrest and recurrent shock refractory ventricular arrhythmias (VT/VF). Amiodarone is generally recommended as first line for shock refractory VT/VF. Lidocaine may be used as an alternative, particularly in patients with evidence of underlying coronary ischaemia. Recommendations for antiarrhythmic drug therapy are summarized in Table 8.8. For management of acute ventricular arrhythmias intravenous preparations (IV) of antiarrhythmic drugs are generally preferred.

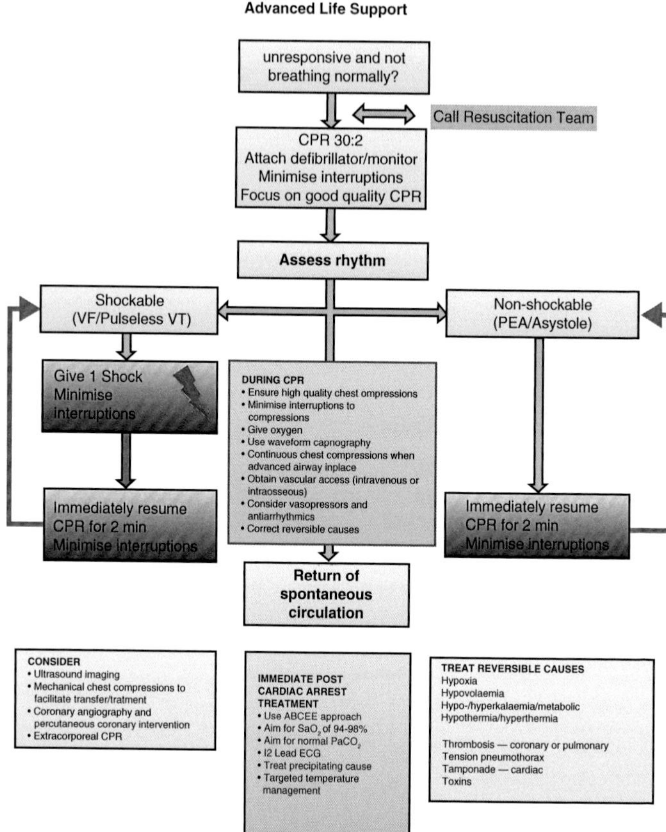


FIGURE 8.10 Algorithm for management of cardiac arrest (based on the 2015 European Resuscitation Council guidelines)

## Acute Management of Ventricular Tachycardia

Any life-threatening ventricular tachyarrhythmia needs immediate termination with cardioversion/defibrillation (Fig. 8.11). Furthermore, the options for management of hemodynamically stable VT include electrical cardioversion with synchronized shock and antiarrhythmic drug therapy (Fig. 8.11 and Table 8.8). It is reasonable to perform electrical cardioversion at any stage in the management of stable VT.

Table 8.8 Antiarrhythmic drugs for the treatment of ventricular tachyarrhythmias

| **Anti-arrhythmic drugs (Vaughan Williams class)**<br>**Oral dose (mg/day)** | **Indication** | **Side effects** | **Contraindications and warnings** |
|---|---|---|---|
| Amiodarone<br>(III)<br>200–400 | VT, VF | Pulmonary, hypothyroidism and hyperthyroidism, neuropathies, corneal deposits, photosensitivity, skin discolouration, hepatotoxicity, sinus bradycardia, QT prolongation, and occasional TdP | Conditions and concomitant treatments associated with QT interval prolongation; inherited LQTS; sinus bradycardia (except in cardiac arrest); sinus node disease (unless a pacemaker is present); severe AV conduction disturbances (unless a pacemaker is present); decompensated HF or cardiomyopathy |
| Beta-blocker<br>(II)<br>Various | PVC, VT, LQTS, CPVT | Bronchospasm, hypotension, sinus bradycardia, AV block, fatigue, depression, sexual disturbances | Severe sinus bradycardia and sinus node disease (unless a pacemaker is present); AV conduction disturbances (unless a pacemaker is present); acute phase of myocardial infarction (avoid if bradycardia, hypotension, LV failure); decompensated HF; Prinzmetal's angina |
| Disopyramide<br>(IA)<br>250–750 | VT, PVC | Negative inotrope, QRS prolongation, AV block, pro-arrhythmia (atrial, monomorphic VT, occasional TdP), anticholinergic effects | Severe sinus node disease (unless a pacemaker is present); severe AV conduction disturbances (unless a pacemaker is present); severe intraventricular conduction disturbances; previous myocardial infarction; CAD; HF; reduced LVEF; hypotension |

(continued)

TABLE 8.8 (continued)

| **Anti-arrhythmic drugs (Vaughan Williams class)** **Oral dose (mg/day)** | **Indication** | **Side effects** | **Contraindications and warnings** |
|---|---|---|---|
| Flecainide (IC) 200–400 | PVC, VT | Negative inotrope, QRS widening, AV block, sinus bradycardia, pro-arrhythmia (atrial, monomorphic VT, occasional TdP), increased incidence of death after myocardial infarction | Sinus node dysfunction (unless a pacemaker is present); (without the concomitant use of AV blocking agents); severe AV conduction disturbances (unless a pacemaker is present); severe intraventricular conduction disturbances; previous myocardial infarction; CAD; HF; reduced LVEF; haemodynamically valvular heart disease; Brugada syndrome; inherited LQTS (other than LQTS3); concomitant treatments associated with QT-interval prolongation |
| Mexiletine (IB) 450–900 | VT, LQT3 | Tremor, dysarthria, dizziness, gastrointestinal disturbance, hypotension, sinus bradycardia | Sinus node dysfunction (unless a pacemaker is present); severeAV conduction disturbances (unless a pacemaker is present); severe HF; reduced LVEF; inherited LQTS (other than LQTS3); concomitant treatments associated with QT-interval prolongation |
| Procainamide (IA) 1000–4000 | VT | Rash, myalgia, vasculitis, hypotension, lupus, agranulocytosis, bradycardia, QT prolongation, TdP | Severe sinus node disease (unless a pacemaker is present); severe AV conduction disturbances (unless a pacemaker is present); severe intraventricular conduction disturbances; previous myocardial infarction; CAD; HF; reduced LVEF; hypotension; reduced LVEF, Brugada syndrome |

| | | | |
|---|---|---|---|
| Propafenone (IC) 450–900 | PVC,VT | Negative inotrope, gastrointestinal disturbance, QRS prolongation, AV block, sinus bradycardia, pro-arrhythmia (atrial monomorphic VT, occasional TdP) | Severe sinus bradycardia and sinus node dysfunction (unless a pacemaker is present); AF or atrial flutter (without the concomitant use of AV-blocking agents); severe AV-conduction disturbances (unless a pacemaker is present); severe intraventricular conduction disturbances; previous myocardial infarction; CAD; HF; reduced LVEF; haemodynamically valvular heart disease; Brugada syndrome; inherited LQTS (other than LQTS3); concomitant treatments associated with QT interval prolongation |
| Quinidine 600–1600 | VT, VF, SQTS, Brugada syndrome | Nausea, diarrhoea, auditory and visual disturbance, confusion, hypotension, thrombocytopenia, haemolytic anaemia, anaphylaxis, QRS and QT prolongation, TdP | Severe sinus node disease (unless a pacemaker is present); severe AV conduction disturbances (unless a pacemaker is present); severe intraventricular conduction disturbances; previous myocardial infarction; CAD; HF; reduced LVEF; hypotension; inherited long QT syndrome; concomitant treatments associated with QT interval prolongation |
| Ranolazine (IB) 750–2000 | LQTS3 | Dizziness, nausea, constipation, hypotension, gastrointestinal disturbance, headache, rash, sinus bradycardia, QT prolongation | Severe sinus bradycardia and sinus node disease; severe HF; inherited long QT syndrome (other than LQTS3); concomitant treatments associated with QT interval prolongation |

(continued)

TABLE 8.8 (continued)

| **Anti-arrhythmic drugs (Vaughan Williams class)** **Oral dose (mg/day)** | **Indication** | **Side effects** | **Contraindications and warnings** |
|---|---|---|---|
| Sotalol (III) 160–320 | VT, (ARVC) | As for other beta-blockers and TdP | Severe sinus bradycardia and sinus node disease (unless a pacemaker is present); AV conduction disturbances (unless a pacemaker is present); severe HF; Prinzmetal's angina; inherited LQTS; concomitant treatments associated with QT interval prolongation |
| Verapamil (IV) 120–480 | LV fascicular tachycardia | Negative inotrope (especially in patients with reduced LVEF), rash, gastrointestinal disturbance, hypotension | Severe sinus bradycardia and sinus node disease (unless a pacemaker is present); severe AV conduction disturbances (unless a pacemaker is present); acute phase of myocardial infarction (avoid if bradycardia, hypotension, left ventricular failure); HF; reduced LVEF; atrial or associated with accessory conducting pathways (e.g. WPW syndrome) |

It is indicated the class of drug (Vaughan Willians classification), the usual adult doses, side-effects, contraindications and warnings of each drug. To note that Ranolazine is only approved for the treatment of chronic stable angina and that Sotalol has been indicated for ARVC but its use has been questioned. Abbreviations: *AF* atrial fibrillation, *ARVC* arrhythmogenic right ventricular cardiomyopathy, *AV* atrio-ventricular, *CAD* coronary artery disease, *CPVT* cathecholaminergic polymorphic ventricular tachycardia, *HF* heart failure, *LQTS3* long QT syndrome type 3, *LQT* long QT syndrome, *LV* left ventricle/ventricular, *LVEF* left ventricular ejection fraction, *PVC* premature ventricular complex, *SQTS* short QT syndrome, *TdP* Torsade de Pointes, *VF* ventricular fibrillation, *VT* ventricular tachycardia, *WPW* Wolff–Parkinson–White

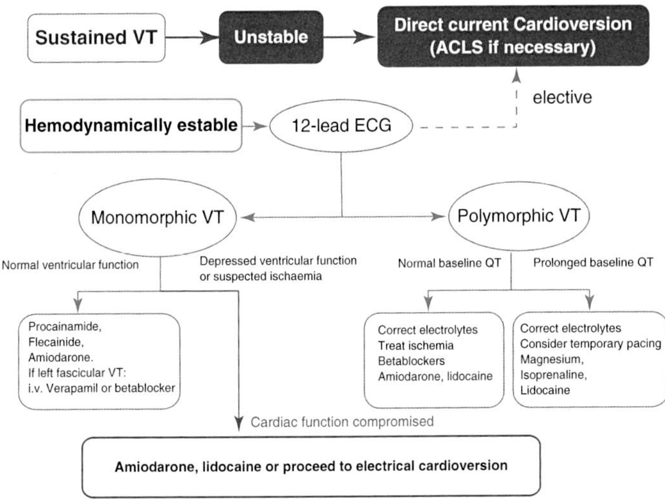


FIGURE 8.11 Treament algorithm guide for the acute management of sustained ventricular tachycardia

For patients with haemodynamically stable sustained monomorphic VT, the options for antiarrhythmic drug therapy include procainamide and flecainide in absence of severe heart failure or acute myocardial infarction. Amiodarone is generally considered first line in patients with sustained monomorphic VT with poor ejection fraction as well as for patients with recurrent shock refractory monomorphic VT (with or without pulse). Lidocaine is an alternative, particularly in patients with underlying coronary ischaemia.

In patients with idiopathic left ventricular fascicular VT (right bundle branch block morphology with left axis deviation) first-line antiarrhythmic therapy includes iv. verapamil or beta-blockers. IV flecainide or amiodarone is alternative in patients with idiopathic VTs.

Temporary cardiac pacing and/or sedation/anesthesia may be considered in certain circumstances for suppression of recurrent VT.

Polymorphic VT with normal basal QT interval is commonly caused by acute coronary ischaemia. IV B-blockers are particularly useful in this setting. Urgent coronary angiography and revascularization should be considered if ischaemia is the suspected cause of the arrhythmia, and if it causes instability urgent cardioversion with high-energy shock is mandatory. In situations with recurrent polymorphic VT, the options for antiarrhythmic drug therapy include IV betablockers, amiodarone and lidocaine. CPVT which is a genetic arrhythmia syndrome usually responds well to B-blockade.

Torsades de pointes is a type of polymorphic VT in patients with LQTS characterized by waxing and waning QRS amplitude, often with twisting image of the QRS and a long-short initiating sequence with long coupling interval to the first VT beat and may present with non-sustained forms. General measures include withdrawal of QT-prolonging drugs and correction of electrolyte abnormalities. Serum potassium should be maintained between 4.5 and 5 mEq/L. IV magnesium sulphate may be effective for acute suppression of torsades de pointes (even when serum magnesium is normal). If torsades de pointes are triggered by bradycardia, temporary pacing is recommended. IV B-blockers may be used in combination with temporary pacing. In patients with drug-induced torsades de pointes, if temporary pacing is not available, IV isoprenaline may be used as an alternative.

## Management of Ventricular Arrhythmias in the Chronic Setting

The longer-term treatment goals for patients with ventricular arrhythmias are prevention of sudden cardiac death and suppression of symptomatic ventricular arrhythmias. Treatment options include implantation of a cardiac defibrillator (ICD), pharmacological therapy, and radiofrequency ablation. Implantation of an ICD is the main strategy for primary and secondary prevention of sudden cardiac death. Indications for ICD include:

- aborted cardiac arrest secondary to VF or VT with no identifiable cause
- spontaneous sustained VT in patients with structural heart disease
- ischaemic heart disease with impaired LV function (ejection fraction ≤35%), NYHA class II or III HF on optimal medical therapy
- dilated cardiomyopathy (non-ischaemic) with severe LV dysfunction (ejection fraction ≤35%) and NYHA class II or III HF on optimal medical therapy ≥3 months of treatment with optimal pharmacological therapy,
- inherited conditions associated with life-threatening ventricular arrhythmias (e.g. LQTS, Brugada syndrome, etc.).

Cardiac resynchronization therapy (CRT), which might improve left ventricular function, is recommended to reduce all-cause mortality in patients with an LVEF ≤35%, left bundle branch block (LBBB) and QRS duration >120 ms, NYHA class III or ambulatory IV HF, ≥3 months of treatment with optimal pharmacological therapy who are expected to survive at least 1 year with good functional status.

CRT should also be considered to reduce all-cause mortality in patients with an LVEF ≤35%, non-LBBB and QRS duration of 120–150 ms (recommendation IIb with evidence B) and with a QRS duration >150 ms (recommendation IIa with level of evidence B), NYHA class III or ambulatory IV HF, ≥3 months of treatment with optimal pharmacological therapy who are expected to survive at least 1 year with good functional status.

Chronic antiarrhythmic drug therapy is aimed mainly at suppression of ventricular arrhythmias in order to reduce the symptom burden. This is because apart from B-blockers, antiarrhythmic drugs have not been demonstrated to reduce the incidence of sudden cardiac death [8, 9]. Antiarrhythmic drugs can be used in isolation or in combination with ICD therapy, or even with catheter ablation in selected cases (e.g. drug resistance or intolerance to drugs). In patients with ICDs, antiarrhythmic drug therapy may reduce the number of shocks and anti-tachycardia pacing episodes delivered by the device.

## *Bradyarrhythmias*

Bradycardia is defined as a low (<60 bpm) heart rate caused by sinus bradycardia or due to AV conduction block.

*Sinus bradycardia* may be physiological (i.e. in trained athletes or at night) or pathological due to intrinsic (sinus node dysfunction) or extrinsic causes (e.g. drugs, metabolic disorders).

Bradycardia due to *AV conduction block* can be classified into first-degree, second-degree, or third-degree heart block, according to the part of the conduction system affected and the appearance on the surface ECG as follows:

1. first-degree heart block: the majority of cases are due to conduction delay at the level of the AV node reflected by a prolonged PR interval (PR interval > 200 ms) in the ECG.
2. second-degree heart block there are two types:
   (a) Mobitz I (or Wenckebach): majority of cases are due to conduction delay at the level of the AV node. The ECG shows progressive prolongation of the PR interval followed by failure to conduct a beat.
   (b) Mobitz II: majority of cases are due to dysfunction of the conduction system distal to the AV node (His–Purkinje system). The ECG shows a constant PR interval with intermittent failure to conduct beats and might progress to third-degree AV block.
3. third-degree heart block: Majority of cases are due to dysfunction of the conduction system distal to the AV node (His–Purkinje system). The ECG shows a complete AV dissociation and an escape rhythm is generated from an accessory pacemaker distal to the AV node. Those patients are at risk of developing haemodynamic compromise due to severe bradycardia or asystolic cardiac arrest.

First-degree and Mobitz I (Wenckebach) heart block are generally considered to be benign conditions and may be physiological (e.g. in patients with high vagal tone) or pathological. Mobitz II second-degree AV block and third-degree AV block are almost always pathological.

The role of pharmacological agents is restricted to management of acute bradycardia since chronic bradycardia must be treated with permanent pacing (e.g. with pacemakers). The acute management depends on the underlying cause, the severity of the bradycardia and the haemodynamic consequence. Correction of reversible underlying causes and, if appropriate, the use of drugs to increase heart rate or temporary cardiac pacing are necessary. In addition to the drugs listed in Table 8.9, drugs such as isoprenaline and glycopyrronium bromide may be used in certain circumstances for management of acute bradycardias. Intravenous isoprenaline has been used as a second-line agent for management of acute symptomatic bradycardia; however, it has fallen out of favour due to adverse side effects such as hypotension and arrhythmias. Glycopyrronium bromide is commonly used during anaesthesia to block vagal inhibitory reflexes.

In the majority of patients with drug-induced bradycardia, the only treatment required is withdrawal of the causing drug. However, in cases of bradycardias due to toxic levels of rate-slowing drugs, in addition to the drugs listed in Table 8.9, specific antidotes may be used in certain circumstances (e.g. sever bradycardia with evidence of end-organ hypoperfusion) (Table 8.10).

## Individualization of Recommendations for Therapy of Arrhythmias Based on Patient's Characteristics

Any therapy in any patient must consider the clinical characteristics of the patient as well as the tolerance and short and long-term risk conferred by the arrhythmia. The final decision is based on a favorable balance to an intervention considering pros and cons of any decision. Some important aspects for individualization of treatment are mentioned.

TABLE 8.9 Drugs to increase heart rate

| Drug | Indications | Comments |
|---|---|---|
| Atropine | First-line drug for treatment of acute symptomatic bradycardia (level of evidence IIa) | Initial dose 0.5 mg IV (repeat to a maximum dose of 3 mg)<br>More useful in patients with:<br>• sinus bradycardia<br>• Mobitz I second-degree heart block<br>• third-degree heart block with high Purkinje or AV nodal escape rhythm<br>Ineffective or less effective in patients with:<br>• sick sinus syndrome<br>• Mobitz II second-degree heart block<br>• third-degree heart block with low Purkinje or ventricular escape rhythm<br>Use with caution in patients with coronary ischaemia:<br>• can precipitate ventricular arrhythmias<br>• in ischaemia-induced conduction block atropine may increase oxygen demand of AV node and worsen block<br>• increase in heart rate may worsen ischaemia or increase the zone of infarction |
| Adrenaline | Second-line agent—May be used for persistent severe bradycardia if atropine or temporary pacing fails (level of evidence IIb) | Can be used as a temporary measure until definitive pacing is instituted or if pacing is not available<br>Particularly useful if hypotension is an issue (due to vasoconstricting effect)<br>Infusion 2–10 mcg/min (titrate against response)<br>Use with caution in patients with coronary ischaemia—Can exacerbate ischaemia |

Table 8.9 (continued)

| Drug | Indications | Comments |
|---|---|---|
| Dopamine | Second-line agent—May be used for persistent severe bradycardia if atropine or temporary pacing fails (level of evidence IIb | Can be used as temporary measure until definitive pacing instituted or if pacing is not available<br>Infusion 5–20 mcg/kg/min (titrate against response)<br>Can be administered alone or added to adrenaline<br>Use with caution in patients with coronary ischaemia—Can exacerbate ischaemia |

Table 8.10 Specific treatment options for bradycardias to drug toxicity

| Drug causing bradycardia | Treatment | Comments |
|---|---|---|
| B-blocker | Glucagon | 1st-line antidote<br>Inotropic effect not mediated by B-receptors; 2–10 mg bolus followed by 2–5 mg/h infusion |
| | Inotropes: Adrenaline, dobutamine, isoprenaline | Competitive B-receptor agonists<br>High doses often required to overcome the effect of B-blockade |
| | Phosphodiesterase inhibitors: Amrinone, milrinone | Inotropic; however, causes peripheral vasodilatation which exacerbates hypotension—Therefore not commonly used<br>Can be used in combination with vasoconstricting inotropes |
| | High-dose insulin | Evidence restricted to case reports<br>Infusion in combination with dextrose—Monitor glucose and potassium |

Table 8.10 (continued)

| Drug causing bradycardia | Treatment | Comments |
|---|---|---|
| CCBs | IV calcium | 1st-line antidote<br>Partially overcomes calcium blockade<br>Calcium chloride or calcium gluconate can be given as boluses or infusion—Monitor levels |
| | Glucagon | Can be used as bolus or infusion: 2–10 mg bolus followed by 2–5 mg/h infusion |
| | High-dose insulin | As with B-blocker, toxicity evidence restricted to case reports |
| Digoxin | Digoxin-specific antibodies (digibind) | First-line antidote<br>Digoxin-specific antibodies (fab fragments)<br>Also indicated for haemodynamically unstable arrhythmias induced by digoxin toxicity |

## *Age*

Practically all types of arrhythmias may occur at any age. However, age critically modulates the probability of different arrhythmic mechanism. Young person with palpitations rarely will suffer of atrial fibrillation which is clearly related to age and to the presence of structural heart disease (often occurs if long-standing significant valvular heart disease or heart failure are present). Excluding well-trained athletes, clinically significant bradyarrhythmias are rare in the young. However, young persons without structural heart disease may suffer not only from supraventricular tachyarrhythmias (the most prevalent in the youth) but also (rarely) from ventricular arrhythmias (e.g. in presence of genetic disorders). In addition, it must be also considered that physiologic changes cause by advanced age may critically influence the pharmacokinetic of drugs altering their absorption, distribution, metabolism or excretion. Therefore, it affects plasmatic levels and their effects (even to toxicity) or interactions with other concomitant drugs.

### *Gender*

Some genetic disorders are gender related and also female gender is more prone to torsade de pointes with some drugs (e.g. Class I and III antiarrhythmic drugs). However, in several situations (e.g. after myocardial infarction) both gender may similarly benefit from diagnostic and therapeutic measures if they are evaluated and treated at same evolutive stages of their pathology [11].

### *Underlying Heart Disease*

Patients suffering of any type of structural heart disease (congenital, valvular, or significant myopathies of any cause) present high risk of arrhythmias (especially ventricular arrhythmias) and of proarrhythmia with drugs (e.g. class IC or class III antiarrhythmic drugs other than amiodarone). Furthermore, actually, only amiodarone is accepted for patients with heart failure who present clinically significant arrhythmias that which cannot be properly managed with betablockers with/without an implantable cardioverter-defibrillator (ICD) (e.g. sustained monomorphic ventricular tachycardia). For the broad majority of patients with structural heart disease, if the patient presents sustained ventricular arrhythmias the most effective treatment for prevention of sudden cardiac death is the ICD [2, 5, 6]. For decreasing the episodes of ventricular arrhythmias, antiarrhythmic class III drugs may be used and catheter ablation might be considered/useful in patients often suffering recurrences or arrhythmic storm.

Some patients might present bradycardia (e.g. sinus node dysfunction) or conduction disturbances and concomitantly intermittent tachyarrhythmias (transient or sustained). Thus, both situations (if clinically relevant) might deserve therapy which typically consist in drugs, ablation or ICD implantation for tachycardia treatment, as well as pacemaker implantation for avoidance of clinically relevant bradycardia (if an ICD has not been used as antitachycardia method). However, if patients present non-severe (or tendency to) bradyarrhythmias, these might be aggravated by antitachycardia drug treatment. Thus, when negative chronotropic drugs are used (e.g. the broad majority of antiarrhythmic drugs), preexisting ECG conditions must be reevaluated (e.g. sinus or AV node function) and treated if necessary.

Unfrequent ventricular ectopic beats usually do not require specific treatment. However, if they cause symptoms betablockers or non-dihydropyridinic calcium-channel blockers (verapamil/diltiazem) in patients with preserved left ventricular function might be useful.

It is known that a high burden of isolated ventricular beats might induce non-previously existing ventricular dysfunction. For its prevention/treatment, betablockers as well as antiarrhythmic drugs (class IC: flecainide and propafenone; class IA: disopyramide) might be used in absence of structural heart disease but ablation is usually more effective and should be considered if the patient suffers invalidating symptoms or a decrease in heart pump function. A similar approach is to be undertaken in presence of recurrent non-sustained ventricular tachycardia, but in this case also amiodarone might be considered if ablation is not possible or unsuccessful.

## *Other Underlying Conditions*

The *kidney function* critically regulates the pharmacokinetic of several drugs and electrolytes. Therefore, alterations in their levels with toxicity may easily develop causing proarrhythmia with even lethal brady- or tachyarrhythmias. Thus, renal function (glomerular filtration rate) should be regularly assessed in all patients treated with drugs (especially with antiarrhythmic drugs) and dosages properly adapted to it [12].

Similarly, *hepatic function* may alter the metabolism of some drugs. In addition, several prodrugs are metabolized in the liver to active metabolites. Thus, if liver present dysfunction is expectable to suffer also changes in drug effects.

*Pregnancy* modifies the mother metabolism and has been traditionally poorly studied with drugs because the teratogenic potential for mother and fetus. Therefore, drugs will be restrictively used when the benefit clearly outweighs the potential harm and always in lowest effective doses. In contrast, vagal manoeuvres should be the first line therapy for supraventricular arrhythmias. If they are unsuccessful for sinus rhythm conversion, then adenosine and if it fails then metoprolol may be used (in absence of preexcited tachycardia). If the mother has long QT syndrome, betablockers can be used and as a second choice sotalol or flecainide can be considered [13]. During pregnancy, as in every arrhythmia causing hemodynamic compromise, also emergent electrical cardioversion should be used. If sustained well tolerated ventricular tachycardia occurs termination with pacing or with lidocaine (intravenous) can be used, and if it fails then procainamide or quinidine can be also considered. Amiodarone should not be used during pregnancy because of relevant fetal side-effects and either propafenone because it has been poorly studied in pregnant period. When drugs fail, catheter ablation with minimal (or without) fluoroscopy can be considered.

During the *post-operative period* of cardiac and non-cardiac surgery often atrial fibrillation occurs. If it is well tolerated, rate control may be sufficient, especially considering that very often it will be self-limiting. In this context, betablockers are helpful for reducing the hyperadrenergic state whereas digoxin is an alternative but usually less effective. The combination of digoxin with betablockers or with non-dihydropyridine calcium channel blockers is possible. If atrial fibrillation is poorly tolerated, electrical cardioversion should be used (like in every critical situation). For elective conversion into sinus rhythm amiodarone can be used in the broad majority of clinical situations. Alternatively, vernakalant is an alternative to amiodarone in absence of contraindications (e.g. severe hypotension, severe systolic left ventricular dysfunction or acute coronary syndrome).

The pre-surgical (>24 h) administration of betablockers, sotalol, amiodarone or magnesium sulfate reduces the incidence of post-operative atrial fibrillation but the decision should be individualized (e.g. it should be avoided in patients prone to bradyarrhythmias).

If poorly tolerated VT or VF occurs then electrical cardioversion/defibrillation should be immediately done. For prevention of recurrences amiodarone, lidocaine and mexiletine can be used. If presence of non-sustained ventricular tachycardia or with ventricular premature beats, a conservative approach with betablockers and proper electrolyte balance is sufficient in the majority of cases. In addition, antiarrhythmic drugs should be avoided if clinically possible.

## Monitoring Drug Effects

Several drugs may facilitate the development of transient arrhythmogenic substrates or substantially modify the properties of chronic substrates facilitating the development of diverse arrhythmias. It is necessary to evaluate the rhythm of patient, the intervals (PR, QRS, QTc) and spatial or temporal dispersion of repolarization as well as comorbidities, concomitant drugs and possible side-effects. A pharmacokinetic evaluation of antiarrhythmic drugs is meaningful after initiation or dose adjustments, if clinically failures, if non-compliance or toxicity is suspected, after clinically relevant changes (e.g. new kidney failure) or changes in concomitant potentially interacting drugs.

## Proarrhythmia: Prevention and Monitoring

Proarrhythmia occurs when new or aggravated arrhythmia develops during drug therapy at clinically usually non-toxic concentration levels. This phenomenon is related to the interaction of drugs with ion-currents that contribute to the action potential of the cardiac cells (at any level). Since there are differences in ionic current contributions between atrial and ventricular action potentials, selective approaches have been proposed for avoidance of proarrhythmia, especially at ventricular level [14].

With the exception of betablockers, antiarrhythmic drugs have not demonstrated to prevent life-threatening ventricular arrhythmias and sudden cardiac death [5, 6, 8, 9]. Controversial results have been presented with amiodarone. However, several antiarrhythmic drugs might cause proarrhythmia [15, 16]. Flecainide, propafenone and quinidine are contraindicated because they increase mortality in patients with previous myocardial infarction. Mexiletine and disopyramide should also be avoided in postmyocardial infarction patients. Dofetilide may provoke TdP in patients with severe heart failure. Amiodarone may also cause TdP although is a very rare effect. Digitalis may cause diverse arrhythmias (e.g. enhanced atrial and ventricular automacity (including sustained ventricular arrhythmias), AV-block). In addition, several drugs (e.g. verapamil, diltiazem, betablockers and digoxin) cause bradycardia and this situation may predispose to severe ventricular arrhythmias in some situations (e.g. hypokalemia) [6, 8, 9, 17].

Therefore, antiarrhythmic drugs should only be used after balancing the risk versus benefits of the treatment. Thus, appropriate use of the drugs for treatment of the appropriate patients is the more effective preventive measure for avoiding proarrhythmia.

Before deciding to use antiarrhythmic drugs in an individual patient the characteristics of the patient (e.g. evaluation of the drug-substrate interaction), the concomitant treatments of the patient (e.g. evaluation of possible drug-to-drug interactions) and the presence of possible proarrhythmia facilitating factors should be carefully evaluated (Table 8.11). Since polypharmacy is very often necessary, drug-drug interactions and their pharmacological consequences (especially QT interval modification) might become crucial. Therefore, careful ECG evaluation previous to and after the administration of the drug is mandatory [17]. Although acquired long QT syndrome and the resulting potentially lethal polymorphic ventricular tachycardia in form of torsade de pointes (TdP) is the most important drug-induced proarrhythmia, other forms as bradycardia might occur. Therefore, all ECG curves, morphologies and intervals must be evaluated before using antiarrhythmic drugs and reevaluated after drug administration for evaluation of electrical tolerability. A full list of drugs implicated in acquired long QT syndrome and TdP may be accessed via internet (www.torsades.org; www.qtdrugs.org; www.longqt.org; www.sads.org).

A drug-induced or facilitated arrhythmia should be suspected in patients treated with drugs that induce electrolyte abnormalities or modify the electrical properties of the heart (e.g. prolonging the QT interval) and after exclusion or inherited or acquired arrhythmogenic substrates.

Always that is suspected or confirmed that a drug induces pro-arrhythmia, the administration of this drug should be interrupted. The rhythm must be monitored and electrolytes must be maintained in normal ranges. In addition, despite a possible correctable cause for serious ventricular arrhythmias (e.g. ventricular tachycardia or fibrillation), the implantation of a cardioverter-defibrillator should be considered based on the individual characteristics of the patient and the future risk of life-threatening ventricular tachyarrhythmias [5, 6, 8, 9].

Importantly, in patients suffering torsade de pointes (TdP) (e.g. those patients with proarrhythmia after action potential prolonging drugs like antiarrhythmic class I or class III drugs) intravenous magnesium should be administered since often suppresses the arrhythmia, even when serum magnesium is normal (Fig. 8.11). In addition, temporary pacing is very effective to stop TdP clusters. Isoproterenol can also be used to increase the heart rate and shorten ventricular action potential duration, to eliminate depolarizations and TdP. Obviously, all correctable cause should be treated (e.g. correction of electrolyte disturbances). Prolonged ECG-monitoring till the proarrhythmic drug/situation has been eliminated is obviously mandatory.

TABLE 8.11 Mechanisms promoting proarrhythmia

*Drug-substrate interaction associated with proarrhythmia*

- Left ventricular hypertrophy: Sotalol, flecainide and propafenone
- Myocardial infarction: Sodium channel blocking agents (antiarrhythmic drugs but also tricyclic antidepressants)
- Structural heart disease: Sodium channel blockers
- Heart failure: Dronedarone, dofetilide

*Drug-drug interaction*

- Inhibitors of potassium channels (e.g. some antibiotics (quinolones, azithromycin, erythromycin, clarithromycin); inhibitors of renin-angiotensin system combined with antibiotics (e.g. cotrimoxazole) and hyperkalemia
- Inhibitors of sodium-channels (e.g. tricyclic antidepressants)
- Cardiotoxics drugs (e.g. anthracycline)
- Toad venom
- Herbal products (e.g. foxglove tea)

*Factors facilitating pro-arrhythmia*

- Hypokalemia
- Rapid rise in extracellular potassium
- Hypomagnesaemia
- Bradycardia
- Pacing
- Myocardial ischemia
- Congestive heart failure
- Left ventricular hypertrophy
- Digitalis therapy
- Rapid intravenous administration of drugs
- Adquired or congenital QT prolongation
- Certain DNA polymorphisms

If mild digitalis toxicity occurs, K+ supplement and clinical observation might be considered whereas in severe intoxications of digitalis, specific antibodies are helpful. Those patients suffering sodium channel block-related proarrhythmia might response to i.v. sodium or sodium bicarbonate, or beta-blockers or other AVN-blocking agents.

## Summary

There are several different arrhythmias, based on diverse mechanisms. The best treatment option for each individual should be evaluated and decided on individual basis which is determined by the substrate (acute or chronic) and the presence of triggers (e.g. extrasistoles) and the modulators (e.g. acute ischemia). Drug therapy (isolated or added to other therapies (e.g. implanted devides)) might be very useful in acute or chronic settings but the potential of proarrhythmia must be considered and decisions must be based in a careful balance of potential risks and benefits.

*Statement of Disclosure*

None

## References

1. Blomström-Lundqvist C, Scheinman MM, Aliot EM, Alpert JS, Calkins H, Camm AJ, et al. ACC/AHA/ESC guidelines for the management of patients with supraventricular arrhythmias—executive summary. A report of the American college of cardiology/American heart association task force on practice guidelines and the European society of cardiology. J Am Coll Cardiol. 2003;42(8):1493–531.
2. Priori SG, Blomstrom-Lundqvist C. 2015 European Society of Cardiology Guidelines for the management of patients with ventricular arrhythmias and the prevention of sudden cardiac death summarized by co-chairs. Eur Heart J. 2015;36(41):2757–9.

3. Soar J, Nolan JP, Bottiger BW, Perkins GD, Lott C, Carli P, Pellis T, Sandroni C, Skrifvars MB, Smith GB, Sunde K, Deakin CD, Adult advanced life support section Collaborators. European Resuscitation Council Guidelines for Resuscitation 2015: Section 3. Adult advanced life support. Resuscitation. 2015;95:100–47.
4. Katritsis DG, Boriani G, Cosio FG, Hindricks G, Jaïs P, Josephson ME, et al. European Heart Rhythm Association (EHRA) consensus document on the management of supraventricular arrhythmias, endorsed by Heart Rhythm Society (HRS), Asia-Pacific Heart Rhythm Society (APHRS), and Sociedad Latinoamericana de Estimulación Cardiaca y Electrofisiología. Eur Heart J. 2018;39(16):1442–5.
5. Al-Khatib SM, Stevenson WG, Ackerman MJ, Bryant wJ, Callans DJ, Curtis AB. 2017 AHA/ACC/HRS guideline for management of patients with ventricular arrhythmias and the prevention of sudden cardiac death. J Am Coll Cardiol. 2018;72(14):e91–220.
6. Dan GA, Martínez-Rubio A, Agewall S, Boriani G, Borggrefe M, Gaita F, et al. Antiarrhythmic drugs–clinical use and clinical decision making: a consensus document from the European Heart Rhythm Association (EHRA) and European Society of Cardiology (ESC) Working Group on Cardiovascular Pharmacology, endorsed by the Heart Rhythm Society (HRS), Asia-Pacific Heart Rhythm Society (APHRS) and International Society of Cardiovascular Pharmacotherapy (ISCP). Europace. 2018;20:731–732an.
7. Kirchhof P, Benussi S, Kotecha D, Ahlsson A, Atar D, Casadei B, et al. 2016 ESC Guidelines for the management of atrial fibrillation developed in collaboration with European Association for Cardio-Thoracic Surgery. Eur Heart J. 2016;37:2893–962.
8. Zipes DP, Camm J, Borggrefe M, Buxton AE, Chaitman B, Fromer M, et al. ACC/AHA/ESC 2006 Guidelines for management of patients with ventricular arrhythmias and the prevention of sudden cardiac death. J Am Coll Cardiol. 2006;48:e247–346.
9. Priori S, Blomström-Lundqvist C, Mazzanti A, Blom N, Borggrefe M, Camm J, et al. 2015 ESC Guidelines for the management of patients with ventricular arrhythmias and the prevention of sudden cardiac death. Eur Heart J. 2015;36:2793–867.
10. Brugada J, Katritsis, DG, Arbelo E, et al. 2019 ESC Guideline for the management of patients with supraventricular tachycardia. Eur Heart J. 2019;00;1–66.
11. Martínez-Rubio A, Borggrefe M, Shenasa M, Chen X, Wichter T, Fetsch T, Reinhardt L, Breithardt G. Are there gender differences in patients with coronary artery disease presenting with

spontaneous ventricular tachycardia and ventricular fibrillation ? Clin Cardiol. 1995;18(3):161–6.
12. Boriani G, Savelieva I, Dan GA, Deharo JC, Ferro C, Israel CW, et al. Chronic kidney disease in patients with cardiac rhythm disturbances or implantable electrical devices: clinical significance and implications for decision making-a position paper of the European Heart Rhythm Association endorsed by the Heart Rhythm Society. Europace. 2015;17:1169–96.
13. Enriquez AD, Economy KE, Tedrow UB. Contemporary management of arrhythmias during pregnancy. Circ Arrhythm Electrophysiol. 2014;7:961–7.
14. Ehrlich JR, Biliczki P, Hohnloser SH, Nattel S. Atrial-selective approaches for the treatment of atrial fibrillation. J Am Coll Cardiol. 2008;51:787–92.
15. Konstantopoulou A, Tsikrikas S, Asvestas D, Korantzopoulos P, Letsas KP. Mechanisms of drug-induced proarrhythmia in clinical practice. World J Cardiol. 2013;5(6):175–85.
16. Roden DM. Pharmacology and toxicology of Nav1.5-class I antiarrhythmic drugs. Card Electrophysiol Clin. 2014;6(4):695–704.
17. Wisniowska B, Tylutki Z, Wyszogrodzka G, Polak S. Drug-drug interactions and QT prolongation as a commonly assessed cardiac effect – comprehensive overview of clinical trials. BMC Pharmacol Toxicol. 2016;17:12. https://doi.org/10.1186/s40360-016-0053-1.

# Index



 
A. Martínez-Rubio et al. (eds.), *Antiarrhythmic Drugs*,
Current Cardiovascular Therapy,
https://doi.org/10.1007/978-3-030-34893-9

**C**